WH170

re the date

Practical Management of Haemoglobinopathies

Practical Management of Haemoglobinopathies

EDITED BY

Iheanyi E Okpala

Department of Haematology
Guy's and St Thomas' Trust
St Thomas' Hospital
London
SE1 7EH

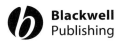

Blackwell
Publishing

First published 2004

Library of Congress Cataloging-in-Publication Data

Practical management of haemoglobinopathies / edited, Iheanyi Okpala.
    p.   ; cm.
  Includes bibliographical references and index.
  ISBN 1-4051-0780-4
  1. Hemoglobinopathy.
  [DNLM: 1. Anemia, Sickle Cell. 2. Thalassemia. WH 170 P895 2004]
I. Okpala, Iheanyi.

  RC641.7.H35P735 2004
  616.1′51–dc22

                   2004008401

A catalogue record for this title is available from the British Library

Set in $9\frac{1}{2}$ / 12 pt Sabon by SNP Best-set Typesetter Ltd., Hong Kong
Printed and bound in India using acid-free paper by Gopsons Paper Ltd, **Noida**

Production Editor: Rebecca Huxley and Deirdre Prinsen
Commissioning Editor: Maria Khan
Editorial Assistant: Claire Bonnett
Production Controller: Mirjana Misina

For further information on Blackwell Publishing, visit our website:
http://www.blackwellpublishing.com

The publisher's policy is to use permanent paper from mills that operate a sustainable forestry policy, and
which has been manufactured from pulp processed using acid-free and elementary chlorine-free practices.
Furthermore, the publisher ensures that the text paper and cover board used have met acceptable environmental accreditation standards.

Contents

Contributors

Ian Abbs, BSc, FRCP, Clinical Director
Directorate of Nephrology & Renal Transplantation, Guy's & St Thomas' Hospitals Trust, London, UK

Elizabeth N Anionwu, Professor, RN, HV, HV Tutor, PhD, CBE, Head of the Mary Seacole Centre for Nursing Practice
Faculty of Health & Human Sciences, Thames Valley University, London, UK

Ikechukwu Obialo Azuonye, BM, BCh, DipMath, MRCPsych, Consultant Psychiatrist/Senior Lecturer
South London & Maudsley NHS Trust, Guy's, King's College & St Thomas' Hospitals, Medical & Dental School of the University of London, and the Research Unit of the Royal College of Psychiatrists

Susan Bewley, MD, MA, FRCOG, Clinical Director
Women's Health Services Directorate, Guy's and St Thomas' Hospitals NHS Trust, St Thomas' Hospital, London, UK

Sadie Daley, RGN, RM, RHV, BSc (Hons), Community Nurse Specialist
South East London Sickle Cell & Thalassaemia Centre, Wooden Spoon House, Kennington, London, UK

Yvonne Daniel, MSc, FIBMS, Chief Medical Laboratory Scientific Officer
Special Haematology Laboratory, Guy's & St Thomas' Hospitals Trust, London, UK

Moira Dick, MB, BCh, BA, DCH, FRCP, FRCPCH, Consultant Community Paediatrician
Lambeth Primary Healthcare Trust, King's College Hospital, London, UK

Christina M Halsey, MB, ChB, MRCP, Specialist Registrar in Haematology
Department of Haematology, Imperial College Faculty of Medicine, London, UK

Cage S Johnson, MD, Professor of Medicine, Director
Comprehensive Sickle Cell Center, Keck School of Medicine, University of Southern California, Los Angeles, CA, USA

Manjiri Khare, MD, MRCOG, Subspecialty trainee in Maternal-Fetal Medicine
Women's and Perinatal Services, University Hospitals of Leicester NHS Trust, Leicester Royal Infirmary, Leicester, UK

Janet Kwiatkowski, MD
Department of Haematology, Children's Hospital of Philadelphia, Philadelphia, PA, USA

Sebastian Lucas, MA, BM, FRCP, FRCPath, Professor of Pathology
King's College London, London, UK

Kwaku Ohene-Frempong, MD, Professor of Paediatric Haematology, University of Pennsylvania, Director
Comprehensive Sickle Cell Centre, Children's Hospital of Philadelphia, Philadelphia, PA, USA

Iheanyi E Okpala, MB, BS (Hons), MSc, FRCPath, FWACP, Consultant Haematologist/Senior Lecturer
St Thomas' Hospital/King's College London, London, UK

Chioma Onyedinma-Ndubueze, RN, BSc, MSc, Senior Lecturer
Faculty of Health, South Bank University, London, UK

Irene AG Roberts, MD, FRCP, FRCPath, Professor of Paediatric Haematology
Department of Haematology, Imperial College Faculty of Medicine, St Mary's and Hammersmith Campus, London, UK

Collis Rochester-Peart, SRN, RM, Dip. in Management, Service Co-ordinator
South East London Sickle & Thalassaemia Centre, London, UK

Adrian Stephens, MD, FRCPath, Consultant Haematologist
Department of Haematological Medicine, King's College Hospital, London, UK

Swee Lay Thein, MA, MB, BS, MRCP, FRCPath, Professor of Molecular Haematology
King's College Hospital, London, UK

Nay Win, FRCP, FRCPath, Consultant Haematologist
National Blood Service, South Thames Centre, London, UK

Beatrix Wonke, MD, FRCP, FRCPath, Consultant Haematologist
Haematology Department, Whittington Hospital, London, UK

Josh Wright, MD, MRCP, MRCPath, Consultant Haematologist
Sheffield University Hospitals Trust, Sheffield, UK

Preface

Haemoglobinopathies are the most prevalent inherited diseases that afflict mankind, and constitute a major health problem in many countries. There is a perceived need among practising health professionals and students for a book on sickle cell disease and thalassaemia designed to fill the gap between the major reference texts and the smaller 'handbooks' on the subjects. Such a book is expected to meet the day-to-day requirements of a growing number of trainees and health-care professionals working in the field. The need for a medium-sized textbook that deals with practical aspects of the laboratory, clinical and community care of people affected by haemoglobinopathies has increased as population screening programmes have been instituted in various countries, and general improvements in medical care have led to longer life expectancy of persons born with the disorders.

In this book, a multidisciplinary group of professionals who work on various aspects of haemoglobinopathy have attempted to share their experiences with colleagues in the field. It begins with an overview of the holistic care required by affected persons, proceeding to practical details of laboratory diagnosis, clinical management, community care, psychosocial support and counselling. The final chapter deals with the challenges faced by health-care professionals who attend to people who have sickle cell disease and thalassaemia, and offers suggestions on how to meet them. It is the profound hope of the contributors that this concise text will go a considerable way towards enabling health-workers to provide optimal care for people with sickle cell disease and thalassaemia.

The authors would like to thank Jackie Marsh and the secretaries who helped in preparing the individual chapters, Elizabeth Callaghan and Maria Khan – editorial staff of Blackwell Publishing Ltd. in Oxford – for all their assistance, Dr Joy Okpala for her comments and support, and Mrs Patricia Moberly, Chairperson of the Management Board of Guy's & St Thomas' Hospitals Trust, London, UK, for kindly writing the foreword to this book.

IE Okpala

Foreword

Guy's & St Thomas' NHS Trust is proud of its annual week-long international conference on sickle cell disease and thalassaemia. The haematologists at the Trust, with the support of the whole organization, are leading the provision of services in Lambeth, Lewisham and Southwark for our many residents who experience these conditions.

We all know that sickle and thalassaemia are among the commonest of mankind's inherited problems, with millions of sufferers across the world. The UK has the highest number of people with sickle cell disease in Europe, and within the UK one of the largest cohorts of patients is in our area of Central London. We estimate that over a quarter of the residents in our three boroughs are at risk of inheriting the sickle cell gene, and numbers are bound to rise. Therefore, we have an immediate and pressing need to ensure that our own local people receive the best possible care and treatment. Those affected by sickle cell disease and thalassaemia include of course the patients and their families and friends who themselves need support and advice. We at Guy's and St Thomas' therefore have not only direct responsibility for a significant group of people but also the opportunity as a famous teaching institution to lead research, to promote better understanding of both the causes and treatment of disease, and to share good practice. Mutual learning between patients, clinicians, researchers and voluntary sec-

tor workers can only be beneficial, and I know that all participants at our conferences leave encouraged by the example and commitment of others.

This book has contributions from many authors and has been compiled in response to requests from those who attended the course in previous years. It will, I hope, reach a wide audience so that many people who did not attend will also benefit from the ideas and discussions generated during the conference. The book demonstrates the co-operative efforts of the multidisciplinary team of health professionals and others who, at various times, have generated ideas during the course. I recommend its contents to everyone who provides services for those who suffer from sickle cell disease and thalassaemia, as it is only through real joint working that comprehensive care can be delivered. This wide-ranging and forward-looking approach, which seeks to understand all the needs of patients, is an approach that this Trust is proud to communicate to others. The example set by the team leading the conference is well demonstrated by this publication, and I am grateful to Dr Okpala and others for their work both in organizing the event and bringing this book together.

Patricia Moberly
Chairperson, Management Board
Guy's & St Thomas' Hospital Trust
London, UK

Chapter 1

The concept of comprehensive care of sickle cell disease

Iheanyi E Okpala

Definition of sickle cell disease

Sickle cell disease (SCD) is a general name for a group of inherited conditions that have two characteristics in common: the presence of sickle- or crescent-shaped red cells in the blood, and development of illness (disease) as a result of having sickle cells. Simply put, sickle cell disease means disease caused by sickle cells. Clinical illness as a result of the presence of sickle red blood cells occurs in various inherited conditions that are types of SCD. These genetic disorders include homozygous (HbSS) sickle cell disease or sickle cell anaemia and compound heterozygous states such as sickle cell haemoglobin C (HbSC) disease, sickle cell thalassaemia (HbSthal), HbS/HbD Punjab (Los Angeles), HbS/HbO-Arab, HbS/HbE, and HbS/Hb Lepore Boston [1]. The carrier state, sickle cell trait (HbAS), is not considered as SCD because it does not cause clinical illness.

What is comprehensive care of SCD?

This is the multidisciplinary, holistic care of people affected by SCD. In addition to individuals who have SCD, the *affected persons* include relatives, friends and others whose lives are significantly affected by the patient's illness. A mother who is absent from work to take her child to the hospital, the brother or sister who suffers maternal deprivation as a result, as well as the patient whose daily schedule could be suddenly interrupted by a sickle cell crisis without forewarning; all these individuals might need psychological support and counselling. The provision of facilities to enhance in-house mobility, and the construction of a ramp to ease access to the house, are non-medical services that improve the quality of life of a person with SCD complicated by stroke.

The medical care of individuals who have SCD is best provided by a team of different specialists because it is a multi-system disease that affects virtually every organ of the body. Although SCD is primarily a blood disorder, its clinical management should not be the sole responsibility of haematologists because, as blood flows to all parts of the body, the fundamental pathological process in SCD – blood vessel occlusion with reduced supply of oxygen and nutrients – can occur in any tissue, resulting in damage and diminished function of affected organs. Thus, effective management of stroke in SCD requires joint treatment by neurologists and haematologists; people with avascular necrosis of the hip joint benefit from a combined orthopaedic and haematology clinic; while expectant mothers who have SCD are best seen by a team of obstetricians, specialist nurses/midwives and haematologists.

The co-operation of people affected by SCD is indispensable for effective provision of the above medical and non-medical services. Without such partnership, comprehensive care cannot be delivered. The affected person is at the apex of the triangle of holistic management of SCD (Fig. 1.1). However efficacious or well-meaning the care plan for an individual is, if it is not presented in an acceptable, culturally appropriate manner that wins the patient's or parent's co-operation, very little may be achieved.

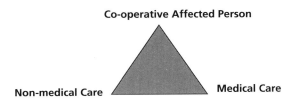

Fig. 1.1 The triangle of comprehensive care of sickle cell disease (SCD).

Components of comprehensive care of SCD

A comprehensive sickle cell service is dynamic, its composition evolves in response to changing situations. The component services discussed below are not meant to be exhaustive. Certain services are so crucial that no comprehensive care system could function without them. Others could be obtained by referral to relevant specialist units. It may not be feasible to provide all the component services within a single comprehensive care system, and appropriate referral should be made when necessary.

Haematology services

As appropriate for a primary genetic abnormality of the blood, the diagnosis and core clinical management of SCD has been the traditional role of haematologists who co-ordinate overall care of affected individuals, and liaise with providers of other component services in comprehensive care. The effectiveness of comprehensive care is critically dependent on efficient co-ordination of the various components to ensure that they work as a whole and provide a seamless service. Close collaboration between the children's and adults' haemoglobinopathy services is crucial. This facilitates accurate planning for the provision of the adult service in the future. A clinic held jointly by the paediatric and adult haematologists for young adults aged 16–18 years fosters this co-operation. Such a transition clinic provides opportunities for children to familiarize themselves with the adult team and their services before they are completely transferred to adult care. The haematologist is in a vantage position to provide initial explanation of the diagnosis

and the nature of SCD to affected individuals. This should be supplemented by further information from sickle cell centres and counsellors.

Information about SCD

Various means of communication in non-technical language are used to share relevant information on SCD with affected individuals. Individual and group discussion, portable cards showing the person's haemoglobin genotype, leaflets, booklets, video or audio cassettes, and posters are effective means of conveying information about the haemoglobinopathy. On a larger scale, public sickle cell awareness events could be held to increase the level of information about the condition in the community. As much as possible, communication should be in lay language, to facilitate understanding. Following the usually unpleasant effect of being told one has SCD, it is helpful to consolidate and further clarify this at a later date when the affected persons would have had time to think about it, and probably have questions about the practical implications of the diagnosis. While this could be carried out by specially trained counsellors or other healthcare professionals, it is crucial that the information provided is consistent, and that this important interaction takes place in a less formal and time-constrained atmosphere than that usually experienced in a busy clinic or ward round. The non-clinical setting of a Sickle Cell and Thalassaemia Centre enables this communication to be informal, and if practicable, a home visit to the affected person is ideal. If the above options are not feasible, consolidation of initial information could be carried out during a follow-up clinic visit.

Subsequent reinforcement and expansion of the initial information should be carried out when appropriate, such as when the child is about to start schooling, during adolescence, before transfer from the childhood to adult comprehensive care, and before starting a family. Genetic counselling, including information about pre-implantation genetic and prenatal diagnoses, is beneficial for couples whose haemoglobin genotypes are such that their offspring could have a clinically significant haemoglobinopathy [2, 3]. For such at-risk couples, genetic counselling is best done pre-conceptually. Failing that, it needs to be done early enough to allow fetal tissue sampling by 11–12 weeks of gestation and possible termination of pregnancy thereafter. Genetic counselling is inextricably linked with antenatal screening. Close co-operation between the haematology laboratory and maternity services ensures that at-risk couples are referred to the medical geneticist at an early stage for assessment, and discussion of the intrinsic risks and error rate of prenatal diagnosis. The consultation is non-directive; it is ultimately the woman's decision whether or not to carry on with an affected pregnancy. When health-care professionals invest time and effort in providing relevant information about SCD to affected individuals, it is very rewarding subsequently. It facilitates bridge-building between both parties, makes a sometimes-uneasy relationship cordial, and helps to win the patient/parent confidence and co-operation that is indispensable in the delivery of comprehensive care.

Prevention of infections

People who have SCD are prone to infection because of reduced splenic function, defective activation of the alternative pathway of complement and impaired ability of neutrophils to kill microbes [4–9]. The infection precipitates a sickle cell crisis, which may be life-threatening or may cause excruciating pain. Therefore, prevention of infection is an essential cornerstone of comprehensive care in SCD. Specific measures include prophylactic antibiotic or antimalarial therapy, and immunization against pneumococcus, meningococcus, *Haemophilus influenzae* type B, and hepatitis B and influenza viruses. A vaccine against parvovirus B19, which causes aplastic crisis, is available in some countries. Commencement of prophylactic penicillin at around the age of 3 months has been shown to reduce mortality from pneumoccocal septicaemia [10].

Social services

The clinical manifestation of sickle cell disease is influenced by the social and economic circumstances of affected persons. The nature of a patient's or parent's occupation, level of general education and specific information about SCD, the suitability or spaciousness of the residential accommodation; all these have an impact on the patient's health. Appropriate heating of the house in which an affected person lives helps to prevent chest infections that can predispose the individual to sickle cell crisis. This reduces the need for hospital attendance or admission, and frees up health-care staff and hospital beds, ultimately saving resources for the health service. Some issues that affected persons have to contend with are not medical. Social workers have very important roles in the comprehensive care of patients with haemoglobinopathies. It is their responsibility to assess the specific social needs of affected persons and ensure that services are provided to meet identified needs. Social services needed by individuals may include registration as disabled, practical help at home, and adaptations to the home such as constructing a ramp or installing a lift to facilitate mobility for people with SCD complicated by stroke or hip damage.

In some countries, currently available regulations for provision of social services are not adequate for the specific needs of people affected by haemoglobinopathies, and need to be reviewed. Some children with SCD fall within the group regarded as being in need. These are children who are disabled, or who require provision of social services to achieve a reasonable standard of health or development, or to prevent impairment of health or development. The Social Services Department has the responsibility to provide the right level of intervention and support that will enable people with haemoglobinopathies to achieve their potential in life.

Psychological support

An immense psychological burden is associated with a chronic illness manifesting as painful episodes that may be life-threatening and occur without forewarning [11, 12]. It is a credit to their resilience that most affected persons cope well with SCD despite this psychological stress. Unvoiced fears about sudden illness or even death, feelings of carrying their burden alone or being depressed as a result, and anxiety about the uncertainty of their future are psychological issues for people who have SCD. These can increase the feeling of pain experienced during crisis or other physical illness [13], and make medical management difficult. As a result, some affected individuals may ask for inappropriate medical intervention such as opiate therapy when this is not really needed. Psychological disturbances could lead to withdrawal from family and friends, communication problems, poor performance at school or work, unemployment, poverty, dependence at an inappropriate age and low self-esteem. Recurrent priapism or prolonged penile erection is a source of anxiety in males who may not volunteer this information or may not even be aware that it is caused by SCD [14]. This can lead to suboptimal sexual function and can affect relationships. Psychological support for persons affected by SCD is needed for chronic pain, challenging behaviour, learning or attention difficulty, transition from paediatric to adult care, depression or anxiety states, and relationship problems. Psychological support may be provided for groups of affected persons, rather than individuals. Such Sickle Cell Support Groups enable people to learn from the experiences of others who have experienced challenges similar to theirs, and to appreciate that they are not alone. An important component of psychological evaluation is to assess the person's quality of life. Cognitive behaviour therapy, a type of psychotherapy, helps affected people to cope with the chronic pain and psychological problems associated with SCD [15].

Drug dependency services

A very small minority of people with SCD become dependent on opiates or other addictive drugs. In most cases this results from use of these drugs in the treatment of SCD. Therefore, the situation calls for understanding, compassion and supportive management. The large amount of health service resources used up by the affected individuals is very much out of proportion to their small number. Health-care personnel have a duty to ensure effective analgesia for people with SCD. However, it is important to recognize when requests for opiates

and other addictive drugs, such as temazepam, exceed the medical needs of the affected individual. The problem might not be obvious, or it may manifest as an apparently unconnected issue such as poor performance at school or work, difficult relationships with family, friends and health-care staff, or unusually frequent sickle cell crises. Affected individuals may use different names and personal details such as date of birth and address, and register with more than one hospital or general practice to enable them to receive prescriptions from different doctors without each one knowing of the other. Whereas differences in (the subjective) impression of the level of pain between doctors and patients are to be expected, a patient's incessant objections to reduction in the dose of opiates considered medically appropriate after clinical review, habitual arguments about the starting dose, frequent requests for increasing the dose (especially if made to doctors-on-call after normal working hours), insistence on directing the dose and frequency of opiates prescribed by doctors without caring as much about antibiotics or other medications; all these should make one consider drug dependence. Opiate addiction is very rare among people with SCD [16, 17]. Addicts may acquire drugs unlawfully, and may commit crimes such as forging and altering prescriptions in attempts to obtain drugs or materials for injecting them. People who misuse drugs may be neither dependent nor addicted, yet they strive to obtain more than their medical needs and dispose of the rest. As opiates and other addictive drugs such as temazepam have street values, SCD might be used as a reason to obtain drugs that are completely disposed of, and it may be that none are taken personally.

The affected person should be referred to the Drug Dependency Unit for expert assessment if drug dependence or addiction is a differential diagnosis. Support from the family and the psychologist is important in management. Treatment requires the co-operation of affected individuals, some of who may not accept that there is an issue because of embarrassment, reluctance to go through treatment, or loss of any personal benefits from disposal of drugs. Only medically required doses of drugs should be prescribed at all times, so that inappropriate use is not encouraged.

Specialty medical care

Although it is primarily a blood disorder, SCD affects virtually every part of the body through vaso-occlusion, ischaemia and infarction. As a result, SCD is a multi-organ disease that requires the co-operation of different medical specialties for optimal management. These include nephrologists for sickle nephropathy, neurologists for stroke, cardiologists for pulmonary hypertension, chest physicians for acute chest syndrome and chronic sickle lung disease, and gastroenterologists for peptic ulcer and liver impairment.

The life expectancy of people with SCD has increased continually with improvements in their medical and non-medical care. As a result an increasing number are surviving long enough to develop long-term complications of SCD such as nephropathy and pulmonary hypertension. The renal manifestations of SCD lead to considerable illness and loss of lives [18–21]. Therefore, proactive management of kidney disease is an essential component of comprehensive care for people with the haemoglobinopathy. Joint clinics run by haematologists and nephrologists facilitate co-operation between the specialties, formulation and implementation of joint treatment protocols, and ultimately, better care of people who have sickle nephropathy. Similar arrangements for joint management could be made with other medical specialties as necessary.

Orthopaedic and other types of surgery

The skeleton is the commonest site of infarction in SCD. The tissue necrosis involves bone and bone marrow, and predisposes to osteomyelitis because dead tissue is less able to resist infection than living cells. Other skeletal manifestations of the haemoglobinopathy include the pathognomonic hand-foot syndrome, bone pain crisis, septic arthritis and avascular necrosis of joints. The hip, shoulder and spine are commonly affected by avascular necrosis; the ankle and knee less frequently. The prevalence of avascular necrosis of joints increases with age; the hip alone is affected in about 41% of adults, although symptomatic in 3–5% [22–26]. Orthopaedic treatment is needed in cases of acute ostomyelitis with subperiosteal fluid collection, chronic osteomyelitis requiring sequestrectomy, avascular necrosis with chronic pain uncontrollable by medications, and other situations advised by the surgeon. Co-operation between haematologists and orthopaedic surgeons is essential for management of such cases, and joint consultation in a comprehensive clinic facilitates delivery of such care.

General surgery input in SCD is required for patients with symptomatic gall bladder stones or acute surgical abdomen. The latter may mimic vaso-occlusive crisis affecting abdominal organs, and may cause difficulty in differential diagnosis [26]. The management of major priapism unresponsive to medical therapy, or erectile dysfunction resulting from this manifestation of SCD, fall into the province of urosurgery [14]. Vaso-occlusive infarction may occur in the mandible or maxilla, predisposing to infection and loosening of the teeth. Dental assessment is beneficial in such cases, and tooth extraction may be necessary. Special measures to reduce the risk of hypoxaemia and red cell sickling are essential during anaesthesia and peri-operative management of people with SCD.

Obstetric care

The clinical severity of sickle cell disease may be increased during pregnancy, and the prevalence of complications of pregnancy is higher in people with SCD compared with HbAA individuals [27–31]. Therefore, pregnancy in SCD is considered high risk and appropriate for specialist obstetric care; preferably by health-care professionals with experience in attending to people who have this blood disorder. The multidisciplinary team of professionals may include obstetricians, genetic counsellors, midwives, specialist sickle cell nurses and haematologists. Monthly reviews in haematology clinics are recommended during pregnancy, and regular exchange blood transfusion for individuals with multiple pregnancy, poor obstetric history and frequent sickle cell crisis. Considering the risks associated with pregnancy in SCD, with a perinatal mortality as high as 15%, it is advisable to refer the expectant mother to a centre with considerable expertise if this is not available locally.

Specialist sickle cell nursing in the hospital and community

In both clinical and community settings, special sickle cell nursing has made increasing contributions to comprehensive care. The role of the clinical sickle cell nurse specialist includes initial assessment of patients in haematology clinics, exchange blood transfusion, desferrioxamine therapy in conjunction with pharmacists, data collection and management for the sickle cell register and database, and general nursing duties as and when necessary. The community sickle cell nurse specialist provides a link between the patient's home, the hospital and community-based services. These include social workers, voluntary agencies, adult disability teams, rehabilitation centres, community occupational therapists and physiotherapists, housing officers, visual impairment teams, council staff who provide help at home, and general practitioners.

Developing and monitoring a comprehensive sickle cell service

A fundamental requirement of a comprehensive haemoglobinopathy service is the multidisciplinary team to deliver it. The team's skill-mix should be appropriate to enable them to provide the various components of comprehensive care outlined above. While it may not be feasible in some circumstances to have the full complement of required professionals, every effort should be made to involve as many as possible. Once assembled, the team's effectiveness and success depend critically on co-operation among its members. This is enhanced by leadership that actively promotes interaction and cohesion within the team, while supporting and encouraging individual roles. Co-ordination between hospital and community-based services is crucial. These two arms, by and large, deliver the bulk of comprehensive care; and it is important that each hand knows what the other is doing. To this end, regular briefing and planning meetings of the team are very useful. The comprehensive care team achieves better results by working in partnership with management staff of the hospital or the community-based services, the local health authority, and non-governmental agencies with similar goals such as the Sickle Cell Society and the Organisation for Sickle Cell Anaemia Research.

A service development that has had a great impact on the provision of holistic care to people affected by SCD is the establishment of a Comprehensive Sickle Clinic. This omnibus clinic provides the opportunity for affected persons to see various professionals in one place during a single hospital visit. Currently, the components of the Comprehensive Sickle Clinic in our centre are the Transition/Adolescent, Antenatal, Orthopaedic, Iron Overload and Renal Clinics. More components could be added in the future as the service evolves. The psychologist, sickle cell nurse specialist, counsellors and haematologist attend to affected persons with the appropriate medical or surgical specialist, depending on the clinic. The presence of a physiotherapist increases the quality of care delivered in the Sickle Orthopaedic Clinic, and a pharmacist dedicated to iron chelation therapy attends the Iron Overload Clinic. The comprehensive sickle clinic makes it possible to provide a wide range of services on an outpatient basis.

A comprehensive sickle cell service can be monitored effectively by regular audit of established practices, management protocols and treatment guidelines. Monitoring is greatly facilitated by having a patients register or a computer database that can, with appropriate controls, talk to regional, national or international networks. The service should be assessed continually, and improvements made to reflect findings from audit, research and suggestions from team members or users of the service.

A multidisciplinary team providing holistic care for people affected by haemoglobinopathies is a rich resource for continuing professional development (CPD) and for raising public awareness of globin gene disorders. Unique opportunities for training and education are available within a comprehensive haemoglobinopathy care system. Resources and protected time should be set aside for lectures and seminars to enhance the professional skills and knowledge of team members and staff of other units or organizations.

Advantages of comprehensive care over episodic treatment of SCD

Holistic care enhances the quality of life for people affected by SCD. A better overall result is achieved by interaction of a co-operative patient with the team of various professionals and organizations working in partnership. Comprehensive care reduces the number of hospital admissions for people with SCD, and shortens the length of hospital stay (Fig. 1.2a,b). These translate to considerable savings in the cost of health care. Complications of SCD such as renal impairment and avascular joint necrosis are detected and treated earlier; so reduc-

ing disease-related morbidity and mortality. The immense psychological burden for affected persons is ameliorated, enabling them to live a fuller life. The holistic approach provides opportunities for health promotion, community-based care and improved communication between various disciplines. When people affected by SCD experience the benefits of holistic care, they are more compliant with medical treatment and co-operate more willingly with professionals providing the non-medical aspects of the care. The advantages of comprehensive care over episodic treatment of SCD have been observed in various centres in different parts of the world, and include the benefits of proactive blood

HOSPITAL ADMISSIONS FOR ADULTS WITH SICKLE CELL DISEASE

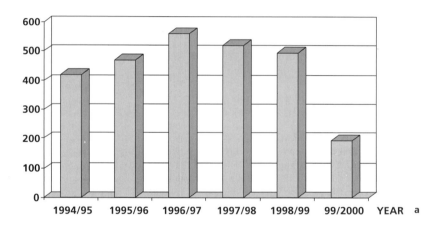

AVERAGE LENGTH OF HOSPITAL ADMISSIONS FOR ADULTS WITH SCD

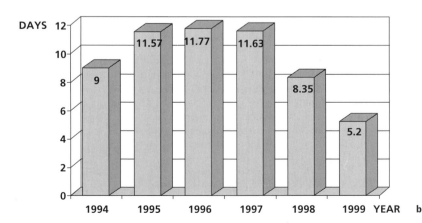

Fig. 1.2 (a) Hospital admissions for adults with sickle cell disease (SCD). Note the fall in admissions following the establishment of a Comprehensive Sickle Clinic in 1999. (b) Average length of hospital admissions for adults with SCD.

transfusion therapy for primary prevention of the devastation brought to the lives of affected persons by stroke [32, 33], a smoother transition from children's to adult care [34], striking reduction in childhood mortality from splenic sequestration crisis achieved by parent education [35] and enhanced ability to secure employment as a result of psychosocial services [36]; all of which are achieved at lower cost to the health service [37].

These positive effects of comprehensive care make it the preferred mode of service delivery to people affected by sickle cell disease.

References

1. Serjeant GR. *Sickle Cell Disease*. Oxford: Oxford University Press, 1992.
2. British Committee for Standards in Haematology. Haemoglobinopathy screening. *Clin Lab Haematol* 1988; **10**: 87–94.
3. British Committee for Standards in Haematology. Fetal diagnosis of globin gene disorders. *J Clin Pathol* 1994; 47: 199–204.
4. Pearson HA. The kidney, hepatobiliary system, and spleen in sickle cell anaemia. *Ann N Y Acad Sci* 1989; **565**: 120–5.
5. Johnston RB Jr, Hewman SL, Struth AC. An abnormality of the alternative pathway of complement activation in sickle cell disease. *N Engl J Med* 1973; **288**: 803–5.
6. Anyaegbu CC, Okpala IE, Aken'Ova AY, Salimonu LS. Complement haemolytic activity, circulating immune complexes and the morbidity of sickle cell anaemia. *Acta Pathol Microbiol Scand* 1999; **107**: 699–702.
7. Anyaegbu CC, Okpala IE, Aken'Ova AY, Salimonu LS. Peripheral blood neutrophil count and candidacidal activity correlate with the clinical severity of sickle cell anaemia. *Eur J Haematol* 1998; **60**: 267–8.
8. Mollapour E, Porter JB, Kaczmarski R, Linch DC, Roberts PJ. Raised neutrophil phospholipase A2 activity and defective priming of NADPH oxidase and phospholipase A2 in sickle cell disease. *Blood* 1998; **91**: 3423–9.
9. Attah EB, Ekere MC. Death patterns in sickle cell anemia. *JAMA* 1975; **233**: 889–90.
10. Gaston MH, Verter JI, Woods G *et al.* for the Prophylactic Penicillin Group. Prophylaxis with oral penicillin in children with sickle cell anaemia: a randomized trial. *N Engl J Med* 1986; **314**: 1593–9.
11. Midence K, Elander J. *The Psychosocial Aspects of Sickle Cell Disease*. Oxford: Radcliffe Medical Press, 1994.
12. Midence K, Fuggle P, Davies SC. Psychosocial aspects of sickle cell disease in childhood and adolescence. *Br J Clin Psychol* 1993; **32**: 271–80.
13. Thomas VJ. Cognitive behavioural therapy in pain management for sickle cell disease. *Int J Palliat Nurs* 2000; **6**: 434–42.
14. Okpala IE, Westerdale N, Jegede T, Cheung B. Etilefrine for the prevention of priapism in adult sickle cell disease. *Br J Haematol* 2002; **118**: 918–21.
15. Thomas VJ, Dixon AL, Milligan P. Cognitive behaviour therapy for the management of sickle cell disease pain: an evaluation of a community-based intervention. *Br J Health Psychol* 1999; **4**: 777–81.
16. Porter J, Jick H. Addiction is rare in patients treated with narcotics. *N Engl J Med* 1980; **302**: 123.
17. Brookoff D, Polomano R. Treating sickle cell pain like cancer pain. *Ann Intern Med* 1992; **116**: 364–8.
18. Ataga KI, Orringer EU. Renal abnormalities in sickle cell disease. *Am J Hematol* 2000; **63**: 205–11.
19. Falk RJ, Scheinmn J, Phillips G *et al.* Prevalence and pathologic features of sickle cell nephropathy and response to inhibition of angiotensin-converting enzyme. *N Engl J Med* 1992; **326**: 910–15.
20. Johnson CS, Giorgio AJ. Arterial blood pressure in adults with sickle cell disease. *Arch Intern Med* 1981; **141**: 891–3.
21. Guasch A, Cua M, Mitch WE. Early detection and the course of glomerular injury in patients with sickle cell anemia. *Kidney Int* 1996; **49**: 786–91.
22. Iwegbu CG, Fleming AF. Avascular necrosis of the femoral head in sickle cell disease. *J Bone Joint Surg* 1985; **67**: 29–32.
23. Moran MC. Osteonecrosis of the hip in sickle cell haemoglobinopathy. *Am J Orthoped* 1995; **24**: 18–24.
24. Milner PF, Kraus AP, Sebes JI. Sickle cell disease as a cause of osteonecrosis of the femoral head. *N Engl J Med* 1991; **21**: 1476–81.
25. Lee RE, Golging JSR, Serjeant GR. The radiological features of avascular necrosis of the femoral head in homozygous sickle cell disease. *Clin Radiol* 1981; **32**: 205–14.
26. Okpala IE. The management of crisis in sickle cell disease (review). *Eur J Haematol* 1998; **60**: 1–6.
27. Hendrikse JPV, Harrison KA, Watson-Williams EJ, Luzzatto L, Ajabor LN. Pregnancy in homozygous sickle cell anaemia. *J Obstet Gynaecol Br Commonwealth* 1972; **79**: 396–409.
28. Anyaegbunam A, Morel MG, Merkatz IR. Antepartum fetal surveillance tests during sickle cell crisis. *Am J Obstet Gynecol* 1991; **165**: 1081–3.
29. Department of Health, Welsh Office, Scottish Home and Health Department, Department of Health & Social Services, Northern Ireland. *Report on Confidential Enquiries into Maternal Deaths in the United Kingdom 1994–1996*. London: HMSO, 1998.
30. Howard RJ, Tuck SM, Pearson TC. Pregnancy in sickle

cell disease in the UK: results of a multicentre survey of the effect of prophylactic blood transfusion on maternal and fetal outcome. *Br J Obstet Gynaecol* 1995; **102**: 947–51.

31. Dare FO, Makinde OO, Fasuba OB. The obstetric performance of sickle cell disease patients and homozygous haemoglobin C patients in Ile-Ife, Nigeria. *Int J Gynaecol Obstet* 1992; **37**: 163–8.

32. Ohene-Frempong K. Indications for red cell transfusion in sickle cell disease. *Semin Hematol* 2001; **38**: 5–13.

33. Adams RJ, McKie VC, Hsu L *et al*. Prevention of a first stroke by transfusions in children with sickle cell anemia and abnormal results on transcranial Doppler ultrasonography. *N Engl J Med* 1998; **339**: 5–11.

34. Kinney TR, Ware RE. The adolescent with sickle cell anemia. *Hematol/Oncol Clin North Am* 1996; **10**: 1255–64.

35. Emond AM, Collis R, Darville D *et al*. Acute splenic sequestration in homozygous sickle cell disease; natural history and management. *J Pediatr* 1985; **107**: 201–6.

36. Koshy M, Dorn L. Continuing care for adult patients with sickle cell disease. *Hematol/Oncol Clin North Am* 1996; **10**: 1265–73.

37. Yang YM, Shah AK, Watson M, Mankad VN. Comparison of costs to the health sector of comprehensive and episodic care of sickle cell disease patients. *Public Health Rep* 1995; **110**: 80–6.

Chapter 2

Haemoglobinopathy diagnostic tests: blood counts, sickle solubility test, haemoglobin electrophoresis and high-performance liquid chromatography

Yvonne Daniel

Introduction

The normal adult red blood cell contains three types of haemoglobin, approximately 95 % haemoglobin A (HbA) with haemoglobin A2 (HbA2) and F (HbF) forming minor fractions. Globin chains of amino acids linked to form a tetramer are an integral part of the haemoglobin molecule. HbA comprises two alpha and two beta chains ($\alpha_2\beta_2$), HbA2 has two alpha and two delta chains ($\alpha_2\delta_2$) and HbF has two alpha and two gamma chains ($\alpha_2\gamma_2$). Variations from normal can be classified into three major categories: structural variants, thalassaemias and hereditary persistence of fetal haemoglobin (HPFH).

Structural haemoglobin variants result from mutations that give rise to the formation of globin with an abnormal structure; the majority are point mutations. HbS is one of the best known of these and results from the substitution of the amino acid valine for glutamic acid at position six of the beta chain [1]. Other documented causes of structural variants include double point mutations, mutations resulting in shortened or lengthened chains and gene fusion [2–8].

Thalassaemias result from mutations that cause a defect in the synthesis of one or more globin chains disturbing the ratio of alpha to non-alpha chains. Beta thalassaemia results from deletional, frameshift and point mutations and can be divided into two types: beta zero in which no beta chains are produced and beta plus in which there is reduced chain production. Alpha thalassaemia is primarily caused by gene deletions. Again the nomenclature of alpha plus and alpha zero is used. This relates to the number of genes which are non-functional and therefore to the amount of alpha chains produced and thus clinical severity. HPFH refers to a benign group of conditions in which the synthesis of fetal haemoglobin remains raised throughout life.

Haemoglobinopathies have arisen in areas where malaria has been endemic and different mutations occur within the same ethnic group. Therefore, an important point to consider when diagnosing haemoglobinopathies is that it is possible for more than one type of abnormality to be co-inherited. It is clear that homozygosity for these abnormalities can lead to clinical disease such as sickle cell disease (SCD) or thalassaemia major. However, it is also possible for different types of beta chain variants, such as HbS and HbC, and for beta and alpha chain variants to be co-inherited. Globin chain variants may also be co-inherited with thalassaemia and/or HPFH. Similarly, alpha and beta thalassaemia may be seen in the same individual.

The purpose of this chapter is to provide an overview of the first-line laboratory tests for the diagnosis of haemoglobinopathies and interpretation of data obtained from these procedures. It is not intended to be comprehensive. If the results of routine laboratory tests do not provide enough information for definitive diagnosis, it may be necessary to determine the haemoglobin genotype by mass spectrometry or DNA analysis.

Blood counts

The full blood count (FBC) and blood film are important primary screening tests in haemoglo-

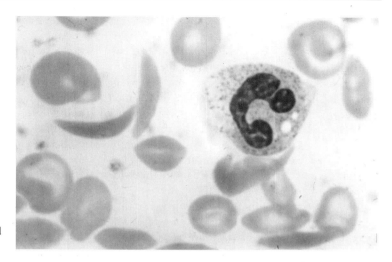

Fig. 2.1 Blood film showing sickle–shaped cells.

binopathy diagnosis. Neonatal screening is the exception, as dried blood spots are frequently used, precluding FBC analysis. If the FBC is available it should be noted that normal ranges are age-dependent. Of particular interest are the red cell indices: red count (RBC), haemoglobin (Hb), mean cell volume (MCV) and mean cell haemoglobin (MCH). These are essential in thalassaemia diagnosis. Classically the picture in thalassaemia trait is described as one with a mildly raised RBC, normal Hb and reduced MCV and MCH; these are referred to as thalassaemic red cell indices. However, this may not always be the case because other conditions, such as concomitant iron deficiency and co-inheritance of alpha and beta thalassaemia trait, will influence the results. Iron deficiency has the effect of lowering the red cell indices and has also been reported to lower the HbA2 value [9, 10]. Co-inheritance of alpha and beta thalassaemia may cause the red cell indices to normalize, as excess alpha chains are partly responsible for the pathology in beta thalassaemia.

Red cell indices are also useful in the differential diagnosis of delta beta thalassaemia trait and HPFH, as those with delta beta thalassaemia will have classically thalassaemic indices while those with HPFH will be normal.

A blood film can provide valuable information in the diagnosis of haemoglobinopathies. There are characteristic red cell features, such as sickle-shaped cells, basophilic stippling and target cells

which may point to the haemoglobin variant present. Figure 2.1 shows a blood film with the characteristic sickle- or crescent-shaped cells seen in sickle cell disease, target cells can also be seen. Nucleated red cells are seen in some states including thalassaemia intermedia and major and SCD. The reticulocyte count should also be performed: with unstable haemoglobin variants and other chronic haemolytic processes, reticulocytes are elevated and the level can relate to the severity of haemolysis [11].

Tests used in haemoglobin analysis

High-performance liquid chromatography (HPLC)

HPLC systems are today the primary haemoglobinopathy screening mechanism in many laboratories. Usually automated, these systems comprise a reservoir for the mobile or liquid phase, pump, injector, chromatographic column, detector and a system for recording and processing data. In common with most other separation systems, HPLC uses the fact that most mutations cause a change in the charge of the molecule. For the analysis of haemoglobin variants, weak cation exchange columns are used. The column is negatively charged and the positively charged globin molecules bind with varying degrees of affinity according to the charge present on the molecule. Buffer of increasing cation concentration is passed through the column, causing competition with bound globin molecules and elution of the globin at a time relative to the positive charge. Within each system the time of elution or as it is more commonly known, the retention time, is characteristic for each normal or variant analysed. The haemoglobins eluted are represented graphically and quantified optically as they pass through the detector. This allows accurate quantification of Hb variants and HbA2 and HbF, a major advantage over screening systems that utilize electrophoresis, as these require secondary methods for quantification of haemoglobins.

HPLC system manufacturers identify variants, which separate from HbA, in different ways. The more common haemoglobin variants, e.g. HbS and HbC, have well characterized retention times. In some systems, the instrument software will identify variants as the haemoglobin into which retention time window they have eluted. Haemoglobins eluting outside of these defined times will be labelled as unknown. Care must be taken when interpreting HPLC plots even when the variant has fallen into a known retention time window. It is possible for variants to overlap and for more than one haemoglobin to elute within a given window. Examples are Hb Lepore and HbE, which elute in the same window as HbA2. Thus all variants should have further confirmatory tests. Despite these limitations it is possible to provisionally identify a greater number of haemoglobin variants than by conventional electrophoresis screening methods. Figure 2.2(a–c) illustrates typical Biorad Variant HPLC

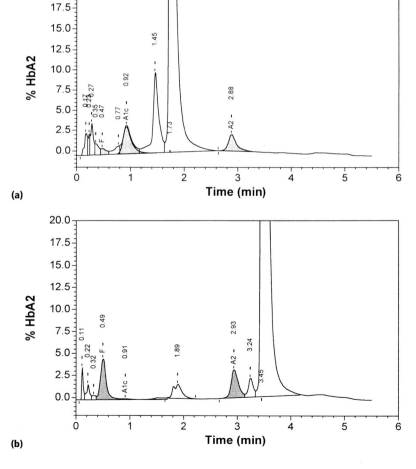

(a)

(b)

Fig. 2.2 Typical Biorad Variant HPLC elution patterns (Biorad Laboratories, Hercules, CA, USA). (a) Normal. (b) Haemoglobin SS (HbSS). (c) Haemoglobin SC (HbSC). (d) Sickle cell trait (haemoglobin AS, HbAS). (e) Haemoglobin G (HbG) Philadelphia trait. (f) Haemoglobin S/G (HbS/G) Philadelphia compound heterozygote.

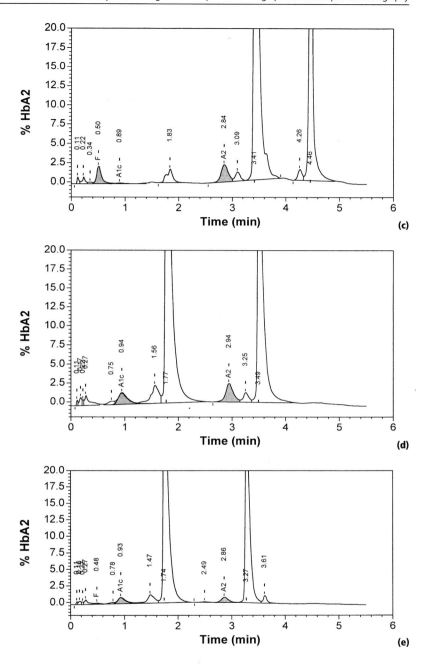

Fig. 2.2 *Continued*

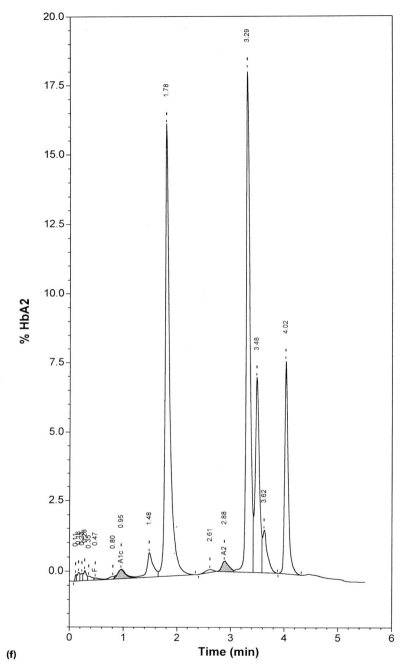

(f)

Fig. 2.2 *Continued*

elution patterns for normal, HbSS and HbSC samples.

The confirmatory tests performed will depend on which variant or variants are detected. Haemoglo-

bins eluting in the HbS window should have a sickle solubility test performed to confirm the presence of a sickling haemoglobin. Because of the evident clinical significance of a sickling haemoglobin, some suggest that a sickle solubility test should probably be performed on all samples with a haemoglobin variant and as a minimum on samples with unidentified variants to ensure that these are not one of the other sickling haemoglobins [12]. HbC can be confirmed by electrophoresis at acid pH, where HbC is clearly separated from other haemoglobin variants. Unidentified variants may require a far greater range of tests such as electrophoresis at alkaline and acid pH, isoelectric focusing and mass spectrometry, before identification can be reached.

Electrophoresis

Electrophoresis enables the separation of different haemoglobins on the basis of charge and, for a long time, has been the most common technique for initial detection and characterization of variant haemoglobins. Today, when not used as a primary screening method, electrophoresis has a valuable place as a confirmatory technique following HPLC screening. Electrophoretic separation at two pH values, alkaline and acid, enables identification of common haemoglobin structural variants A/F/S/D/G, C/E/O-Arab, H, as well as other less common variants. Most mutations cause a change in the charge of the molecule and thus a change in electrophoretic behaviour. HbA is negatively charged at alkaline pH and moves towards the positive electrode during electrophoresis. Other haemoglobins are interpreted according to their movement relative to HbA. If a variant haemoglobin is detected at alkaline pH, it is necessary to confirm its identity by an alternative technique such as electrophoresis at acid pH using either citrate agar or agarose gel. In this case the separation of the haemoglobin depends not only on the electrical charge but also on interaction with components in the gel medium, particularly agaropectin [13]. Use of both acid and alkaline techniques will allow differentiation of HbS from HbD/G but will not usually differentiate HbD from HbG. HbC is also separated from HbE, HbC Harlem and HbO-Arab. If electrophoresis is used as a primary screening method additional techniques are required for accurate quantification of haemoglobins.

Solubility test

Red cells that contain a sickling haemoglobin form a characteristic sickle shape at low oxygen pressure [14]. Sickle solubility tests utilize this principle to induce sickling in red cells by subjecting them to low oxygen tension using a buffer containing a reducing agent such as sodium dithionite. Under such conditions HbS or other sickling haemoglobins will sickle and precipitate within the red cells, preventing lysis and leading to a turbid solution. While HbS is the best known sickling haemoglobin, there are others, which include HbC Harlem, HbS Travis, HbC Zignixchor, HbS Antilles, HbS-Oman and HbS Providence [15].

The sickle solubility test is not reliable at HbS levels below 15–20%, the minimum proportion required to give a positive result. This means that it is not reliable in neonates, and may be unreliable in infants and people with HbS who have recently been transfused with normal (HbAA) blood. In such circumstances it is possible to use an alternative method in which freshly made sodium bisulphate is used to induce sickling with subsequent micro-scopic examination of the preparation [16]. This may enable detection of sickling haemoglobins present at reduced levels.

It should be noted that a positive test indicates only that a sickling haemoglobin is present and does not enable definitive diagnosis of what the haemoglobin is or which other haemoglobins may be present.

Identification of haemoglobin variants

Combined data from HPLC, electrophoresis at alkaline and acid pH, and the sickle solubility test enable definitive identification of HbA, HbF, HbS, HbC, and several others. They differentiate HbC, HbE and HbO and distinguish HbS from variants that migrate like HbS at alkaline pH. Data must be interpreted with appropriate control samples to ensure that techniques are working and to provide a reference for unknowns. As a minimum all electrophoretic strips should have a control, which contains HbA, HbS and HbF.

HPLC data interpretation can be complicated by the fact that the separation of glycosylated and acetylated haemoglobins is different from that of non-glycosylated and acetylated forms. Glycosylated HbA elutes before HbA, and is usually observed as a series of small peaks preceding the HbA peak. However, the levels of glycosylated haemoglobin are usually elevated in individuals with diabetes and in addition some haemoglobin variants such as HbJ can elute at the same time as the glycosylated HbA fraction.

Some clinically significant mutations are referred to as electrophoretically silent in that there is no alteration in electrical charge. While some may be separated at acid pH or by HPLC but not at alkaline pH, others are not detected by any of these techniques. One group of clinically significant haemoglobins, which are frequently electrophoretically silent, are high-affinity haemoglobins such as Hb Johnston [17]. If such haemoglobins are suspected other techniques such as an oxygen affinity curve or mass spectrometry are recommended.

Quantification and interpretation of HbA2 levels

Accurate quantification of HbA2 is required for the diagnosis of alpha and beta thalassaemia. HbF levels can be useful in these circumstances but are essential for diagnosis of delta beta thalassaemia trait and HPFH. Each laboratory should establish relevant reference ranges, but an HbA2 value between 4% and 7% with the classical thalassaemic red cell indices is usually considered diagnostic of beta thalassaemia trait.

Mutations or combinations of mutations that present without the classical phenotype can cause some problems with the diagnosis of beta thalassaemia trait. The phenotypes are: normal red cell indices with a raised HbA2, normal red cell indices with a normal or borderline normal HbA2 and abnormal red cell indices with a normal HbA2 [12]. One advantage of using HPLC as a primary screening method for beta thalassaemia is that a HbA2 value is provided on all samples. This allows diagnosis of beta thalassaemia trait in samples with normal red cell indices and will also identify borderline normal values. Such situations may be missed if criteria such as low red cell indices are used to select samples for secondary HbA2 and/or HbF quantification following electrophoresis.

A normal HbA2 value with reduced MCV and MCH may be due to several factors and establishing the exact cause can be difficult using standard screening procedures. The most common causes of such a picture are iron deficiency and/or alpha thalassaemia trait. The ethnic background of the individual being tested will influence the frequency of alpha thalassaemia and the underlying genotype. The diagnosis and significance of alpha thalassaemia are discussed in more detail in Chapter 5.

Quantification and interpretation of HbF levels

There are various underlying mechanisms for increased HbF production; increased values may be due to a genetic disorder of haemoglobin production or may be acquired in a variety of different haematological conditions [18, 19].

Delta beta thalassaemia results from a failure of delta and beta chain synthesis and the heterozygous phenotype is classically described as having thalassaemic red cell indices, a normal HbA2 with HbF levels of 5–20%. As a clinically significant mutation, which can lead to a thalassaemia major phenotype, it is important to distinguish this from HPFH. This can be difficult using only phenotypic data because individuals do not always present with the classical picture. Furthermore it is suggested that because these mutations occur within the same locus they are in fact, overlapping syndromes [19]. For this reason genetic analysis may be required to obtain a correct diagnosis.

HbF values can also be of value in the monitoring of hydroxyurea therapy, which raises the HbF level [20]. Care should be taken when interpreting results of SCD individuals with raised HbF levels as this may be caused by therapy and may not be innate.

Distinguishing between alpha and beta chain variants

When identifying a haemoglobin variant it is important to determine whether the variant present is alpha or beta chain. This is of particular importance for the purposes of genetic counselling. With universal neonatal screening this may become simpler because alpha chain production is activated early in fetal life, while beta chain production is not fully activated until the neonatal period. Thus inherited alpha chain abnormalities will be expressed throughout life in both fetal and adult haemoglobins while beta chain variants will not become apparent until the fetal to adult haemoglobin switch is made. The ratio of normal to abnormal haemoglobin reflects the genetic composition, each person having two beta globin chain genes and four alpha globin chain genes. In a normal adult each beta gene produces approximately 50% of the beta chains while each alpha gene produces approximately 25%. When a beta chain variant is present, these proportions alter such that heterozygosity for a beta chain mutation will result in approximately 40% variant haemoglobin detected. Figure 2.2(d) shows a Biorad Variant HPLC analysis plot for an individual heterozygous for HbS with HbA and HbS in the appropriate ratio. If there is a single alpha gene mutation, the quantity of variant detected will be approximately 25%, with the remaining haemoglobins being HbA, HbA2 and HbF.

There are three situations in which this does not apply: variants produced in thalassaemic quantities, such as HbE and Hb Constant Spring, concomitant thalassaemia and unstable haemoglobins. HbE, a beta chain variant, is usually present at about 30% of the total haemoglobin. The mutation results in reduced beta globin chain production and this is reflected in the red cell indices. However, values up to 45% with normal red cell indices have been reported [21].

Co-inheritance of thalassaemia should also give the classical picture of thalassaemic red cell indices. A compound heterozygote for a beta chain variant and beta zero thalassaemia will lead to the absence of HbA with the variant haemoglobin being the predominant haemoglobin detected. HbA2 is often raised. Co-inheritance of a beta plus thalassaemia mutation and a beta chain variant classically results in 15–20% HbA with the remainder being the variant haemoglobin. Again, HbA2 is often raised. In situations where the variant haemoglobins co-elute with HbA2, such as HbC or HbE, HbA2 quantification by conventional methods will not be possible.

Co-inheritance of a beta chain variant with alpha thalassaemia has the effect of lowering the amount of the variant present to 25–30%. In this situation it may be possible to confuse a beta chain variant with an alpha chain variant. When an alpha chain variant is present, all alpha chain-containing haemoglobins will be affected by the variant. Therefore, samples containing alpha chain variants will not only show a variant band but will also have a split HbA2 and HbF. These are frequently more easily visualized on HPLC plots, particularly the split HbA2 with slow alpha chain variants, than by electrophoretic methods. An example of an alpha chain variant, HbG Philadelphia analysed by Biorad Variant HPLC is shown in Fig. 2.2(e). The reduced quantity of variant haemoglobin and the split HbA2 can be noted. Delta chain variants also show a split HbA2. These are usually regarded as clinically insignificant and in these cases there will be no other variant bands. Where there is a split HbA2 due to a delta chain variant, the two peaks must be added to give a total HbA2 or beta thalassaemia trait may be missed. A further point to be noted with the HbA2 is that in some HPLC systems a falsely elevated value can be seen with haemoglobin variants that elute soon after HbA2. This is most frequently observed with HbS, and is thought to be due to gylcosylated HbS [22, 23].

Complicated HPLC plots will be seen when both alpha and beta chain variants are co-inherited. There will always be four haemoglobins: normal HbA ($\alpha_2\beta_2$), haemoglobin containing the alpha chain variant ($\alpha\alpha_{(variant)2}\beta_2$), haemoglobin containing the beta chain variant ($\alpha_2\beta\beta_{(variant)}$) and haemoglobin comprising both the alpha and beta chain variant ($\alpha\alpha_{(variant)}\beta\beta_{(variant)}$). These may not all elute separately. However, when multiple peaks are seen, co-inheritance of alpha and beta chain variants should be suspected. Figure 2.2(f) shows a Biorad Variant HPLC analysis of a compound heterozygote for HbS and HbG Philadelphia. The four haemoglobins described can be visualized; normal HbA ($\alpha_2\beta_2$), HbS ($\alpha_2\beta\beta_{(S)}$), HbG Philadelphia ($\alpha\alpha_{(G\ Philadelphia)}\beta_2$) and the hybrid haemoglobin ($\alpha\alpha_{(G\ Philadelphia)}\beta\beta_{(S)}$).

Homo-tetramer haemoglobins

Haemoglobins such as HbH and Hb Barts elute very quickly from HPLC columns; this may occur before the programmed analysis period. They can be seen as a sharp peak at the beginning of the HPLC trace but may not be recognized by the software and thus not labelled. When reviewing plots care should be taken to check for such peaks. In adults the characteristic thalassaemic red cell indices should be present and a HbH preparation should confirm the presence of HbH bodies.

Fusion haemoglobins

Hb Lepore is a structural variant in which the non-alpha chains consist of part delta and part beta chains termed delta beta fusion chains. The affected chromosome is unable to synthesize normal delta or beta chains [24]. Hb Lepore is clinically significant and can lead to a thalassaemia major phenotype. Hb Lepore trait shows a phenotype of thalassaemic red cell indices, the variant is present at 5–10% of total haemoglobin and elutes near HbA2 on HPLC and HbS on alkaline gel. There are also a group of beta delta fusion haemoglobins sometimes referred to as the anti-lepores such as Hb Miyada. These have normal haematology and are not clinically significant [25].

Haemoglobins resulting from fusion of other chains also exist such as Hb Kenya, which is the result of a beta gamma fusion [26, 27].

Unstable haemoglobins

Unstable haemoglobin variants may occur in all globin chains and have varying degrees of instability. Some haemoglobin variants are so unstable that they almost completely precipitate in the red cells shortly after synthesis, e.g. Hb Indianapolis [28]. Other haemoglobin variants may be mildly unstable and present in reduced quantities on the HPLC plot. The amount of variant present usually relates to the instability. However, some unstable haemoglobin variants cause no change in charge and therefore do not separate from HbA, such as Hb Bushwick [29]. Care should be taken not to confuse mildly unstable beta chain variants with alpha chain variants, nor should small peaks be disregarded. If the unstable haemoglobin is a beta chain variant the HbA2 may be slightly increased. Further tests for unstable haemoglobins include the isopropanol stability test and heat instability test [16].

Elongated alpha chain variants

There are a group of haemoglobin variants such as Hb Constant Spring, Hb Icaria and Hb Koya Dora that are produced by a mutation in the stop codon of the alpha chain. This results in elongated alpha chains and gives rise to a phenotype of mild alpha thalassaemia trait. The elongated chains tend to degrade, particularly with storage, as there are several sites susceptible to proteolytic attack; consequently they present as slow variants in trace amounts with very small peaks or electrophoretic bands [30, 31]. There are frequently two fractions; however, the number depends on the degree of degradation. These haemoglobins are always found in relatively low quantities and, as the haematology tends to be nearly normal, they may easily be missed.

Conclusion

Owing to the diverse nature of haemoglobinopathies and the limitations of many of the procedures, no single phenotypic screening test can provide a diagnosis. Most routine techniques are based on the physicochemical properties of the haemoglobin and therefore can only provide presumptive identification. If an accurate diagnosis is to be reached the results of several investigations must be interpreted with the appropriate clinical data. Misdiagnosis may occur if the correct data are not obtained or the data are not correctly interpreted. It is important to remember that classical pictures are not always seen in practice, as many factors may combine to influence the results. Currently only techniques such as mass spectrometry or DNA analysis will provide a definitive understanding of the nature of the mutation.

References

1. Ingram VM. A case of sickle-cell anaemia: a commentary on 'Abnormal Human Haemoglobins'. I. The Comparison of Normal Human and Sickle-Cell Haemoglobins by 'Fingerprinting' with II. The Chymotryptic Digestion of the Trypsin-resistant 'Core' of Haemoglobins A and S and III. The Chemical Difference Between Normal and

Sickle Cell Haemoglobins. *Biochim Biophys Acta* 1989; **1000**: 147–50.

2. Michelson AM, Orkin SH. The 3' untranslated regions of the duplicated human alpha-globin genes are unexpectedly divergent. *Cell* 1980; **22**: 371–7.

3. Seid-Akhavan M, Winter WP, Abramson RK, Rucknagel DL. Hemoglobin Wayne: a frameshift mutation detected in human hemoglobin alpha chains. *Proc Natl Acad Sci U S A* 1976; **73**: 882–6.

4. Bunn HF, Schmidt GJ, Haney DN, Dluhy RG. Hemoglobin Cranston, an unstable variant having an elongated beta chain due to nonhomologous cross over between two normal beta chain genes. *Proc Natl Acad Sci U S A* 1975; **72**: 3609–13.

5. Imai K, Lehmann H. The oxygen affinity of haemoglobin Tak, a variant with an elongated beta chain. *Biochim Biophys Acta* 1975; **412**: 288–94.

6. Bradley TB Jr, Wohl RC, Rieder RF. Hemoglobin Gunn Hill: deletion of five amino acid residues and impaired heme-globin binding. *Science* 1967; **157**: 1581–3.

7. Huisman TH, Wilson JB, Gravely M, Hubbard M. Hemoglobin Grady: the first example of a variant with elongated chains due to an insertion of residues. *Proc Natl Acad Sci U S A* 1974; **71**: 3270–3.

8. Baglioni C. The fusion of two polypeptide chains in hemoglobin Lepore and its interpretation as a genetic deletion. *Proc Natl Acad Sci U S A* 1962; **48**: 1880–6.

9. Wasi P, Disthasongchan P, Na-Nakorn S. The effect of iron deficiency on the levels of hemoglobins A2 and E. *J Lab Clin Med* 1968; **71**: 85–91.

10. Kattamis C, Lagos P, Metaxotou-Mavromati A, Matsoniatis N. Serum iron and unsaturated iron-binding capacity in the thalassaemia trait: their relation to the levels of haemoglobins A, A2 and F. *J Med Genet* 1972; **9**: 154–9.

11. White JM. The unstable haemoglobins. *Br Med Bull* 1976; **32**: 219–22.

12. The laboratory diagnosis of haemoglobinopathies. *Br J Haematol* 1998; **101**: 783–92.

13. Schneider RG, Hosty TS, Tomlin G, Atkins R. Identification of hemoglobins and hemoglobinopathies by electrophoresis on cellulose acetate plates impregnated with citrate agar. *Clin Chem* 1974; **20**: 74–7.

14. Itano HA. Solubilities of naturally occurring mixtures of human hemoglobin. *Arch Biochem Biophys* 1953; **47**: 148–52.

15. Weatherall DJ, Clegg JB. *The Thalassaemia Syndromes*, 3rd edn. Oxford: Blackwell Scientific Publications, 1981.

16. Dacie JV, Lewis SM. *Practical Haematology*. London: Churchill Livingstone, 1995: 249–86.

17. Huisman THJ, Carver MFH, Efremov GD. *A Syllabus of Human Hemoglobin Variants*, 2nd edn. Augusta, GA: Sickle Cell Anemia Foundation, 1999.

18. Leonova JYe, Kazanetz EG, Smetanina NS *et al.* Variability in the fetal hemoglobin level of the normal adult. *Am J Hematol* 1996; **53**: 59–65.

19. Rochette J, Craig JE, Thein SL. Fetal hemoglobin levels in adults. *Blood Rev* 1994; **8**: 213–24.

20. Atweh GG, Loukopoulos D. Pharmacological induction of fetal hemoglobin in sickle cell disease and beta-thalassemia. *Semin Hematol* 2001; **38**: 367–73.

21. Fairbanks VF, Gilchrist GS, Brimhall B, Jereb JA, Goldston EC. Hemoglobin E trait reexamined: a cause of microcytosis and erthrocytosis. *Blood* 1979; **53**: 109–15.

22. Shokrani M, Terrell F, Turner EA, Aguinaga MD. Chromatographic measurements of hemoglobin A2 in blood samples that contain sickle hemoglobin. *Ann Clin Lab Sci* 2000; **30**: 191–4.

23. Craver RD, Abermanis JG, Warrier RP, Ode DL, Hempe JM. Hemoglobin A2 levels in healthy persons, sickle cell disease, sickle cell trait, and beta-thalassemia by capillary isoelectric focusing *Am J Clin Pathol* 1997; **107**: 88–91.

24. Marinucci M, Mavilio F, Massa A *et al.* Haemoglobin Lepore trait: haematological and structural studies on the Italian population. *Br J Haematol* 1979; **42**: 557–65.

25. Driscoll MC, Ohta Y, Nakamura F, Bloom A, Bank A. Hemoglobin Miyada: DNA analysis of the anti-Lepore beta delta fusion gene. *Am J Hematol* 1984; **17**: 355–62.

26. Kendall AG, Ojwang PJ, Schroeder WA, Huisman TH. Hemoglobin Kenya, the product of a gamma-beta fusion gene: studies of the family. *Am J Hum Genet* 1973; **25**: 548–63.

27. Huisman TH, Wrightstone RN, Wilson JB, Schroeder WA, Kendall AG. Hemoglobin Kenya, the product of fusion of amd polypeptide chains. *Arch Biochem Biophys* 1972; **153**: 850–3.

28. Adams JG 3rd, Boxer LA, Baehner RL *et al.* Hemoglobin Indianapolis (beta 112[G14] arginine). An unstable beta-chain variant producing the phenotype of severe beta-thalassemia. *J Clin Invest* 1979; **63**: 931–8.

29. Ohba Y, Miyaji T, Ihzumi T, Shibata A. Hb Bushwick, an unstable hemoglobin with tendency to lose heme. *Hemoglobin* 1985; **9**: 517–23.

30. Derry S, Wood WG, Pippard M *et al.* Hematologic and biosynthetic studies in homozygous hemoglobin Constant Spring. *J Clin Invest* 1984; **73**: 1673–82.

31. Hunt DM, Higgs DR, Winichagoon P, Clegg JB, Weatherall DJ. Haemoglobin Constant Spring has an unstable alpha chain messenger RNA. *Br J Haematol* 1982; **51**: 405–13.

32. Bain BJ. *Haemoglobinopathy Diagnosis*. London: Blackwell Science, 2001.

33. Rowan RM, Assendelft OWV, Preston FE. Haemoglobin A2, F and the abnormal haemoglobins. In: *Advanced Laboratory Methods in Haematology*. London: Arnold Publishers, 2002: 193–221.

Chapter 3
Epidemiology, genetics and pathophysiology of sickle cell disease

Iheanyi E Okpala

History and epidemiology

Oral history passed down the generations in Africa gives account of an inherited chronic disease characterized by recurrent episodes of bone pain associated with cold weather [1]. The first written account of the condition was published in 1874 by Africanus Horton [2]. Born in 1835 of Igbo parents from Nigeria who lived in Sierra Leone, Africanus Horton qualified from the medical school of King's College London, UK, at the young age of 24 years. Postgraduate medical training and research earned him a Doctor of Medicine degree from the University of Edinburgh, after which he worked as a clinician in West Africa. In his book, *The Diseases of Tropical Climates and their Treatment*, Africanus Horton described various features of the inherited disease – including persistent abnormality of blood, painful crisis associated with fever and increased frequency of the painful episodes during the rainy season. In 1910, Dr James Herrick working in Chicago, USA, reported 'Peculiar elongated and sickle shaped red blood corpuscles in a case of severe anemia' [3]. The inherited disease was subsequently called sickle cell anaemia, and has continued to attract the attention of medical scientists to the present day. The sustained interest of the scientific community led to a major breakthrough in 1949 when Linus Pauling and colleagues discovered that sickle cell anaemia is caused by a mutation in the gene for beta globin [4]. So, three-quarters of a century after the original documentation by Africanus Horton, sickle cell anaemia became the first human disease to be described at the molecular level. The Nobel Prize for Medicine was awarded to Pauling in honour of this seminal work that marked the dawn of an era of studies on the pathophysiology of sickle cell disease (SCD). It soon became apparent that SCD affects every part of the body and has protean clinical manifestations [5].

The feasibility of accurate molecular diagnosis encouraged epidemiological studies which revealed that SCD was more prevalent than was initially appreciated. The inherited condition affects people of European, Arabian, Indian, Oriental and African ancestry [6]. About 300 000 children are born annually with SCD and millions of people are affected across the continents; making it a major public health problem on a global scale, and the commonest inherited blood disorder that afflicts mankind [7]. The paradox of how the gene for a multi-organ disease that led to death in childhood not only survived natural selection over the generations, but also became very widespread, was initially not understood. Insight came from the observation that the original geographical distribution of SCD was identical to that of malaria [8]. Children heterozygous for the sickle cell gene (HbAS) are less likely than HbAA or HbSS homozygotes to have cerebral malaria – the commonest cause of childhood mortality in malaria endemic regions [9]. So, HbAS heterozygotes have a survival advantage over HbAA or HbSS homozygotes in parts of the world where malaria occurs. This phenomenon, called balanced polymorphism, has ensured the selection and spread of the sickle cell gene through the generations. The variable severity of SCD among homozygous (HbSS) individuals led to the discovery of other genetic factors that modulate its manifestation [10]. Today, the challenge is to translate the wealth of information on the pathophysiology of SCD into effective, safe and affordable treatment for the benefit of affected individuals.

Genetics and inheritance

The sickle cell gene is the result of a point mutation (G<u>A</u>G→G<u>T</u>G) in the sixth codon of the gene for beta globin [4]. So, the sixth amino acid in the beta chain of haemoglobin S (HbS) is valine, instead of glutamic acid as found in the usual adult haemoglobin (HbA). This amino acid substitution is expressed as β6 glu→val. Some, but not all, the haemoglobin variants that interact with HbS to cause clinical illness (i.e. sickle cell disease, SCD) in the compound heterozygous state also have amino acid substitutions in the beta globin chain. HbC, a result of the mutation <u>G</u>AG→<u>A</u>AG in the sixth codon, has lysine as the sixth amino acid of the beta chain; β6 glu→lys. In HbD Punjab (Los Angeles) glutamine replaces glutamic acid in position 121; β121 glu→gln. HbE is the result of a similar mutation that gave rise to HbC, but in the 26th codon: β26 glu→lys. HbO-Arab has a similar amino acid substitution in position 121, β121 glu→lys, and migrates like HbC on electrophoresis. Some of the variants that result from mutations in codon 121, such as HbO-Arab, cause clinical disease because they stabilize the HbS polymer. Lepore haemoglobins result from unequal cross-over between the genes for beta and delta globin chains; both genes are replaced by a δβ hybrid gene. This Hb Lepore gene is not well expressed and the condition is a form of thalassaemia.

The frequency of sickle cell gene varies considerably between different populations. The carrier state (HbAS) occurs in 1 in 4 Nigerians, 1 in 5 Ghanaians, and 1 in 10 Afro-Caribbeans. HbC gene is most prevalent in a region of West Africa including Northern Ghana and Burkina Fasso, where it is thought to have originated. HbC is most common among people whose ancestry can be traced to that geographical area. It is less common in regions of West Africa east of the River Niger, which was a natural barrier to migration of people with high prevalence of HbC. Similarly, the low prevalence of HbS (< 1%) in the part of Africa south of the River

Zambesi is considered the result of such a natural barrier to population movements from Central Africa where the carrier rate is about 25%. The frequency of β^s gene also varies according to geographical and historical factors in North and South America, the Mediterranean region, Northern Europe, the Middle East, India and the Far East. Whereas haemoglobin genotype is the type of globin genes a person has (SS or S/thal), the β^s haplotype (literally type of chromosome) could be viewed as the genetic background in which the gene exists. Haplotype studies in different populations suggest that the GAG→GTG mutation which results in HbS has probably occurred at least five times in human history; corresponding to the Bantu, Benin, Cameroon, Senegalese and Saudi-Indian β^s haplotypes [11]. This is of practical importance because Bantu and Benin haplotypes are associated with clinically severe SCD, Senegalese with moderate, and Saudi-Indian with mild disease.

As each person has two genes for beta globin, the possible haemoglobin genotypes in children of parents with sickle cell trait (HbAS) are shown in Fig. 3.1. From the pattern of inheritance of beta globin genes, it can be seen that for each pregnancy, there is a 1 in 4 chance of having a normal child, 1 in 2 chance of having a child with sickle cell trait, and 1 in 4 chance of having a child with sickle cell anaemia. Using the same method, it can be worked out that if one parent has Hb genotype AA and the other SS, all the children will have sickle cell trait. If one parent has sickle cell trait and the other sickle cell anaemia, the chances are 1 in 2, respectively, that the child will have sickle cell trait, or sickle cell anaemia. In the unusual event of both parents having sickle cell anaemia, all their children will have sickle cell anaemia.

HbC is inherited in the same way as HbS. The possible Hb genotypes of a child if one parent has haemoglobin C trait (HbAC), and the other has

Parents	Mother A S			Father A S
Offspring	A A Normal	A S Sickle cell trait	A S	S S Sickle cell anaemia

Fig. 3.1 Inheritance of sickle cell anaemia.

Parents	Mother A S			Father A C	
Offspring	A A Normal	A S Sickle cell trait	A C HbC trait	S C Sickle cell haemoglobin C disease	**Fig. 3.2** Inheritance of sickle cell haemoglobin C (HbSC) disease.

sickle cell trait, are shown in Fig. 3.2. For each pregnancy, there is a 1 in 4 chance, respectively, that the child will be normal, have haemoglobin C trait, sickle cell trait, or sickle cell haemoglobin C (HbSC) disease. If one parent is normal and the other has HbSC disease, the chances are 1 in 2 that their child will have sickle cell trait, and 1 in 2 of having haemoglobin C trait. In the unlikely event of one parent having sickle cell anaemia, and the other HbSC disease; there is a 1 in 2 chance in each pregnancy that the child will have sickle cell anaemia, or HbSC disease. If both parents are carriers of HbC gene, the situation is analogous to that of parents who have sickle cell trait illustrated in Fig. 3.1. The possible Hb genotypes in the offspring of parents both of whom have HbC trait are: AA (1 in 4 chances), AC (1 in 2) and homozygous haemoglobin C (HbCC) disease (1 in 4 chances). If one parent has sickle cell trait and the other has beta thalassaemia trait, there is a 1 in 4 chance, respectively, that each pregnancy results in a normal child or one with sickle cell beta thalassaemia (HbSβthal), and 1 in 2 chances of a child who has beta thalassaemia trait (HbA/βthal).

Pathophysiology

The mechanisms of SCD include three fundamental pathological processes: vaso-occlusion, sickling of red blood cells and susceptibility to infections. SCD is associated with proneness to infections because of hyposplenism [12], a defect in the alternative pathway of complement activation [13, 14], and reduced ability of neutrophils to kill pathogenic organisms [15, 16]. Hyposplenism results from repeated infarction of splenic tissue, leading to virtual absence of the spleen in most adults (autosplenectomy). Also, even in childhood before autosplenectomy occurs, splenic function is reduced although the spleen may be enlarged

(functional asplenia). The basis of reduced neutrophil function in SCD is not clear. Similarly, the cause of the defect in activation of the alternative pathway of complement has not been elucidated. The serum concentration of factor B, the C3 convertase in the alternative pathway, was not reduced in a study of people with homozygous SCD [14]. Although the exact cause of the complement defect is unknown, it is of such clinical importance that the frequency of sickle cell crisis increases with the degree of the defect [14]. The overall susceptibility to infections has even greater clinical relevance in SCD. Infection is the most common precipitating factor for sickle cell crisis, and the leading cause of mortality in SCD [17].

When haemoglobin S loses oxygen, it crystallizes within the erythrocytes. The affected red blood cells develop various abnormal shapes [18], including the characteristic crescent or sickle shape that gave SCD its name. Sickled erythrocytes are more rigid than normal red cells, and are more readily destroyed by the reticulo-endothelial system. This process of haemolysis is the cause of anaemia in SCD. It is mostly extravascular, although some intravascular haemolysis occurs in people with the haemoglobinopathy. Intravascular haemolysis appears to be important in the pathogenesis of pulmonary hypertension secondary to SCD and other chronic haemolytic conditions, such as thalassaemia and paroxysmal nocturnal haemoglobinuria. This is discussed in greater detail in Chapter 14.

Occlusion of blood vessels is the most important pathological process in SCD. The parts of the body so deprived of blood and nutrients suffer from ischaemia and infarction. Recurrent and widespread vaso-occlusion is the cause of the multi-organ organ damage and loss of functional parenchymal tissue in SCD. A process that is fairly simple in conception, blood vessel occlusion in SCD is devilishly complex in pathogenesis; and the details are not fully understood. The current model of vaso-occlusion in SCD views the process as a result of interaction of erythrocytes, leucocytes, platelets, plasma proteins and vascular endothelium [19]. The pathophysiology of microvascular (small vessel) occlusion is different from that of macrovascular (large vessel) occlusion. Interaction of blood cells with vascular endothelium is more important in microvascular occlusion, and typically results in generalized painful crisis. Occlusion of larger blood vessels such as the carotid and cerebral arteries, which leads to stroke, results from hyperplasia of the tunica intima of the vessel wall. Both types of vaso-occlusion could occur in the same organ and increase the likelihood of ischaemic tissue damage.

The role of erythrocytes in vaso-occlusion

Early workers recognized that sickled red cells are rigid, could obstruct the lumen of small blood vessels, and so contribute to the vaso-occlusive process in SCD [5]. More recent studies have shown that both sickled and unsickled erythrocytes attach to the vascular endothelium via adhesion molecules such as phosphatidylserine, $\alpha_4\beta_1$ integrin, CD36 and the Lutheran blood group antigen [20–24]. In this way, red blood cells contribute to vaso-occlusion in SCD through an active process distinct from passive mechanical obstruction. Both sickle and unsickled red blood cells also attach to leucocytes or platelets and form cell aggregates that could obstruct the lumen of blood vessels more easily than single cells [19, 25–27]. Although it is difficult to ascertain the relative contribution of erythrocytes in this multicellular process, the clinical importance of the role of red cells that contain HbS (and could sickle) in SCD is underlined by the efficacy of exchange blood transfusion in the prevention and treatment of vaso-occlusive manifestations such as stroke, acute chest syndrome and sickle cell crisis [28]. Conditions that promote erythrocyte sickling include dehydration, acidosis, slow blood flow, high plasma osmolality and high metabolic rate in a tissue with resultant hypoxia. These conditions also predispose to sickle cell crisis, and occur in the sinusoidal circulations of the placenta, bone marrow and penis, but are particularly

marked in the kidneys, where even the red cells of people with sickle cell trait undergo sickling [29, 30].

The role of leucocytes in vaso-occlusion

It is intriguing to consider the contribution of white blood cells to vaso-occlusion in SCD – a condition traditionally regarded as a disorder of red blood cells. Similar to the contribution of erythrocytes containing HbS, the clinical significance of the role of white blood cells in vaso-occlusion is illustrated by observations that the number of vaso-occlusive events in SCD increases with leucocyte count [15, 31], and reducing white blood cell count by hydroxyurea therapy decreases the frequency of vaso-occlusive crisis, even when there is no increase in fetal haemoglobin [32–34]. White blood cells contribute to vaso-occlusion in SCD by adhering to the wall of blood vessels, and by forming cell aggregates with each other as well as other blood cells [19]. Leucocyte adherence to vascular endothelium and aggregation with other blood cells are mediated by adhesion molecules. People with high expression of the leucocyte adhesion molecules $\alpha M\beta 2$ integrin and L-selectin have severe manifestations of SCD [35]. The importance of leucocyte–endothelial interaction in the pathogenesis of vessel occlusion is supported by observations that the post-capillary venule where leucocytes normally attach to vascular endothelium before entering the extravascular space [36] is the same site at which microvascular occlusion occurs in SCD [37–39].

Leucocytes indirectly enhance vaso-occlusion in SCD by activating vascular endothelium, as demonstrated for peripheral blood monocytes [40]. Monocytes activate vascular endothelium by secreting the inflammatory cytokines tumour necrosis factor-alpha (TNF-α) and interleukin-1β [40]. Activated endothelial cells increase their expression of ligands for adhesion molecules on leucocytes and erythrocytes, such as intercellular adhesion molecule-1 (ICAM-1) and vascular cell adhesion molecule-1 (VCAM-1) [41, 42]. In this manner, monocytes facilitate adherence of circulating blood cells to the vessel wall and enhance vaso-occlusion. Infection precipitates vaso-occlusive crisis partly by increasing the interaction of leucocytes with vascular endothelium. The number of white blood cells is increased, they are activated and express more adhesion molecules; vascular endothelial cells are also activated and express more ligands (receptors) for adhesion molecules on leucocytes. Increased numbers of activated leucocytes attach to the endo-thelium at several sites in the microvasculature, in attempts to enter the tissues and kill the infecting organisms. This facilitates occlusion of small blood vessels in several parts of the body, with ischaemia and infarction in the affected tissues, leading to generalized painful crisis.

The roles of platelets and plasma proteins

In contrast to the established clinical relevance of the contributions of erythrocytes and leucocytes, the role of platelets in the vaso-occlusive process that characterizes SCD is not clear. Although a role for platelets in vaso-occlusion is suggested by *in vitro* observations that activated platelets promote sickle erythrocyte adherence to vascular endo-thelium by releasing thrombospondin and other adhesive plasma proteins [43], clinical studies give variable reports on the relationship between steady-state platelet count and the occurrence of vaso-occlusive manifestations of SCD [44, 45].

While our understanding of the pathophysiology of sickle cell disorders continually improves, a major challenge is to translate the immense body of knowledge on the mechanisms of these diseases into clinically efficacious therapy for affected individuals.

References

1. Konotey-Ahulu FID. Hereditary qualitative and quantitative erythrocyte defects in Ghana: an historical and geographical survey. *Ghana Med J* 1968; 7: 118–19.
2. Africanus Horton JB. *The Diseases of Tropical Climates and their Treatment*. London: Churchill, 1874.
3. Herrick JB. Peculiar elongated and sickled red blood corpuscles in a case of severe anaemia. *Arch Intern Med* 1910; 6: 517–21.
4. Pauling L, Itano HA, Singer SJ, Wells IC. Sickle cell anaemia, a molecular disease. *Science* 1949; 10: 543–8.
5. Attah EB. The pathophysiology of sickle cell disease. In: Fleming AF, ed. *Sickle Cell Disease: A Handbook for the General Clinician*. Edinburgh: Churchill Livingstone, 1982: 43–56.
6. Weatherall DJ, Clegg JB. Inherited haemoglobin disorders: an increasing global health problem. *Bull World Health Organ* 2001; 79: 704–12.
7. Serjeant GR. Sickle cell disease. *Lancet* 1997; 350: 725–30.
8. Allison AC. The distribution of sickle cell trait in East Africa and elsewhere, and its apparent relationship to the incidence of subtertian malaria. *Trans R Soc Trop Med Hyg* 1954; 48: 312–18.
9. Edington GM, Watson-Williams EJ. Sickling, haemoglobin C, glucose-6-phosphate dehydrogenase deficiency and malaria in Western Nigeria. In: Jonix JHP, ed. *Abnormal Haemoglobins in Africa*. Oxford: Blackwell Scientific Publications, 1965: 393–401.
10. Steinberg MH, Rodgers GP. Pathophysiology of sickle cell disease: role of genetic and cellular modifiers. *Semin Hematol* 2001; 38: 229–306.
11. Powars DR. βs – Gene-cluster haplotypes in sickle cell anemia: clinical and hematologic features. *Hematol Oncol Clin North Am* 1991; 5: 475–93.
12. Pearson HA. The kidney, hepatobiliary system, and spleen in sickle cell anaemia. *Ann N Y Acad Sci* 1989; 565: 120–5.
13. Johnston RB Jr, Hewman SL, Struth AC. An abnormality of the alternative pathway of complement activation in sickle cell disease. *N Engl J Med* 1973; 288: 803–5.
14. Anyaegbu CC, Okpala IE, Aken'Ova AY, Salimonu LS. Complement haemolytic activity, circulating immune complexes and the morbidity of sickle cell anaemia. *Acta Pathol Microbiol Scand* 1999; 107: 699–702.
15. Anyaegbu CC, Okpala IE, Aken'Ova AY, Salimonu LS. Peripheral blood neutrophil count and candidacidal activity correlate with the clinical severity of sickle cell anaemia. *Eur J Haematol* 1998; 60: 267–8.
16. Mollapour E, Porter JB, Kacmarski R, Linch D, Roberts PJ. Raised neutrophil phospholipase A2 activity and defective priming of NADPH oxidase and phospholipase A2 in sickle cell disease. *Blood* 1998; 91: 3423–9.
17. Attah Ed B, Ekere MC. Death patterns in sickle cell anemia. *JAMA* 1975; 233: 889–90.
18. Rodgers GP. Overview of pathophysiology and rationale for treatment of sickle cell anemia. *Semin Hematol* 1997; 34: 2–7.
19. Frenette PS. Sickle cell vaso-occlusion: multistep and multicellular paradigm. *Curr Opin Hematol* 2002; 9: 101–6.
20. Joneckis CC, Ackley RL, Orringer EP, Wayner EA, Parise LV. Integrin $\alpha_4\beta_1$ and glycoprotein IV (CD36) are expressed on circulating reticulocytes in sickle cell anemia. *Blood* 1993; 82: 3548–55.
21. Swerlick RA, Eckman JR, Kumar A, Jeitler M, Wick TM. $\alpha_4\beta_1$ integrin expression in sickle reticulocytes: vascular

cell adhesion molecule-1 dependent binding to endothelium. *Blood* 1993; **82**: 1891–9.

22. Udani M, Zen Q, Cottman M *et al*. Basal cell adhesion molecule/Lutheran protein. The receptor critical for sickle cell adhesion to laminin. *J Clin Invest* 1997; **99**: 2561–4.

23. Setty YBN, Kulkami S, Stuart MJ. Role of erythrocyte phosphatidylserine in sickle red cell–endothelial adhesion. *Blood* 2002; **99**: 1564–71.

24. Manodori AB, Barabino GA, Lubin BH, Kuypers FA. Adherence of phosphatidyl-exposing erythrocytes to endothelial matrix thrombospondin. *Blood* 2000; **95**: 1293–300.

25. Walcheck B, Moore KL, McEver RP, Kishimoto TK. Neutrophil–neutrophil interactions under hydrodynamic shear stress involve L-selectin and PSGL-1. A mechanism that amplifies initial leukocyte accumulation of P-selectin in vitro. *J Clin Invest* 1996; **98**: 1081–7.

26. Patel KD, Moore KL, Nollert MU, McEver RP. Neutrophils use both shared and distinct mechanisms to adhere to selectins under static and flow conditions. *J Clin Invest* 1996; **96**: 1887–96.

27. Silverstein RL, Asch AS, Nachman RL. Glycoprotein IV mediates thrombospondin-dependent platelet–monocyte and platelet–U937 cell adhesion. *J Clin Invest* 1989; **84**: 546–52.

28. Ohene-Frempong K. Indications for red cell transfusion in sickle cell disease. *Semin Hematol* 2001; **38** (Suppl 1): 5–13.

29. Herard A, Colin J, Youinou Y, Drancourt E, Brandt B. Massive hematuria in a sickle cell trait patient with renal papillary necrosis. *Eur Urol* 1998; **34**: 161–2.

30. Ataga KI, Orringer EU. Renal abnormalities in sickle cell disease. *Am J Hematol* 2000; **63**: 205–11.

31. Platt OS, Brambilla DJ, Rosse WF *et al*. Mortality in sickle cell disease – life expectancy and risk factors for early death. *N Engl J Med* 1994; **330**: 1639–43.

32. Charache S, Terrin ML, Moore RD *et al*. Effect of hydroxyurea on the frequency of painful crisis in sickle cell anemia. *N Engl J Med* 1995; **322**: 1314–22.

33. Charache S. The mechanism of action of hydroxyurea in the management of sickle cell anaemia in adults. *Semin Hematol* 1997; **34** (Suppl 3):15–21.

34. Abboud MR, Laver J, Blau CA. Elevation of neutrophil count after G-CSF therapy leads to vaso-occlusive crisis and acute chest syndrome in a patient with sickle cell anaemia. *Blood* 1996; **88** (Suppl): 15b.

35. Okpala IE, Daniel Y, Haynes R, Odoemene D, Goldman JM. Relationship between the clinical manifestations of sickle cell disease and the expression of adhesion molecules on white blood cells. *Eur J Haematol* 2002; **69**: 135–44.

36. Tan P, Luscinkas FW, Homer-Vanniasinkams S. Cellular and molecular mechanisms of inflammation and thrombosis (review). *Eur J Vasc Endovasc Surg* 1999; **17**: 373–89.

37. Kaul DK, Fabry ME, Nagel RL. Microvasculature sites and characteristics of sickle cell adhesion to vascular endothelium in shear flow conditions. Pathophysiologic implications. *Proc Natl Acad Sci U S A* 1989; **86**: 3356–60.

38. Kaul DK, Fabry ME, Constantini F, Rubin EM, Nagel RL. In vivo demonstration of red cell–endothelial interaction, sickling and altered microvascular response to oxygen in the sickle transgenic mouse. *J Clin Invest* 1995; **96**: 2845–53.

39. Nagel RL, Platt OS. General pathophysiology of sickle cell anemia. In: Steinberg MH, Forget BG, Higgs RD, Nagel RL, eds. *Disorders of Hemoglobin: Genetics, Pathophysiology and Clinical Management.* Cambridge: Cambridge University Press, 2001: 494–526.

40. Belcher JD, Marker PH, Weber JP, Hebbel RP, Vercellotti GM. Activated monocytes in sickle cell disease: potential role in the activation of vascular endothelium and vaso-occlusion. *Blood* 2000; **96**: 2451–9.

41. Springer T. Traffic signals for lymphocyte recirculation and leukocyte emigration: the multistep paradigm. *Cell* 1994; **76**: 301–14.

42. Carlos TM, Harlan JM. Leukocyte-endothelial adhesion molecules. *Blood* 1994; **84**: 2068–101.

43. Britain HA, Eckman JR, Swerlick *et al*. Thrombospondin from activated platelets promotes sickle erythrocyte adherence to human microvascular endothelium under physiologic flow: a potential for platelet activation in sickle cell vaso-occlusion. *Blood* 1993; **81**: 2137–53.

44. Miller ST, Sleeper LA, Pegalow CH *et al*. Prediction of adverse outcomes in children with sickle cell disease: a report from the cooperative study (CSSCD). *N Engl J Med* 2000; **342**: 83–9.

45. Okpala IE. Steady-state platelet count and complications of sickle cell disease. *Hematol J* 2002; **3**: 214–15.

Chapter 4
The genetics and multiple phenotypes of beta thalassaemia

Swee Lay Thein

Introduction

Beta thalassaemia can be broadly defined as a syndrome of inherited haemoglobin disorders characterized by a quantitative deficiency of functional beta globin chains. The keywords here are quantitative and functional, and the definitive diagnostic test is an imbalanced alpha/non-alpha globin synthesis ratio. Although it is defined as a reduction in the synthesis of beta globin, some forms result from structural haemoglobin variants that are ineffectively synthesized or are so unstable that they result in a functional deficiency of the beta chains and a thalassaemia phenotype [1]. The most common forms are those that are prevalent in the malarial tropical and subtropical regions where a few mutations have reached high gene frequencies because of the protection they provide against malaria. In these countries where beta thalassaemia is prevalent, a limited number of alleles (four to five) account for 90% or more of the beta thalassaemia, such that a focused molecular diagnostic approach can be undertaken [2]. In other countries such as the UK, where there is an ethnic mix, a screening approach may be more appropriate and effective. This chapter reviews the clinical and haematological diversity encountered in beta thalassaemia and their relationships with the underlying genotypes.

The beta globin gene – structure, function and expression

Beta globin is encoded by a structural gene found in a cluster with the other beta-like genes on the short arm of chromosome 11, band 11p15.4 (Fig. 4.1). The cluster contains five functional genes, $5'$-ε-$^G\gamma$-$^A\gamma$-$\psi\beta$-δ-β-$3'$, which are arranged in the order of their developmental expression. The two fetal gamma genes lie 15 and 20 kb downstream of the embryonic epsilon gene, followed by the adult delta and beta genes at 35 and 43 kb further downstream. Upstream of the entire beta globin complex is the locus control region (LCR) which consists of five DNase 1 hypersensitive (HS) sites (designated HS1–5) distributed between 6 and 20 kb $5'$ of the epsilon gene. There is one other hypersensitive site ~20 kb $3'$ to the beta gene. The two extreme HS sites flanking the beta complex have been suggested to mark the boundaries of the beta globin gene domain. The beta globin complex is embedded in a cluster of olfactory receptor genes (ORG), part of the family of ~1000 genes that are widely distributed throughout the genome, and expressed in the olfactory epithelium [3].

The entire beta globin complex has been sequenced, and many of the regulatory sequences have been defined (http://ncbi.nlm.nih.gov). Two categories of repetitive sequences have been identified in the complex. One category consists of short sequence repeats – a microsatellite of $(CA)_n$, where n is usually 17, and another of $(ATTTT)_n$ between the delta and beta genes. The other category consists of long stretches of interspersed repetitive DNA – the *Alu* and L1 families of repeat DNA sequences. *Alu* repeats occur $5'$ of the epsilon gene (inverted pairs) and on either side of the gamma gene pair; inverted pairs also occur upstream of the delta gene and downstream of the beta gene. There are two long stretches (~6 kb each) of L1 repeat

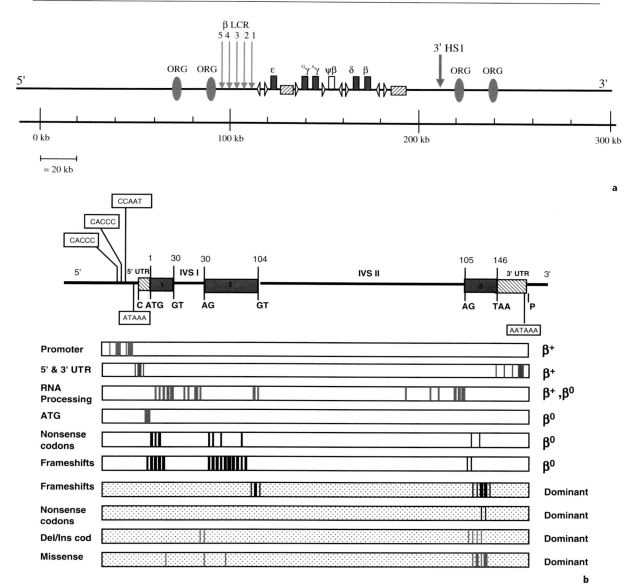

Fig. 4.1 (a) The beta globin gene cluster flanked by olfactory receptor genes (ORG). The downward arrows indicate the hypersensitive site (HS). HS1–5 denote the βLCR. The triangles indicate the *Alu*1, and hatched boxes the L1 repetitive sequences. Globin genes are shown as boxes, and the ORGs as ovals. (b) General structure of the beta globin gene with the exons, introns and conserved sequences as indicated. Below the gene structure are the sites of the different classes of beta thalassaemia mutations; those that are dominantly inherited are indicated in the four stippled boxes.

sequences, one between the epsilon and $^{G}\gamma$ genes, and the other downstream of the beta gene. The precise role of these repetitive DNA sequences is not known. *Alu*1 and L1 repeats may be contributory to the generation of the various deletions of the beta

globin cluster, while the microsatellites have been proposed as candidates for the recombination 'hot spot' between the delta and beta genes.

The cluster also contains numerous single nucleotide polymorphisms (SNPs), many of which affect cleavage sites for restriction endonucleases (REs) giving rise to restriction fragment length polymorphisms (RFLPs). Each of the RE sites can be present (+) or absent (−) and are combined in a limited number of haplotypes, that are in linkage disequilibrium with the beta globin gene mutations [4]. Beta haplotype analysis provides information on the chromosomal background on which the beta thalassaemia mutations have occurred and has been of considerable value in population studies and prenatal diagnosis (PND) before direct detection of the mutations became a practical reality [5]. Based on haplotype analysis, it became apparent that non-random association of the RFLPs occurs within two regions; a 5′ segment, from the epsilon gene to the 5′ end of the delta gene, and a 3′ segment extending 19 kb in a 3′ direction from the 5′ end of the beta gene. Between the 5′ and 3′ clusters, there is a 9-kb region that displays random association with either segment, and has therefore been proposed as a recombination 'hot spot' [6]. To date, five families with recombination within this region have been observed [7–11].

The general structure of the beta globin gene is typical of the other globin loci. The genomic sequence which codes for 146 amino acids spans 1600 bp; the transcribed region is contained in three exons separated by two introns or intervening sequences (IVSs) (Fig. 4.1b). The first exon encodes amino acids 1–29 together with the first two bases for codon 30; exon 2 encodes part of residue 30 together with amino acids 31–104; and exon 3 encodes amino acids 105–146. Exon 2 encodes the residues involved in haem binding and αβ dimer formation, while exons 1 and 3 encode for the non-haem-binding regions of the beta globin chain. Many of the amino acids involved in globin subunit interactions required for the Bohr effect, and 2,3-DPG (diphosphoglycerate) binding, are found in exon 3. Conserved sequences important for gene function are found in the 5′ promoter region, at the exon–intron junctions, and in the 3′ untranslated region (3′-UTR) at the end of the mRNA sequences. The beta globin gene promoter includes three positive cis-acting elements: TATA box (positions −28 to −31), a CCAAT box (positions −72 to −76) and duplicated CACCC motifs (proximal at positions −86 to −90, and distal at position −101 to −105).

While the CCAAT and TATA elements are found in many eukaryotic promoters, the CACCC sequence is found predominantly in erythroid cell-specific promoters. Binding of the erythroid Krüppel-like factor (EKLF) to the CACCC motif appears to be crucial for normal adult beta globin expression. In addition to these motifs, the region upstream of the beta globin promoter contains two binding motifs for the erythroid transcription factor GATA-1. The importance of these various 5′-flanking sequences for normal gene expression is underscored by beta thalassaemia arising from point mutations in these sequences specifically in and around the TATA box and the CACCC motifs in the −80 to −100 region. An enhancer is also found in intron 2 and 3′ of the globin gene, 600–900 bp downstream of the poly (A) site.

The 5′ untranslated region (5′-UTR) occupies a region of 50 nucleotides between the CAP site, the start of transcription and the initiation (ATG) codon. There are two prominently conserved sequences in the 5′-UTR of the various globin genes (both alpha and beta). One is the CTTCTG hexanucleotide found 8–13 nucleotides downstream from the CAP site, i.e. at positions +8 to +13. The second conserved sequence is CACCATG, in which the last three nucleotides form the initiation codon (ATG). Again, the importance of these sequences in the regulation of the beta gene expression is exemplified by the several mutations in the 5′-UTR causing beta thalassaemia.

The 3′-UTR constitutes the region between the termination codon (TAA) and the poly (A) tail. It consists of 132 nucleotides with one conserved sequence, AATAAA, located 20 nucleotides upstream of the poly (A) tail. This consensus hexanucleotide serves as a signal for the cleavage of the 3′ end of the primary transcript and addition of a poly (A) tract, which confers stability on the processed mRNA and enhances translation. Several mutations affecting the AATAAA sequence and other sequences in the 3′-UTR causing beta thalassaemia have been described.

The LCR plays a critical role in beta globin gene expression, it maintains an 'open' globin locus domain and acts as a powerful enhancer of globin gene transcription, in the absence of which the level of gene expression is low. Four of the sites (HS 1–4) are erythroid-specific, encompassing binding sequences for erythroid-restricted transcription factors (GATA-1 and NF-E2), while HS5 is ubiquitous and is thought to form the 5′ boundary of the beta globin domain.

The developmental regulation of the globin genes reflects their sequential activation in a 5′–3′ direction. While the alpha-like genes undergo a single developmental 'switch' (embryonic → fetal/adult), the beta-like genes undergo two 'switches' (embryonic → fetal→ adult). Transcription of the epsilon gene in the embryonic yolk gene switches after the sixth week of gestation to the transcription of the two gamma genes in the fetal liver, and then around the prenatal period, to that of the delta (minor adult) and beta (major adult) genes. At 6 months after birth, HbF comprises < 5% of the total haemoglobin and continues to fall; reaching the adult level of < 1% at 2 years of age. It is at this stage that mutations affecting the beta gene become clinically apparent. The 'switch' from fetal (gamma) to adult (beta) haemoglobin production is not total, in that small amounts of gamma expression persist in adult life. The residual amount of fetal haemoglobin ($\alpha_2\gamma_2$) is present in a subset of erythrocytes called F cells which also contain adult ($\alpha_2\beta_2$) haemoglobin.

The tissue- and developmental-specific expression of the individual globin genes is governed by the direct physical interactions between the globin promoters and the βLCR [12, 13], the interaction is mediated through binding of tissue-restricted and ubiquitous transcription factors. This precise developmental expression relies on two mechanisms, gene silencing and gene competition, mediated by the different transcription factors in embryonic, fetal and adult cells. While the epsilon and gamma globin genes are autonomously silenced at the appropriate developmental stage, expression of the adult beta globin gene depends on lack of competition from the gamma gene for the LCR sequences. This is supported by the down-regulation of the *cis* beta gene when gamma gene is up-regulated by point mutations in their promoters as illustrated by the non-deletional hereditary persistence of fetal haemoglobin (HPFH) [14]. Also, mutations which affect the beta promoter, which remove competition for the βLCR, tend to be associated with variable increases in the gamma and delta gene expression.

Pathophysiology and clinical diversity of beta thalassaemia

The underlying pathophysiology of beta thalassaemia relates to the deficiency of functional beta globin chains, which leads to an unbalanced globin chain production and an excess of alpha globin chains [1, 15]. The latter aggregate in red cell precursors forming inclusion bodies, causing mechanical damage and their premature destruction in the bone marrow, i.e. ineffective erythropoiesis. Red cells that survive to reach the peripheral circulation are prematurely destroyed. Anaemia in beta thalassaemia thus results from a combination of ineffective erythropoiesis, peripheral haemolysis and an overall reduction in haemoglobin synthesis. It is quite clear that the severity of beta thalassaemia is directly related to the severity of chain imbalance. Thus factors that reduce the degree of chain imbalance and the magnitude of alpha chain excess in the red cell precursors will have an ameliorating effect on the phenotype. At the primary level, this is related directly to the nature of the beta thalassaemia mutation itself. At the secondary level, the severity of globin chain imbalance is influenced by variability at two loci: alpha globin and gamma globin genes. Co-inheritance of alpha thalassaemia reduces the amount of redundant alpha globin and alpha/beta chain imbalance with an ameliorating effect, while the presence of extra alpha globin genes will have an adverse effect. Similarly an inherent capacity for producing gamma chain which combines with the excess alpha to form HbF ($\alpha_2\gamma_2$), will have an ameliorating effect.

A direct effect of the anaemia is the increased production of erythropoietin, which leads to intense proliferation and expansion of the bone marrow with the resulting skeletal deformities. To a large extent these secondary complications of bone disease – splenomegaly, endocrine and cardiac damage – can be related to the severity of anaemia and the iron loading that results from the increased gastrointestinal absorption and the blood transfusions. Recently, it has become apparent that these compli-

29

cations of beta thalassaemia may be genetically modified by variability at other loci (tertiary modifiers).

The clinical manifestations of beta thalassaemia are extremely diverse, spanning a broad spectrum from the transfusion-dependent state of thalassaemia major to the asymptomatic state of thalassaemia trait. The most severe end of the spectrum is characterized by the complete absence of beta globin production and results from the inheritance of two β^0 thalassaemia alleles, homozygous or compound heterozygous states. This condition is referred to as beta thalassaemia major and, at their worst, the patients present within 6 months of life, and if not treated with regular blood transfusions, die within their first 2 years. Conversely, many patients who have inherited two beta thalassaemia alleles may have a milder disease, ranging from a condition that is only slightly less severe than transfusion dependence through a spectrum of decreasing severity to one that is asymptomatic and often mistaken for beta thalassaemia trait. This diverse collection of phenotypes between the two extremes of thalassaemia major and trait constitute the clinical syndrome of thalassaemia intermedia. The underlying genotypes are equally heterogeneous, resulting from the interaction of other genetic variables with the inheritance of one or two beta thalassaemia alleles.

Beta thalassaemia trait, which forms the other end of the phenotypic spectrum of beta thalassaemia, is usually associated with the inheritance of a single beta thalassaemia allele, β^0 or β^+. Carriers for beta thalassaemia are clinically asymptomatic; they may have a mild anaemia with characteristic hypochromic microcytic red blood cells, elevated levels of HbA2 and variable levels of HbF. However, even the heterozygous states for beta thalassaemia show a phenotypic diversity comparable to that of thalassaemia major. In some cases, the beta thalassaemia allele can be phenotypically 'silent', with no anaemia or haematological abnormalities. In others, the heterozygous state causes a phenotype almost as severe as the major forms, i.e. the beta thalassaemia allele is dominantly inherited.

Although definition of the two extremes of the clinical spectrum of beta thalassaemia is easy, assigning the severity of the intermediate form can be problematic. Criteria such as age and level of haemoglobin at presentation, transfusion history and the requirements for intermittent blood transfusion have been used, but these have their inherent limitations and are highly clinician-dependent.

Mechanisms underlying phenotypic diversity of beta thalassaemia

Progress in our understanding of the mechanisms underlying the remarkable phenotypic variability of beta thalassaemia has been made possible by a combination of the analysis of the molecular basis of the different forms of thalassaemia, family studies and analysis of the genotype/phenotype relationship of the thalassaemia intermedias.

Heterogeneity and variable severity of beta thalassaemia alleles

The most common forms of beta thalassaemia alleles are those that are prevalent in the Mediterranean, tropical and subtropical regions including the Middle East, parts of Africa, the Indian subcontinent and South-East Asia, but they are by no means confined to those regions [2]. With the exception of a few deletions, the vast majority of beta thalassaemias are caused by point mutations within the gene or its immediate flanking sequences. A few beta thalassaemia mutations which segregate independently of the beta globin cluster have been described in several families [16]; in such cases, *trans*-acting regulatory factors have been implicated. Examples of reduced beta globin production caused by mutations in loci outside the beta globin complex include those arising in the general transcription factor TF11H [17] and the erythroid-specific transcription factor GATA-1 [18].

β^0 vs β^+ and β^{++} thalassaemia alleles

Functionally, the beta thalassaemia alleles can be classified as β^0 or β^+ reflecting the resulting phenotype: β^0 thalassaemia in which there is a complete absence of beta globin production and the most severe possible, and β^+ thalassaemia in which there is some, although reduced beta globin product. There is very mild reduction of beta chain production with β^{++} alleles.

Deletions causing beta thalassaemia are rare and result in a complete absence of beta globin product. Fourteen deletions which involve the structural beta globin gene alone, have been described [16]; only the 619-bp deletion at the 3′ end of the beta gene is common, but even that is restricted to the Sind and Punjab populations of India and Pakistan where it accounts for ~20% of the beta thalassaemia alleles. The other deletions, although extremely rare, are of particular functional and phenotypic interest because they are associated with an unusually high level of HbA2 in heterozygotes. These deletions differ widely in size, but remove in common a region (from positions −125 to +78 relative to the mRNA cap site) in the beta promoter, which includes the CACCC, CCAAT and TATA elements. The mechanism underlying the markedly elevated levels of HbA2 and the variable increase in HbF in heterozygotes for these deletions appears to be related to the removal of the 5′ promoter region of the beta gene. This removes competition for the upstream LCR leading to its increased interaction with the gamma and delta genes in *cis*, enhancing their expression. Although the increases in HbF are variable, and moderate in heterozygotes, they are adequate to compensate for the complete absence of beta globin in homozygotes for these deletions [19, 20]. This mechanism may also explain the unusually high HbA2 levels that accompany point mutations affecting the promoter regions.

Other deletions affecting the beta globin cluster are much more extensive; they down-regulate the beta gene as part of $(\varepsilon\gamma\delta\beta)^0$ thalassaemia. They can be classified into two groups: three upstream deletions remove all or part of the βLCR but leave the beta gene itself intact, and eight extensive deletions that remove the entire beta globin cluster [21].

Transposable elements may occasionally disrupt human genes and result in their inactivation. The insertion of such an element, a retrotransposon of the family called L1, has been reported with the phenotype of β^+ thalassaemia. Despite the insertion of 6–7 kb DNA into its IVS2, the affected gene expresses full-length beta globin transcripts at a level corresponding to about 15% of normal beta globin mRNA [22].

The point mutations causing beta thalassaemia result from single base substitutions, minor inser-

tions or deletions of a few bases within the gene or its immediate flanking sequences [16]. They may affect any level of genetic regulation and they are classified according to the mechanism by which they affect gene function: transcription, RNA processing or RNA translation. Mutations affecting transcription can either involve the conserved DNA sequences that form the beta globin promoter or the stretch of 50 nucleotides in the 5′-UTR. Generally they result in a mild to minimal deficit of beta globin output reflecting the relatively mild phenotype of these β^+ thalassaemias. The C-T mutation at position −101 to the beta globin gene appears to cause an extremely mild deficit of beta globin such that it is 'silent' in heterozygotes who have normal HbA2 levels and normal red cell indices. Several mutations in the 5′-UTR, e.g. CAP+1A-C, also have a 'silent' phenotype.

Mutations that affect RNA processing can involve either of the invariant dinucleotides (GT at 5′ and AG at 3′) in the splice junction, in which case normal splicing is completely abolished with the resulting phenotype of β^0 thalassaemia. Mutations within the consensus sequences at the splice junctions reduce the efficiency of normal splicing to varying degrees and produce a β^+ phenotype that ranges from mild to severe. Mutations within introns or exons might also affect the splicing pattern of the pre-mRNAs. For example, a cryptic splice site that contains the sequence GT GGT GAG G has been found in exon 1 of the beta globin gene, spanning codons 24–27. Three mutations within this region activate this cryptic site, which acts as an alternative donor site in RNA processing. The mutation in codon 26 (GAC → AAE) that gives rise to HbE (β26 Gln → Lys) is one such mutation that activates this cryptic splice site, with a reduction of the normal splicing that produces the HbE variant. As HbE production is also quantitatively reduced, the compound heterozygous state, HbE/beta thalassaemia results in a clinical picture closely resembling homozygous beta thalassaemia – ranging from severe anaemia and transfusion dependency to thalassaemia intermedia. Other RNA processing mutants affect the polyadenylation signal (AATAAA) and the 3′-UTR. These are generally mild β^+ thalassaemia alleles.

Mutations that are expressed at the level of

31

mRNA translation involve either the initiation or extension phases of globin synthesis and are all associated with a β^0 phenotype. Approximately half of the beta thalassaemia alleles are characterized by premature termination of beta chain extension. They result from the introduction of premature termination codons due to frameshifts or nonsense mutations and nearly all terminate within exon 1 and 2. Mutations that result in premature termination early in the sequence (in exons 1 and 2) are associated with minimal steady-state levels of β-mRNA in erythroid cells, owing to an accelerated decay of the abnormal mRNA referred to as non-sense-mediated mRNA decay (NMD) [23]. In heterozygotes for such cases, no beta chain is produced from the mutant allele and only half the normal beta globin is present, resulting in a typical asymptomatic phenotype. By contrast, mutations that produce in-phase termination later in the beta sequence (in exon 3) are not subjected to NMD, resulting in substantial amounts of abnormal β-mRNA comparable to that of the normal allele [24, 25]. The abnormal mRNA is presumably translated into variant beta chains that are not only non-functional but deleterious, causing a dominant negative phenotype. Hence, these mutants are usually dominantly inherited (see later).

The variable severity of the different beta thalassaemia alleles is reflected in their phenotypic effect in heterozygotes, in the degree of hypochromia and microcytosis as indicated by the mean cell haemoglobin (MCH) and mean cell volume (MCV) values, respectively. Rund et al. [26] showed that the β^0 thalassaemia alleles, which are associated with the most severe phenotype, demonstrated a fairly tight range of MCVs (63.1 fl, SD = 3.4), while the β^+ alleles were associated with a wider range of MCVs (69.3 fl, SD = 5.6). The cut-off point between the β^0 and β^+ thalassaemias was 67 fl. The broader range of MCV in β^+ thalassaemia, when compared with β^0 thalassaemia, is not surprising given the broad range in the deficit of beta globin production, from barely detectable levels at the severe end, to just a little less than normal in the very mild or 'silent' alleles.

A more recent study has taken the correlation between the severity of beta thalassaemia alleles with haematological parameters to a finer level.

Skarmoutsou et al. [27] measured a series of haematological parameters, including reticulocyte haemoglobin content (CHr), soluble transferrin receptor (sTfR), reticulocytes and HbA2 and HbF levels in 57 iron-replete individuals with heterozygous beta thalassaemia. There was a negative correlation between the values of sTfR, a reliable quantitative assessment of the erythropoietic activity, and the severity of the beta thalassaemia alleles; the values were lowest in the very mild beta thalassaemia (β^{silent}), and highest in β^0 thalassaemia heterozygotes. CHr, a product of reticulocyte haemoglobin and volume, was lower in β^{silent} thalassaemia compared with normals but the difference was not statistically significant. However, the CHr values between the β^{silent} and the severe groups (β^+ and β^0 thalassaemia alleles) was significant, being much higher (27.0–32.0 pg) in the former, compared with the latter group (19.5–25.3 pg). Furthermore, while sTfR values showed a positive correlation with HbA2, there was a significant negative correlation between CHr and HbA2 levels. This study confirms that all heterozygous beta thalassaemias have some degree of ineffective erythropoiesis that varies with the severity of the beta thalassaemia mutation.

The 'silent' mutations are normally identified in the compound heterozygous states with a severe beta thalassaemia allele, which results in thalassaemia intermedia, or in homozygotes who have a typical phenotype of beta thalassaemia trait. The 'silent' beta thalassaemia alleles are not common, except for the −101 C-T, which accounts for a large number of the milder forms of beta thalassaemia in the Mediterranean [28].

The mild beta thalassaemia alleles are associated with clearly defined changes in heterozygotes and result in disorders of intermediate severity in homozygotes. Interactions with the severe alleles are less predictable because of the wider range of beta globin output, and extend from transfusion dependence to intermediate forms of beta thalassaemia at the mild end of the spectrum [29, 30].

Ameliorating effect of HbF owing to nature of beta thalassaemia alleles

Although some of the phenotypic variability of beta thalassaemia can be explained by the differing severity of the beta thalassaemia alleles, it does not explain why identical mutations in different ethnic groups sometimes produce a different phenotype or why individuals with β^0 thalassaemia deletions have milder disease despite the complete absence of beta chain production. Both situations can be explained by an inherent propensity to produce HbF for different reasons. Although a given mutation is generally found within one ethnic group, a number of identical mutations have been described in different racial groups. In these cases the mutations may have arisen on different beta chromosomal backgrounds, some of which contain the common genetic variant, C-T at position −158 of the gamma globin gene, also referred to as the *Xmn*1-Gγ polymorphism. Although *Xmn*1-Gγ polymorphism has little effect in normal individuals, under haematopoietic stress, the presence of this site can have the effect of increasing HbF levels, resulting in a milder disease in homozygous beta thalassaemia [31]. The increased HbF output observed in deletions or mutations that involve the promoter sequence of the beta globin gene reflect the competition between the gamma and beta globin gene promoters for interaction with the LCR or rate-limiting transcription factors. Hence, although such deletions cause a complete absence of beta globin product, the severity of the phenotype is offset by the concomitant increase in HbF [19].

Dominantly inherited beta thalassaemia

The common beta thalassaemia alleles that are prevalent in the malarious regions are inherited typically as Mendelian recessives; heterozygotes are clinically asymptomatic and the inheritance of two mutant alleles – as homozygotes or compound heterozygotes – is required to produce clinical disease. However, some forms of beta thalassaemia are dominantly inherited, in that inheritance of a single beta thalassaemia allele in the presence of a normal alpha globin genotype results in a clinically detectable disease [32, 33]. Heterozygotes have a thalassaemia intermedia phenotype with moderate anaemia, splenomegaly and a thalassaemic blood picture. Apart from the usual features of heterozygous beta thalassaemia, such as increased levels of HbA2 and the unbalanced alpha/beta globin

biosynthesis, large inclusion bodies similar to those seen in thalassaemia major are often observed in the red cell precursors, hence the original term of 'inclusion body beta thalassaemia' [34].

This unusual form of beta thalassaemia was probably first described in an Irish family in 1973 [35]; several members of the family spanning three generations had a thalassaemia intermedia phenotype that was clearly inherited as a Mendelian dominant. Since the first description, more than 30 dominantly inherited beta thalassaemia alleles have now been described [32, 36]; they include missense mutations, minor deletions leading to the loss of intact codons, frameshifts arising from minor insertions and deletions resulting in elongated beta variants with abnormal carboxy-terminal ends, and truncated beta variants resulting from nonsense mutations. The common denominator of these mutations is the predicted synthesis of highly unstable beta chain variants, so unstable that in many cases they are not detectable and only implicated from the DNA sequence. The predicted synthesis is supported by the presence of substantial amounts of abnormal β-mRNA in the peripheral reticulocytes [25], comparable in amount to that produced from the normal beta allele. Indeed, the large intra-erythroblastic inclusions, that are so characteristic of this form of beta thalassaemia, have subsequently been shown to be composed of both alpha and beta globin chains [37]. In contrast, the inclusion bodies in homozygous beta thalassaemia consisted only of precipitated alpha globin.

How is it that some premature termination mutations cause thalassaemia intermedia while the majority are clinically asymptomatic in the heterozygous state? The answer appears to lie in the differential effects of these in-phase termination mutants on the accumulation of mutant mRNA. The in-phase termination mutations that are recessively inherited terminate in exon 1 or 2, while those that are dominantly inherited terminate much later in the sequence of the beta globin gene, in exon 3 or beyond. Premature stop codons near the 3′ end of the gene, in exon 3 of beta gene, are less likely to trigger the surveillance mechanism of NMD, leading to an accumulation of the mutant β-mRNA and to the synthesis of truncated beta chain variants [38]. These in-phase termination mutations exemplify how shifting the position of a nonsense codon can alter the phenotype of recessive inheritance caused by haplo-insufficiency, to a dominant negative effect caused by the synthesis of an abnormal and deleterious protein.

The pathophysiology of these beta chain variants relates to their hyper-instability caused by the nature and position of the mutations [33]. The molecular mechanisms include: substitution of the critical amino acids in the hydrophobic haem pocket displacing haem, leading to aggregation of the globin variant; disruption of secondary structure due to replacement of critical amino acids; substitution or deletion of amino acids involved in $\alpha\beta$ dimer formation; and elongation of subunits by a hydrophobic tail [39]. Again, a spectrum in phenotypic severity of this class of beta thalassaemia variants is observed, that can be related to variation in the degree of instability of the beta globin products. The dominantly inherited beta thalassaemias, characterized by the synthesis of highly unstable beta chain variants, resembles the intermediate forms of beta thalassaemia by virtue of the ineffective erythropoiesis, but there is also a variable degree of peripheral haemolysis.

Unlike recessive beta thalassaemia, which is prevalent in malaria-endemic regions, dominant beta thalassaemias are rare, occurring in dispersed geographical regions where the gene frequency for beta thalassaemia is very low. The vast majority of the dominant beta thalassaemia alleles have been described in single families, many as *de novo* events. It is likely that the low frequency of the dominant beta thalassaemia alleles is due to the lack of positive selection that occurs in the recessive forms. Clinically, since spontaneous mutations are common in dominant beta thalassaemia, it is important that the disorder should be suspected in any patient with a thalassaemia intermedia phenotype even if both parents are haematologically normal and the patient is from an ethnic background where beta thalassaemia is rare.

Secondary modifiers

The severity of anaemia in beta thalassaemia reflects the degree of globin chain imbalance and the excess of alpha globin chains with all their deleteri-

ous effects on the red cell precursors. This globin chain imbalance can be genetically modified by two factors – variation in the amount of alpha globin production and variation in fetal haemoglobin response.

Alpha globin genotype

In many populations in which beta thalassaemia is prevalent, alpha thalassaemia also occurs at a high frequency and hence it is not uncommon to co-inherit both conditions. Homozygotes or compound heterozygotes for beta thalassaemia who co-inherit alpha thalassaemia will have less redundant alpha globin and tend to have a less severe condition. As with beta thalassaemia, the different alpha thalassaemias that predominate in different racial groups display a wide range of severity. This interaction alone provides the basis for considerable clinical heterogeneity; the degree of amelioration depends on the severity of the beta thalassaemia alleles and the number of functional alpha globin genes [29, 30]. Co-inheritance of a single alpha gene deletion has very little effect on the phenotype of β^0 thalassaemia, while individuals with two alpha gene deletions and homozygous β^+ thalassaemia may have a mild form of thalassaemia intermedia. At the other extreme, patients who have co-inherited HbH (equivalent of only one functioning alpha gene) and homozygous beta thalassaemia, also have thalassaemia intermedia.

Just as co-inheritance of alpha thalassaemia can reduce the clinical severity of homozygous beta thalassaemia, the presence of increased alpha globin product in beta thalassaemia heterozygotes tips the globin chain imbalance further, converting a typically clinically asymptomatic state to that of thalassaemia intermedia. In the majority of cases, this is related to the co-inheritance of triplicated alpha globin genes. Triplicated alpha genes ($\alpha\alpha\alpha/$) occur in most populations at a low frequency. The co-inheritance of two extra alpha globin genes ($\alpha\alpha\alpha/\alpha\alpha\alpha$) or ($\alpha\alpha\alpha\alpha/\alpha\alpha$) with heterozygous beta thalassaemia results in the thalassaemia intermedia [40, 41]. However, the phenotype of a single extra gene ($\alpha\alpha\alpha/\alpha\alpha$) with heterozygous beta thalassaemia is more variable and depends on the severity of the beta thalassaemia allele [42, 43]. There appears to be a critical threshold of globin chain imbalance in each individual above which clinical symptoms appear. This may be related to the efficiency of the proteolytic mechanism of the erythroid precursors or perhaps to the level of the newly discovered alpha haemoglobin-stabilizing protein (AHSP), a chaperone of alpha globin [44].

Variation in fetal haemoglobin production

The role of increased HbF response as an ameliorating factor becomes evident in the group of homozygous β^0 thalassaemia patients who have a mild disease and are able to maintain a reasonable level of haemoglobin all of which is HbF. Production of fetal haemoglobin after the neonatal period in beta thalassaemia is an extremely complex process and still poorly understood. There appears to be a genuine increase in gamma chain synthesis, presumably reflecting the expansion of the ineffective erythroid mass. The effect is augmented by the selective survival of the erythroid precursors that synthesize relatively more gamma chains. Hence all beta thalassaemias, heterozygous or homozygous, have variable increases in their levels of HbF. Against this background, there are undoubtedly genetic factors involved. Recent studies have shown that the level of HbF and F cells (a subset of erythrocytes that contain HbF) are overwhelmingly genetically controlled [45]. About one-third of the genetic variance is due to determinants linked to the beta globin gene complex but more than 50% of the genetic variance in F cell levels is due to factors not linked to the beta chromosome [46]. These *trans*-acting factors presumably play an important role in the fine-tuning of gamma globin production in adult life. Linkage studies have mapped loci controlling HbF and F cell levels to three regions of the genome – chromosomes 6q23, Xp22 and 8q (see below).

There are several determinants within the beta globin gene cluster that are associated with a defect in the normal switch from fetal to adult haemoglobin production leading to increased HbF levels in adult life. They constitute the group of hereditary persistence of fetal haemoglobin (HPFH) and delta beta thalassaemias. These are caused by large deletions of the beta globin complex or point mutations in the gamma globin promoters and are clearly inherited as alleles of the beta globin complex in a Mendelian fashion with HbF levels of 5–35% in the heterozygous state [14]. These variants, however, are rare. Much more common is a genetic variant, C-T polymorphism, at position −158 of the Gγ globin gene, also referred to as *Xmn*1-Gγ polymorphism. The *Xmn*1-Gγ site is common in all population groups and is present at a frequency of 0.32–0.35 [46]. Our linkage studies indicate that it accounts for up to 35% of the F cell variance in the general population [46]. Although the increases in HbF and F cells are minimal in normal people, clinical studies have shown that, under conditions of haematopoietic stress, for example, in homozygous beta thalassaemia and sickle cell disease (SCD), the presence of the *Xmn*1-Gγ site favours a higher HbF response [47, 48]. This could explain why the same mutations on different beta chromosomal backgrounds (some with and others without the *Xmn*1-Gγ site) are associated with different clinical severity.

Although the presence of the *cis Xmn*1-Gγ site is a modulating factor, clearly there are some patients who have enhanced HbF response despite being *Xmn*1-Gγ−/− [29, 48]. In many cases, family studies have shown that there is an inherent capacity for producing HbF and that the genetic determinant is not linked to the beta globin cluster. This is in keeping with our sib-pair studies which showed that > 50% of the F cell variance in the general population is accounted for by *trans*-acting factors. Indeed, analysis of a single large family spanning seven generations has assigned one such quantitative trait locus (QTL) for F cell to chromosome 6q23 [50]. Analyses of similar families indicate that there are other QTLs for HbF and F cells and that they are not linked to 6q or the beta globin gene complex [51]. A genetic determinant which is associated with F cell variance in SCD has been assigned to chromosome Xp [52] but its role, if any, in determining the level of HbF in beta thalassaemia is not clear. Recently, another QTL for F cell levels has been assigned to chromosome 8q; the effects of this locus are conditional on the *Xmn*1-Gγ site [53]. As the genetic basis of the propensity to produce HbF becomes unravelled it is becoming clear that the conglomeration of the Xmn1-Gγ polymorphism, the QTLs on 6q, Xp and 8q and others, linked and unlinked to the beta globin complex, constitute the loosely defined syndrome of heterocellular HPFH [54]. Until the different entities become better defined, detection of an inherent capacity for increased HbF production is, at present, difficult and usually inferred from family studies.

Mosaicism due to somatic deletion of beta globin gene

This novel mechanism was recently described in an individual who had moderately severe thalassaemia intermedia despite being constitutionally heterozygous for β^0 thalassaemia with a normal alpha genotype [55]. Subsequent investigations revealed that he had a somatic deletion of a region of chromosome 11p15 including the beta globin complex giving rise to a mosaic of cells, 50% with one and 50% without any beta globin gene. The sum total of the beta globin product is ~25% less than the normally asymptomatic beta thalassaemia trait.

This unusual case once again illustrates that the severity of anaemia of beta thalassaemia reflects the defective beta globin chain production. Furthermore, with respect to potential gene therapy, expression of a single beta globin gene in a proportion of the red blood cells appears to be sufficient to redress the chain imbalance to produce a condition mild enough not to need major medical intervention.

Tertiary modifiers

With the increasing lifespan of the beta thalassaemia patients, subtle variations in the phenotype with regard to some of the complications have become apparent and evidence suggests that they may be affected by genetic variants.

Hyperbilirubinaemia and a propensity to gallstone formation is a common complication of beta thalassaemia and is attributed to the rapid turnover of the red blood cells, bilirubin being a break-down product of haemoglobin. Varying degrees of jaundice have often been observed in the thalassaemia syndromes – from thalassaemia trait through to thalassaemia major [56–58]. Studies have shown that the levels of bilirubin and the incidence of gallstones in beta thalassaemia are related to a polymorphic variant (seven TA repeats) in the promoter of the uridine diphosphate-glucoronyltransferase IA (UGTIA) gene, also referred to as Gilbert's syndrome. Normal individuals who are homozygous for the $[TA]_7$ variant instead of the usual six, tend to have higher levels of bilirubin [59]. The $[TA]_7$ variant has also been shown to be associated with increased bilirubin levels in SCD and other haemolytic anaemias [60]. In vitro studies indicate that the variant causes a reduced expression of the UGTIA gene [59].

A common complication of beta thalassaemia involves organ damage from iron overload, not just from blood transfusions but also from increased absorption. Preliminary studies suggest that the common mutation C282Y in the HFE gene that causes hereditary haemochromatosis, predisposes to iron loading in thalassaemia intermedia [61]. The co-existence of beta thalassaemia trait aggravates and accentuates iron loading in C282Y HFE homozygotes [62]. As the C282Y mutation is rare in populations in which beta thalassaemia is common it has a limited role in iron loading among these patients [63]. Much more common is the HFE gene polymorphism, H63D, whose functional role is still being investigated. None the less, a recent study showed that beta thalassaemia carriers who are homozygotes for H63D have higher serum ferritin levels than carriers without the polymorphism, suggesting that the H63D polymorphism may have a modulating effect on iron absorption [64]. As other genes in iron homeostasis become uncovered, it is likely there will be genetic variants in these loci that influence the different degrees of iron loading in beta thalassaemia [65].

Similarly, there is increasing evidence that progressive osteoporosis and osteopenia, another increasingly common complication encountered in young adults with beta thalassaemia [66], may be modified by polymorphisms in the genes for the vitamin D and oestrogen receptor, and the COLIA1 gene that regulates synthesis of type 1 collagen [67]. Genetic variants implicated in other complications of beta thalassaemia include the apolipoprotein E (APOE) ε4 allele in cardiac damage [68]; specific HLA alleles in the tendency to hepatitis and liver cirrhosis; genetic variants in factor V, prothrombin and MTHFR; and the tendency to thrombosis.

Conclusion

There is a spectrum of phenotypes in beta thalassaemia, the severity of which relates directly to the degree of chain imbalance and the alpha globin excess. Much of the variation can be explained by heterogeneity of the molecular lesions affecting the beta globin gene itself but it is also clear that variability at the two loci – alpha and gamma globin genes – is important in determining the phenotype, which is extremely encouraging for genetic counselling. However, while genotyping at the beta globin and alpha globin loci is relatively easy to incorporate into the prenatal diagnosis and counselling programme, detecting an inherent ability to increase HbF in response to haematopoietic stress is still difficult. The presence of such heterocellular HPFH determinants is usually implicated from studies of family members who are often not available. Until the quantitative trait loci for HbF are better defined, it would appear that it is still not possible to consistently predict phenotype from genotype apart from the two categories of extra alpha globin genes with heterozygous beta thalassaemia, and the inheritance of mild β^+ thalassaemia alleles. Ethnicity and environment are important factors in the analysis of genotype/phenotype relationships. Studies have shown that all three categories of genetic modifiers – primary, secondary and tertiary – are population-specific. The tertiary locus includes the many different genetic polymorphisms that form the background genes, some of which have been co-selected with the thalassaemias.

Acknowledgement

I thank Claire Steward for help in preparation of the manuscript and Helen Hunt for Fig. 4.1a.

References

1. Weatherall DJ, Clegg JB. *The Thalassaemia Syndromes.* Oxford: Blackwell Science, 2001.

2. Flint J, Harding RM, Boyce AJ, Clegg JB. The population genetics of the haemoglobinopathies. In: Rodgers GP, ed. *Baillière's Clinical Haematology*, Vol. 11. London: Bailliere Tindall, 1998: 1–52.

3. Bulger M, Bender MA, van Doorninck JH *et al.* Comparative structural and functional analysis of the olfactory receptor genes flanking the human and mouse b-globin gene clusters. *Proc Natl Acad Sci U S A* 2000; **97**: 14560–5.

4. Antonarakis SE, Boehm CD, Giardinia PJV, Kazazian HHJ. Non-random association of polymorphic restriction sites in the β-globin gene cluster. *Proc Natl Acad Sci U S A* 1982; **79**: 137–41.

5. Orkin SH, Kazazian HHJ, Antonarakis SE *et al.* Linkage of β-thalassaemia mutations and β-globin gene polymorphisms with DNA polymorphisms in human β-globin gene cluster. *Nature* 1982; **296**: 627–31.

6. Chakravarti A, Buetow KH, Antonarakis SE *et al.* Nonuniform recombination within the human β-globin gene cluster. *Am J Hum Genet* 1984; **36**: 1239–58.

7. Gerhard DS, Kidd KK, Kidd JR, Egeland JA, Housman DE. Identification of a recent recombination event within the human β-globin gene cluster. *Proc Natl Acad Sci U S A* 1984; **81**: 7875–9.

8. Old JM, Heath C, Fitches A *et al.* Meiotic recombination between two polymorphic restriction sites within the β globin gene cluster. *J Med Genet* 1986; **23**: 14–18.

9. Camaschella C, Serra A, Saglio G *et al.* Meiotic recombination in the β globin gene cluster causing an error in prenatal diagnosis of β thalassaemia. *J Med Genet* 1988; **25**: 307–10.

10. Hall GW, Sampietro M, Barnetson R *et al.* Meiotic recombination in an Irish family with beta-thalassaemia. *Hum Genet* 1993; **92**: 28–32.

11. Smith RA, Ho PJ, Clegg JB, Kidd JR, Thein SL. Recombination breakpoints in the human beta-globin gene cluster. *Blood* 1998; **92**: 4415–21.

12. Carter D, Chakalova L, Osborne CS, Dai YF, Fraser P. Long-range chromatin regulatory interactions in vivo. *Nat Genet* 2002; **32**: 623–6.

13. Tolhuis B, Palstra RJ, Splinter E, Grosveld F, de Laat W. Looping and interaction between hypersensitive sites in the active beta-globin locus. *Mol Cell* 2002; **10**: 1453–65.

14. Wood WG. Hereditary persistence of fetal hemoglobin and δβ thalassaemia. In: Steinberg MH, Forget BG, Higgs DR, Nagel RL, eds. *Disorders of Hemoglobin: Genetics, Pathophysiology, and Clinical Management.* Cambridge, UK: Cambridge University Press, 2001: 356–88.

15. Schrier SL. Pathophysiology of thalassemia. *Curr Opin Hematol* 2002; **9**: 123–6.

16. Thein SL. Beta thalassaemia. In: Rodgers GP, ed. *Baillière's Clinical Haematology, Sickle Cell Disease and Thalassaemia*, Vol. 11:1. London: Baillière Tindall, 1998: 91–126.

17. Viprakasit V, Gibbons RJ, Broughton BC et al. Mutations in the general transcription factor TFIIH result in
beta-thalassaemia in individuals with trichothiodystro-
phy. Hum Mol Genet 2001; 10: 2797–802.
18. Yu C, Niakan KK, Matsushita M et al. X-linked thrombocytopenia with thalassaemia from a mutation in the
amino finger of GATA-1 affecting DNA binding rather
than a FOG-1 interaction. Blood 2002; 100: 2040–5.
19. Craig JE, Kelly SJ, Barnetson R, Thein SL. Molecular
characterization of a novel 10.3 kb deletion causing β-
thalassaemia with unusually high Hb A$_2$. Br J Haematol
1992; 82: 735–44.
20. Schokker RC, Went LN, Bok J. A new genetic variant of
β-thalassaemia. Nature 1966; 209: 44–6.
21. Game L, Bergounioux J, Close JP, Marzouka BE, Thein
SL. A novel deletion causing (egdb)zero thalassemia in a
Chilean family. Br J Haematol 2003; 122: 1–6.
22. Divoky V, Indrak K, Mrug M et al. A novel mechanism of
β thalassemia: the insertion of L1 retrotransposable element into β globin IVS II. Blood 1996; 88:148a.
23. Maquat LE. When cells stop making sense: effects of
nonsense codons on RNA metabolism in vertebrate cells.
RNA 1995; 1: 453–65.
24. Maquat LE, Carmichael GG. Quality control of mRNA
function. Cell 2001; 104: 173–6.
25. Hall GW, Thein SL. Nonsense codon mutations in the
terminal exon of the β-globin gene are not associated
with a reduction in β-mRNA accumulation: a mechanism for the phenotype of dominant β-thalassaemia.
Blood 1994; 83: 2031–7.
26. Rund D, Filon D, Strauss N, Rachmilewitz EA,
Oppenheim A. Mean corpuscular volume of heterozygotes for β-thalassaemia correlates with the severity of
mutations. Blood 1991; 79: 238–43.
27. Skarmoutsou C, Papassotiriou I, Traeger-Synodinos
J et al. Erythroid bone marrow activity and red cell
hemoglobinization in iron sufficient b-thalassaemia heterozygotes as reflected by soluble transferrin receptor
and reticulocyte hemoglobin in content. Correlation
with genotypes and Hb A2 levels. Haematologica 2003;
88: 631–6.
28. Maragoudaki E, Kanavakis E, Trager-Synodinos J et al.
Molecular, haematological and clinical studies of the
−101 C–>T substitution in the β-globin gene promoter in
25 β-thalassaemia intermedia patients and 45 heterozygotes. Br J Haematol 1999; 107: 699–706.
29. Ho PJ, Hall GW, Luo LY, Weatherall DJ, Thein SL. Beta
thalassemia intermedia: is it possible to consistently predict phenotype from genotype? Br J Haematol 1998;
100: 70–8.
30. Camaschella C, Maza U, Roetto A et al. Genetic interactions in thalassemia intermedia: analysis of β-mutations,
α-genotype, γ-promoters, and β-LCR hypersensitive
sites 2 and 4 in Italian patients. Am J Hematol 1995; 48:
82–7.
31. Thein SL, Hesketh C, Wallace RB, Weatherall DJ. The
molecular basis of thalassaemia major and thalassaemia
intermedia in Asian Indians: application to prenatal
diagnosis. Br J Haematol 1988; 70: 225–31.
32. Thein SL. Is it dominantly inherited β thalassaemia or
just a β-chain variant that is highly unstable? Br J
Haematol 1999; 107: 12–21.
33. Thein SL. Structural variants with a β-thalassemia phenotype. In: Steinberg MH, Forget BG, Higgs DR, Nagel
R L, eds. Disorders of Hemoglobin: Genetics, Pathophysiology, and Clinical Management. Cambridge, UK:
Cambridge University Press, 2001: 342–55.
34. Fei YJ, Stoming TA, Kutlar A, Huisman THJ, Stamatoy-
annopoulos G. One form of inclusion body β-
thalassaemia is due to a GAA->TAA mutation at codon
121 of the β chain. Blood 1989; 73: 1075–7.
35. Weatherall DJ, Clegg JB, Knox-Macaulay HHM et al. A
genetically determined disorder with features both of
thalassaemia and congenital dyserythropoietic anaemia.
Br J Haematol 1973; 24: 681–702.
36. Thein SL. Dominant β thalassaemia: molecular basis and
pathophysiology. Br J Haematol 1992; 80: 273–7.
37. Ho PJ, Wickramasinghe SN, Rees DC et al. Erythroblas-
tic inclusions in dominantly inherited β thalassaemias.
Blood 1997; 89: 322–8.
38. Hentze MW, Kulozik AE. A perfect message: RNA surveillance and nonsense-mediated decay. Cell 1999; 96:
307–10.
39. Bunn HF, Forget BG. Hemoglobin: Molecular, Genetic
and Clinical Aspects. Philadelphia, PA: WB Saunders,
1986.
40. Thein SL, Al-Hakim I, Hoffbrand AV. Thalassaemia
intermedia: a new molecular basis. Br J Haematol 1984;
56: 333–7.
41. Galanello R, Ruggeri R, Paglietti E et al. A family with
segregating triplicated alpha globin loci and beta thalassaemia. Blood 1983; 62: 1035–40.
42. Camaschella C, Kattamis AC, Petroni D et al. Different
hematological phenotypes caused by the interaction
of triplicated α-globin genes and heterozygous β-
thalassaemia. Am J Hematol 1997; 55: 83–8.
43. Traeger-Synodinos J, Kanavakis E, Vrettou C et al.
The triplicated α-globin gene locus in β-thalassaemia
heterozygotes: clinical, haematological, biosynthetic
and molecular studies. Br J Haematol 1996; 95:
467–71.
44. Kihm AJ, Kong Y, Hong W et al. An abundant erythroid
protein that stabilizes free alpha-haemoglobin. Nature
2002; 417: 758–63.
45. Garner C, Tatu T, Reittie JE et al. Genetic influences on F
cells and other hematological variables: a twin heritability study. Blood 2000; 95: 342–6.
46. Garner C, Tatu T, Game L et al. A candidate gene study of
F cell levels in sibling pairs using a joint linkage and association analysis. GeneScreen 2000; 1: 9–14.

47. Thein SL, Wainscoat JS, Sampietro M *et al.* Association of thalassaemia intermedia with a beta-globin gene haplotype. *Br J Haematol* 1987; **65**: 367–73.

48. Labie D, Pagnier J, Lapoumeroulie C *et al.* Common haplotype dependency of high $^G\gamma$-globin gene expression and high Hb F levels in β-thalassaemia and sickle cell anemia patients. *Proc Natl Acad Sci U S A* 1985; **82**: 2111–14.

49. Galanello R, Dessi E, Melis MA *et al.* Molecular analysis of β^o-thalassemia intermedia in Sardinia. *Blood* 1989; **74**: 823–7.

50. Craig JE, Rochette J, Fisher CA *et al.* Dissecting the loci controlling fetal haemoglobin production on chromosomes 11p and 6q by the regressive approach. *Nat Genet* 1996; **12**: 58–64.

51. Craig JE, Rochette J, Sampietro M *et al.* Genetic heterogeneity in heterocellular hereditary persistence of fetal hemoglobin. *Blood* 1997; **90**: 428–34.

52. Dover GJ, Smith KD, Chang YC *et al.* Fetal hemoglobin levels in sickle cell disease and normal individuals are partially controlled by an X-linked gene located at Xp22.2. *Blood* 1992; **80**: 816–24.

53. Garner CP, Tatu T, Best S, Creary L, Thein SL. Evidence for genetic interaction between the beta-globin complex and chromosome 8q in the expression of fetal hemoglobin. *Am J Hum Genet* 2002; **70**: 793–9.

54. Thein SL, Craig JE. Genetics of Hb F/F cell variance in adults and heterocellular hereditary persistence of fetal hemoglobin. *Hemoglobin* 1998; **22**: 401–14.

55. Badens C, Mattei MG, Imbert AM *et al.* A novel mechanism for thalassaemia intermedia. *Lancet* 2002; **359**: 132–3.

56. Galanello R, Perseu L, Melis MA *et al.* Hyperbilirubinaemia in heterozygous β-thalassaemia is related to co-inherited Gilbert's syndrome. *Br J Haematol* 1997; **99**: 433–6.

57. Sampietro M, Lupica L, Perrero L, Comino A, Martinez di Montemuros F. The expression of uridine diphosphate glucuronosyltransferase gene is a major determinant of bilirubin level in heterozygous β-thalassaemia and in glucose-6-phosphate. *Br J Haematol* 1997; **99**: 437–9.

58. Galanello R, Piras S, Barella S *et al.* Cholelithiasis and Gilbert's syndrome in homozygous β-thalassaemia. *Br J Haematol* 2001; **115**: 926–8.

59. Bosma PJ, Chowdhury JR, Bakker C *et al.* The genetic basis of the reduced expression of bilirubin UDP-glucuronosyltransferase 1 in Gilbert's syndrome. *N Engl J Med* 1995; **333**: 1171–5.

60. Passon RG, Howard TA, Zimmerman SA, Schultz WH, Ware RE. Influence of bilirubin uridine diphosphate-glucuronosyltransferase 1A promoter polymorphisms on serum bilirubin levels and cholelithiasis in children with sickle cell anemia. *Am J Pediatr Hematol Oncol* 2001; **23**: 448–51.

61. Rees DC, Luo LY, Thein SL, Sing BM, Wickramasinghe S. Nontransfusional iron overload in thalassemia: association with hereditary hemochromatosis. *Blood* 1997; **90**: 3234–6.

62. Piperno A, Mariani R, Arosio C *et al.* Haemochromatosis in patients with beta-thalassaemia trait. *Br J Haematol* 2000; **111**: 908–14.

63. Merryweather-Clarke AT, Pointon JJ, Shearman JD, Robson KJH. Global prevalence of putative haemochromatosis mutations. *J Med Genet* 1997; **34**: 275–8.

64. Melis MA, Cau M, Deidda F *et al.* H63D mutation in the HFE gene increases iron overload in beta-thalassaemia carriers. *Haematologica* 2002; **87**: 242–5.

65. Andrews N. Iron homeostasis: insights from genetics and animal models. *Nature Rev Genet* 2000; **1**: 208–16.

66. Wonke B. Bone disease in β-thalassaemia major. *Br J Haematol* 1998; **103**: 897–901.

67. Dresner Pollack R, Rachmilewitz E, Blumenfeld A, Idelson M, Goldfarb AW. Bone mineral metabolism in adults with beta-thalassaemia major and intermedia. *Br J Haematol* 2000; **111**: 902–7.

68. Economou-Peterson E, Aesspopos A, Kladi A *et al.* Apolipoprotein E ε4 allele as a genetic risk factor for left ventricular failure in homozygous β-thalassaemia. *Blood* 1998; **92**: 3455–9.

Chapter 5
The diagnosis and significance of alpha thalassaemia

AD Stephens

Introduction

Alpha thalassaemia occurs because of inadequate production of alpha globin chains and this is usually caused by an inherited abnormality of the genes responsible for the production of alpha globin. Two allelic pairs of genes situated on chromosome 16 control the alpha globin chains, whereas a single allelic pair of genes on chromosome 11 controls the beta globin chains. Therefore, there are four genes which code for the alpha globin chain and the so-called 'classical' alpha thalassaemia is due to deletion of one or more of these four genes and this results in four different phenotypes. There are also some rarer non-deletional mutations, which can cause alpha thalassaemia. The reduced synthesis of alpha chains leads to chain imbalance with excess gamma chains in the fetus and neonate and excess beta chains in later life. These excess chains form γ_4 and β_4 tetramers, respectively. The haematological consequence of reduced alpha globin chain production is a reduced production of haemoglobin, which reduces both the mean corpuscular haemoglobin (MCH) and the mean corpuscular volume (MCV). The γ_4 and β_4 tetramers have a high affinity for oxygen, making it difficult to deliver oxygen to the tissues; they are also unstable, leading to ineffective erythropoiesis and haemolysis. The extent of these changes is very variable depending on how many of the alpha genes have been deleted, or are otherwise ineffective. In the mildest situation the changes are so small that they may not be detected by the full blood count, whereas the most severe case where no alpha chains are made is incompatible with postnatal life and

affected fetuses usually die *in utero* by 30 weeks of gestation.

Although there are now more than 100 mutations known to cause alpha thalassaemia, the deletional mutations can usefully be divided into two groups: those where two genes are deleted on the same chromosome are called alpha zero (α^0), whereas those where only one gene is deleted on a chromosome are called alpha plus (α^+), so that the α^0 deletions cause a more marked reduction in a globin production than the α^+ deletions. Both α^+ and α^0 can occur as the heterozygous or homozygous state or there may be the compound heterozygous state of α^+/α^0 (see Fig. 5.1). The rarer non-deletional forms of alpha thalassaemia are denoted by α^T and these vary in severity from α^+ to α^0 depending on how many alpha chains are produced by that gene. There is also a very rare form of α^0 thalassaemia associated with mental retardation known as ATR. Over the years various names have been given to different combinations of mutations and these are summarized in Table 5.1. It may seem confusing that the two-gene deletion is called alpha thalassaemia-1 and the one-gene deletion is called alpha thalassaemia-2, but like much in medicine there is a good historical reason in that the clinically more severe condition was found first and when the milder condition was found they were called types 1 and 2, respectively. It was only later that gene analyses showed the underlying causes.

Similarly, the clinical condition associated with deletion of three alpha globin genes is called HbH disease, because when it was first investigated an unusual haemoglobin was found to be present and

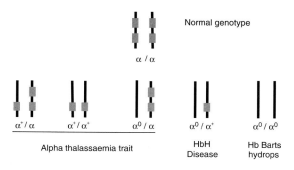

α / α

Normal genotype

α^+/α α^+/α^+ α^0/α α^0/α^+ α^0/α^0

Alpha thalassaemia trait

HbH Disease

Hb Barts hydrops

Fig. 5.1 Deletional ('classical') alpha thalassaemia.

Table 5.1 Classification of alpha thalassaemia

Inherited deletional (α^+, α^0)		
Alpha thalassaemia-2 trait	$-\alpha/\alpha\alpha$ or	α^+/α
Alpha thalassaemia-1 trait	$-\alpha/-\alpha$ or	α^+/α^+
	$\alpha\alpha/-$ or	α/α^0
HbH disease	$-\alpha/-$ or	α^+/α^0
Hb Barts hydrops	$-/-$ or	α^0/α^0
Inherited non-deletional (α^T)		
Alpha thalassaemia with mental retardation (ATR-16 and ATR-X)		
Acquired alpha thalassaemia with MDS (ATMDS)		

named HbH. It was only later shown that HbH was composed of a tetramer of four normal beta chains. Similarly when blood was examined from a dead, hydropic fetus, no fetal haemoglobin (HbF) and no adult haemoglobin (HbA) were present, only an unusual haemoglobin that had previously been called haemoglobin Barts. Hb Barts had first been described in a young Chinese girl with HbH disease and it was only later shown that Hb Barts was composed of a γ_4 tetramer.

Clinical significance

The clinical syndrome of alpha thalassaemia trait (deletion of one or two alpha globin genes) is very similar to beta thalassaemia trait in that the MCH and MCV will be reduced, the haemoglobin concentration may be slightly reduced but the red count will be higher than expected for the haemoglobin level. Various mathematical formulae have been derived to make use of these changes and these are often called discriminatory functions, but unfortunately they are only a guide and are not diagnostic and they do not differentiate alpha from beta thalassaemia. At first sight, the red cell indices can be confused with iron deficiency but people with alpha or beta thalassaemia trait should only be treated with iron if they are also shown to be iron-deficient. Alpha thalassaemia trait will never do the affected individual any harm but can be confused with both beta thalassaemia trait and iron deficiency. However, some people may have two, or even three, of these conditions; for instance, one individual may have both alpha and beta thalassaemia and iron

deficiency at the same time. HbH disease is associated with a moderate anaemia of 7–8 g/dl, a reduced MCH and MCV and a very abnormal blood film, which can best be described as bizarre with microcytes, macrocytes, fragmented cells, target cells, polychromasia and occasional nucleated red cells and splenomegaly. In spite of these abnormalities affected people usually lead quite normal lives with full exercise tolerance and no treatment is needed. Occasionally hypersplenism occurs and if so splenectomy will be necessary. Sometimes blood transfusion is required and this is most likely to occur during pregnancy. HbH disease is sometimes confused with severe iron deficiency but affected people should only receive iron supplements if iron deficiency has been documented. Occasionally HbH disease is clinically more severe and these individuals have usually inherited one of the non-deletional (α^T) forms of alpha thalassaemia (Table 5.1).

As stated earlier, homozygous α^0 thalassaemia leads to 'Hb Barts hydrops' in which the developing fetus is unable to make any alpha globin chains and hence cannot make any fetal or adult haemoglobin. The only 'normal' haemoglobins that can be made are the embryonic haemoglobins: Hb Portland ($\zeta_2\gamma_2$) and Hb Gower 1 ($\zeta_2\epsilon_2$). Some Hb Barts (γ_4) is also present, but it has very little capacity to deliver oxygen to the fetal tissues. By approximately 16 weeks of gestation the fetus becomes oedematous (hydropic) and this can be detected by ultrasound. The pregnant mother often suffers from severe pre-eclampsia and the fetus usually dies at about 30 weeks gestation. A few untreated fetuses have survived a few minutes after delivery. It is hard to understand how the fetus can survive so long *in utero* without any fetal haemoglobin. As stated above the only haemoglobins present are Hb Barts and small amounts of two embryonic haemoglobins.

Geographical distribution

Alpha thalassaemia occurs in all populations, but it is only common in those areas of the world where malaria used to be, and may still be, a common killer disease. It is now known that the distribution of alpha thalassaemia, like sickle cell disease and G6PD deficiency, is linked to malaria. Neither heterozygous nor homozygous α^+ thalassaemia causes clinical problems, although homozygous α^0 or the compound heterozygote of α^+ with α^0 do so. It is therefore very important to know which people are at risk of having α^0 thalassaemia. The latter is only common in South-East Asia, although it also occurs in the Eastern Mediterranean and it is therefore only people whose ancestors came from these areas that are at risk of having HbH disease or Hb Barts hydrops. Conversely, as the α^0 gene is extremely rare in people whose ancestors came from Africa or South Asia (India, Pakistan and Bangladesh) such people can be reassured that they are highly unlikely to have children with HbH disease or Hb Barts hydrops. With increasing mixing of populations there will come a time in the future when it will be harder, or even impossible, to make such predictions on the geographical origins of people's ancestors. As stated earlier, sporadic cases of α^+ and α^0 thalassaemia can occur anywhere in the world and so no absolute predictions can be made on the knowledge of ancestral origins. α^+ Thalassaemia is common in people of African descent and studies in Jamaica have shown that approximately 20% of the population are heterozygous for α^+ thalassaemia and 3% are homozygous for this mutation. In some East Indian islands the incidence is even higher, with levels of > 80% being reported, so in situations like this it can hardly be called abnormal. α^0 and α^T thalassaemia are very much rarer but as stated above α^0 thalassaemia is most common in parts of South-East Asia.

Diagnosis of alpha thalassaemia trait

In routine clinical laboratories alpha thalassaemia trait is much more difficult to diagnose than beta thalassaemia trait, as there is no reliable marker for alpha thalassaemia such as the raised HbA2 level which can be used to diagnose beta thalassaemia trait. The diagnosis is usually one of 'exclusion', which is similar to most medical diagnoses. The first step in diagnosis is to examine the blood count. If the haemoglobin and red cell indices are within normal limits it is highly unlikely that the individual has alpha thalassaemia trait. If the blood count shows hypochromic, microcytic red cell indices and the red cell count is relatively high for the haemoglobin level, then the individual probably has one of the forms of thalassaemia trait and the HbA2 level should be measured. If the HbA2 is raised the individual has beta thalassaemia trait, but if it is normal or low, then iron deficiency and/or alpha thalassaemia should be considered. If both the HbA2 and the iron status are normal then it is reasonable to infer that the individual has alpha thalassaemia trait. If the full blood count (FBC), iron status and HbA2 are all measured at the same time the process will be expedited. HbH 'bodies' can be detected in some cases of two-gene deletion but this is a very time-consuming test and so many laboratories in the UK have given up looking for HbH bodies in suspected alpha thalassaemia trait; however if they are seen it confirms the diagnosis. As only one HbH-containing red cell may be seen in 1000–10 000 cells examined, a laboratory worker has to inspect each microscope slide for 15–20 minutes and even then alpha thalassaemia trait cannot be excluded if HbH bodies are not seen.

The only definitive way to diagnose alpha thalassaemia trait is to analyse the DNA for the common mutations from some nucleated cells – mature red cells cannot be used, as they have no nuclei. Currently, such techniques are only available to confirm or exclude a provisional diagnosis of alpha thalassaemia in people considering prenatal diagnosis of a fetus at risk of having a clinically significant form of alpha thalassaemia. The techniques of DNA analysis have not yet reached a stage where very large numbers of samples can be tested on a daily basis in routine laboratories. Therefore in most situations the diagnosis of alpha thalassaemia has to be made by exclusion of iron deficiency or beta thalassaemia trait in someone with low red cell indices. However, real life is even more complicated, because as stated above one individual can have alpha thalassaemia, beta thalassaemia and iron deficiency, but the elucidation of such a diagnosis is beyond the scope of this chapter. In the future it may be possible to test any individual with low red cell indices for alpha thalassaemia trait by DNA techniques.

HbH disease

This is much more easily accomplished than the diagnosis of alpha thalassaemia trait. The Hb, red blood cell (RBC) count, MCH and MCV will all be reduced but the RBC count will be higher than expected for the haemoglobin level. As stated earlier the red cells have a very bizarre appearance on the stained blood film. Haemoglobin electrophoresis should reveal a band (HbH) anodal to HbA. However, it may be necessary to watch the haemoglobin migration very carefully and reduce the electrophoresis 'run time' by up to 20%, as HbH migrates so quickly that it may run off the anodal end of the electrophoresis strip and be lost onto the electrophoresis wick. High-performance liquid chromatography (HPLC) can be used, but the peak detector may not recognize the peak, as the peak elutes very quickly and often during a period when the peak detector is switched off in order to exclude non-haemoglobin artefacts that elute with, or shortly after, the void volume. It is therefore essential to examine the chromatogram carefully and not rely on electronic interfaces. If HbH disease is suspected it is important to examine both the blood film and HbH preparation carefully, as the blood film will be very abnormal; and the HbH preparation will reveal 20–80% of the red cells to contain HbH bodies. It will therefore only take a few moments to examine the HbH preparation in this situation.

Alpha thalassaemia associated with mental retardation

There are two very rare conditions known as ATR-16 and ATR-X in which there is genetic linkage between alpha thalassaemia and mental retardation. In ATR-16 the condition is due to a large deletion of several genes at the tip of chromosome 16 and this is associated with a variable phenotype probably related to the extent of the deletion in a particular individual. In ATR-X there is no apparent abnormality on chromosome 16, but the condition appears to be caused by an abnormality on the X chromosome, which affects the expression of the alpha globin genes. In this condition there is a uniform phenotype of severe mental retardation.

Acquired alpha thalassaemia with myelodysplasia (ATMDS)

This is a rare condition and can affect an individual from any racial group. Males are affected more commonly than females. Although it was thought to occur in several bone marrow disorders, it is now known that almost all cases are associated with myelodysplasia (MDS) where up to 20% of the red cells may contain HbH bodies. The proportion of HbH tends to reduce when the MDS is in remission.

Treatment

No treatment is needed for any of the alpha thalassaemia traits caused by one- or two-gene deletions. Such alpha thalassaemia traits should not cause any clinical symptoms and usually the only problem that occurs is of confusion with iron deficiency or some other form of thalassaemia. Affected people should not be given iron supplements unless they are first shown to be iron-deficient. They may of course have iron deficiency as well as alpha thalassaemia; if so it will need investigation and treatment like any other cause of iron deficiency.

No treatment is usually necessary for people with HbH disease, but like people with alpha thalassaemia trait it may also be confused with iron deficiency. Occasionally folic acid supplements are needed but this usually only happens in mal-nourished individuals. Blood transfusion may be required, although most affected individuals complete their lives without needing any blood transfusion. A few people with HbH disease develop hypersplenism and require splenectomy. Rarer forms of HbH disease due to non-deletional alpha thalassaemia (α^T) may have a more severe clinical outcome and require frequent blood transfusions.

Most fetuses with Hb Barts hydrops are so anaemic that they become anoxic and oedematous and then die during the mid-trimester, with very few surviving beyond 30 weeks gestation. In a few cases intrauterine transfusions have been tried, but the outcome is often extremely poor, with many congenital abnormalities being reported.

Screening, DNA diagnosis and counselling

When should we look for alpha thalassaemia? The most severe form of alpha thalassaemia is Hb Barts hydrops, which is due to homozygous α^0 thalassaemia and usually leads to intrauterine death of the fetus and often to severe pre-eclampsia in the mother. This situation most often occurs in people whose ancestors came from South-East Asia, but occasionally occurs in people from the Eastern Mediterranean, especially in those from Greece and Cyprus. If the ancestors of both members of a couple who are expecting or planning for a baby came from these areas, and they have hypochromic, microcytic red cell indices, it is important that they are referred as soon as possible to a unit where the precise genotype can be identified by DNA techniques. If the woman is pregnant, the couple should be referred, if at all possible, before 9 weeks of gestation. This will then allow time for the parental diagnosis to be elucidated and the couple can be offered prenatal diagnosis if indicated, followed by the offer of a first trimester termination if the fetus has homozygous alpha thalassaemia.

Alpha thalassaemia should also be considered in people with a blood count and red cell morphology typical of HbH disease. If people have thalassaemic red cell indices, it is important to consider both alpha and beta thalassaemia trait and to measure the HbA2 and iron status. If these two tests are normal then it is reasonable to assume that the person has alpha thalassaemia trait.

As with any other medical diagnosis and especially with inherited conditions it is very important to explain the results of laboratory tests and their clinical significance to the couple and to any children they may have.

Conclusion

Alpha thalassaemia has a very high incidence throughout the world, which is largely in people whose ancestors came from those parts of the Old World where malaria was a common killer disease, although sporadic cases can occur in any population. However, severe clinical symptoms (Hb Barts hydrops in homozygous α^0) are very uncommon except in people of South-East Asian origin. The other genotypes rarely cause significant clinical disability but can cause confusion with iron deficiency. At the time of writing (2003), precise genetic diagnosis is only available for a few cases and therefore usually has to be restricted to couples at risk of having a pregnancy affected by homozygous α^0 thalassaemia. At present, diagnosis in other situations is therefore largely one of 'exclusion' following the exclusion of iron deficiency and beta thalassaemia in an individual with hypochromic, microcytic red cell indices.

Further reading

British Committee for Standardization in Haematology. Guidelines for the fetal diagnosis of globin gene disorders. *J Clin Pathol* 1994; **47**: 199–204.

British Committee for Standardization in Haematology. Guidelines for the investigation of the α and β thalassaemia traits. *J Clin Pathol* 1994; **47**: 289–95.

Chui DHK, Waye JS. Hydrops fetalis caused by α-thalassaemia: an emerging health care problem. *Blood* 1998; **91**: 2213–22.

Higgs DR. Alpha thalassaemia. In: Higgs DR, Weatherall DJ, eds. *The Haemoglobinopathies. Clinical Haematology, 6/1*. London: Bailliere Tindall, 1993: 117–50.

Weatherall DJ, Clegg JB. *The Thalassaemia Syndromes*, 4th edn. Oxford: Blackwell Scientific, 2001.

Chapter 6

The morbid anatomy of sickle cell disease and sickle cell trait

Sebastian Lucas

Introduction

This chapter describes the main pathological aspects of sickle cell disease (SCD) and sickle cell trait. It is intended for clinicians and others who care for sickle cell patients and particularly for pathologists wishing to have an account of the disease, to help interpret the autopsy findings following a death in such a patient. Therefore the focus is limited to the most important organs in which damage from the disease processes can produce significant morbidity and mortality. The term 'morbid anatomy' is used because the great majority of studies on the morphology of SCD take place on the dead, rather than on biopsies of the living. Incidental identification of the disease process is made by diagnostic histopathologists (e.g. examining maternal sinus red cells in the placenta). But depiction of the most of the life-threatening complications of the haemoglobinopathy (e.g. the acute chest syndrome) is rarely effected on biopsies; they are elucidated when a patient dies unexpectedly and the autopsy suggests the underlying processes. As the management of SCD improves with more effective neonatal screening and proactive treatment including blood transfusion, hydroxyurea therapy and haemopoietic stem cell transplantation, the incidence, patterns, morbidity and mortality of the disease-related pathologies are bound to alter. The message for pathologists is to communicate with clinicians in order to correlate the complex pathological findings in patients with clinical manifestations and treatment.

SCD

Sickle cell disease includes:
- Homozygous (HbSS) sickle cell disease, or sickle cell anaemia
- HbSC disease
- Other compound heterozygous states in which the presence of HbS in the blood leads to development of clinical disease, e.g. HbS/beta thalassaemia and HbS/hereditary persistence of fetal haemoglobin (HPFH).

Although sickle cell trait (HbAS) can lead to organ damage in some individuals, it is traditionally not included in the definition of SCD. Homozygous (HbSS) sickle cell disease is the commonest, and most of the following descriptions pertain to this entity. In varying proportions, the same processes can occur in HbSC disease, HbS-beta thalassaemia, and other compound heterozygous states. HbSC individuals are the more likely to present with acute sickle-related clinical pathology having had little or no previous problems, and often having retained their spleen intact [1]. Sickle cell trait is, of course, more frequent in populations with the sickle cell gene, but rarely causes disease; when it does, the critical pathological processes are similar.

The sickling process

Table 6.1 shows the major general pathological processes that take place in SCD. Evidently, the most important is the phenomenon of red cell sickling in small vessels – small arteries, arterioles,

Table 6.1 Factors influencing the tendency to intravascular sickling

1. Local temperature – cooling
2. Local pO$_2$ – hypoxia
3. Local pH – acidity
4. Local hypertonicity
5. Immature larger red cells
6. Fat/marrow embolism
7. Endothelial adhesion molecule expression
8. Red cell membrane ligand expression
9. Neutrophil adhesion to endothelial cells
10. Rate of blood flow in vessel – delay time
11. Concentrations of HbA2 and HbF in red cells

capillaries and venules. A critical factor is the relative time it takes for red cells to undergo the internal changes that result in morphological elongation (i.e. sickling) compared to the time it takes (the delay time) for the cells to traverse the segments of the vessel where internal and external factors may promote sickling. The many factors that predispose to intravascular sickling are summarized in Table 6.1, and their consequent direct organ damage is illustrated in Fig. 6.1. It is increasingly evident that genetic factors that influence the expression of endothelial cell adhesion molecules, red cell membrane ligand expression, local inflammatory cell responses, as well as the ambient levels of red cell

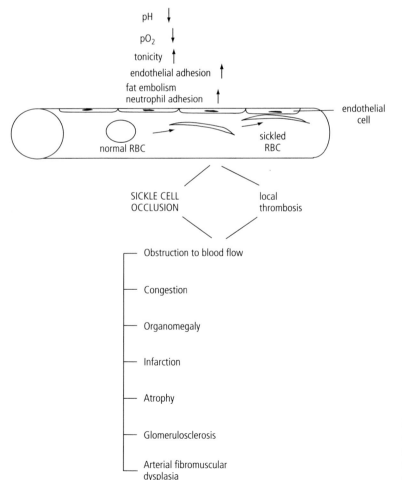

Fig. 6.1 Simplified diagram of the sickling process: predisposing factors, sickle–endothelial cell adhesion, and the local pathological sequelae. RBC, red blood cells.

HbF and HbA2, all play a role in determining the variation in the tendency to sickle at a given time. Thus the clinical and pathological manifestations of SCD in individual patients, how they progress through life, and their susceptibility to sudden and potentially fatal disease-related events are variable [2, 3]. This is considered in more detail in Chapter 18. Further pathophysiological information may come from *in vivo* microscopic studies of small vessels, e.g. in the conjunctiva [4]. These show reduced vascularity and blood flow velocity in SCD patients compared with HbAA controls, even when they are not in clinically overt sickle cell crisis. During crisis, there is further decrease in small vessel diameter and red cell flow.

Histopathology and sickling

Interpretation of histopathology in understanding how microvascular sickling develops and affects tissues is obviously limited by being a snapshot in time (and often post-mortem) and subject to the necessary artefacts of tissue processing, as well as sickling continuing as a post-vital phenomenon. As with HbSS-containing cells, HbAS red cells can sickle where there is hypoxia and acidosis, but have a higher threshold before doing so. Observed sickled red cells in biopsy material are not necessarily sickling at the time of sampling or (in the case of placentae) delivery. Most formalin (the standard tissue fixative) solutions used for histopathological fixation do not include buffers, and are acidotic; further, the tissue milieu becomes progressively hypoxic after immersion in fixative. Thus the sickling process takes place during fixation. Similar processes occur in tissues after death and can cause confusion at autopsy. After death, tissues undergo autolysis and become progressively hypoxic and acidotic, thus encouraging sickle trait (as well as HbSS and HbSC) cells to sickle. Anecdotally, confusing phenomena may occur, such as the unsickling of red cells in lung and other tissues during the interval of several days between the first and second autopsy of a sickle trait person, and absence of sickling in liver sinusoids in HbSS patients when blood vessels in all other organs do show erythrocyte sickling.

Causation of sickle cell crisis

The factors that induce sickle cell crises (such as bone infarction, acute chest syndrome) are many, complex and, in many instances, unknown. The classical Jamaican study documented skin cooling, emotional stress, physical exertion, pregnancy, and infection [5]; other factors include dehydration, drug-induced metabolic acidosis, high altitude, sleep and sleep apnoea [1]. For the autopsy pathologist, it is often impossible, without pre-crisis clinical data, to be certain what might have been the relevant factors, if known. An epidemiologically recent factor that could prove important is anti-retroviral therapy for HIV disease. Highly active anti-retroviral therapy (HAART) was considered a likely precipitator of repeated bone pain crises in a patient with HbSC disease. The proposed pathogenesis is altered cytokine status from HAART and consequent impact on endothelial–red cell interactions [6].

Bone and bone marrow

The volume of bone marrow that is actively haemopoietic is markedly increased in SCD as compensation for haemolysis. In adults, haemopoiesis extends beyond the normal central zones of vertebral bones and proximal femur. Thus the skull marrow space may be markedly thickened, and the middle and distal femur marrow may contain not just fat but active red marrow. Histologically there is relative erythroid hyperplasia. If there is folic acid deficiency, megaloblastic change in erythroid and myeloid precursor cells is evident.

Parvovirus B19 infection

The aplastic crisis in SCD is now firmly recognized as the result of infection with parvovirus B19 [7, 8], and is more common in children compared with adults. The infection is temporary and the virus infects erythroblasts, causing them to stop maturating to reticulocytes, and die. In survivors, there is a reactive proliferation of erythroblasts, and only in the immunosuppressed patient is there chronic infection. Examination of the marrow at time of crisis shows unaffected myeloid and megakaryocyte series but depleted erythroid precursors; those remaining have prominent intranuclear eosinophilic viral inclusion bodies with the nuclear chromatin pushed to the periphery of the nuclei [9]. Detection of serum antibodies to parvovirus B19 can confirm the infection, as can electron microscopy of the infected cells, and use of the polymerase chain reaction to identify the viral genomic material in biological samples.

Bone and marrow necrosis

The bone marrow and associated bony trabeculae are the site of avascular necrosis, which is the morphological basis of the classic painful crisis (Plate 1, shown in colour between pp. 54 and 55). Any bones with hyperplastic marrow can be affected, but pathologists are most likely to see necrotic femoral heads when removed surgically, vertebrae and the femur at autopsy, and iliac crest at biopsy. The cause of necrosis is occlusion of the vasculature in the marrow by sickling, with resultant anoxia [10]. Necrotic marrow, fat and bone trabeculae are distributed in small or large areas, together with repair processes of new bone formation and fibrosis. The embolism of fat and necrotic marrow to the lungs is a result of this necrosis.

Osteomyelitis

Children and young adults are the most susceptible to osteomyelitis. The long bones of the humerus, radius, tibia, femur and ulna are the most commonly affected, the mandible sometimes. Infection occurs in the diaphysis as well as the epiphyseal–meta-physeal junctions. The organisms most frequently responsible are *Staphylococcus aureus*, followed by non-typhoid *Salmonella* spp., and *Strepto-coccus pneumoniae*. The pathogenesis is usually haematogenous seeding into bone at the sites of avascular necrosis, which renders them particularly vulnerable to infection [1]. Healing with antibiotic therapy is often protracted, leaving densely sclerosed bone and associated joint irregularity. It is not clear why *Salmonella* spp. are signifi-

cant causes of bone infection and bacteraemia in SCD. The association of salmonella bacteraemia with SCD might be explained by an increased rate of carriage of the organisms in diseased gall bladders. However, no positive evidence is yet available for this hypothesis [11], nor is there evidence of prolonged intestinal carriage of *Salmonella* spp. in people with SCD [12].

Liver and gall bladder

The hepatobiliary lesions associated with SCD may be classified as direct, and indirect or secondary. The indirect pathologies are:
1 haemosiderosis – excess iron storage following repeated blood transfusions
2 viral hepatitis B and C – from contaminated blood products or other routes
3 gallstones and cholestasis
4 extramedullary haemopoiesis.

While haemosiderosis is commonly seen in sickle cell patients' livers, it is not as severe as that encountered in patients with beta thalassaemia major, and rarely appears to present as the end-fibrotic stage of haemochromatosis. Increased quantities of stainable iron are seen in the Kupffer cells and portal macrophages. None the less, mortality among SCD patients is higher in those with iron overload [13]. Hepatitis caused by hepatitis B and C viruses is no different in sickle patients from usual [14]. It may lead to cirrhosis and sometimes hepatocarcinoma, not different from that in the non-SCD population [15]. SCD does not per se result in cirrhosis, so causes such as alcoholism should be sought in such patients who do have viral infections. Gallstones, due to precipitation of the high levels of excreted bilirubin, are common in SCD [1]; they often present at an early age, in children. The stones are pigment-type and radiological studies indicate a prevalence of cholelithiasis of between 40% and 80% of patients [16]. Acute and chronic cholecystitis are the expected complications, frequently requiring cholecystectomy. There is no meta-analysis in the literature but peri-operative complications (open or laparoscopic procedure) may occur more frequently – and with higher mortality – than in the normal population [17–19]. Acute large bile duct obstruction by a stone causes cholestasis and sometimes ascending cholangitis. Compensatory extramedullary haemopoiesis is frequently observed in the liver sinusoids.

The direct liver pathologies are:
1 congestion and sequestration of sickled red cells
2 intrahepatic cholestasis.

Chronic sinusoidal congestion in the liver probably accounts for the repeated observations that the liver is enlarged in SCD [1]. At autopsy, it is usual for the liver to be enlarged and dark red in colour, with sickled red cells packed in the sinusoids. Perisinusoidal fibrosis is described as a consequence of chronic sinusoidal congestion [20]. Some patients suffer an acute sequestration crisis of the liver, with abnormally severe congestion and sickling within the sinusoids (i.e. sequestration), with a resultant fall in haemoglobin level and sometimes death. In some cases, this is associated with a painful crisis. In a few patients, thrombosis occurs in the hepatic vein (presumably the result of red cell–endothelial cell interaction, as in the pulmonary arteries), so precipitating sequestration [21]. Another common autopsy finding is centri-acinar ischaemic-type degeneration. As these are not generally found on liver biopsies [14], they represent terminal changes of shock and/or cardio-pulmonary failure. Percutaneous liver biopsy in patients undergoing an acute crisis shows the expected sequestration and sinusoidal dilatation. However, a recent study suggests that this procedure is unwarranted: it provides little new clinico-pathological information and is associated with significant mortality through intractable bleeding from the liver [22]. Cholestasis, with bile plugs in the canaliculi but no significant portal tract changes, is a result of acute hepatic damage from erythrocyte sickling and blood vessel occlusion.

Spleen

The major pathologies affecting the spleen are:
1 progressive shrinkage, infarction and asplenia
2 acute sequestration crisis

3 hypersplenism
4 hyperhaemolysis syndrome.

Shrinkage and infarction

The spleen in classical HbSS disease undergoes a sequence of predictable changes [23]. In early life there is progressive enlargement through expansion of the red pulp. There is congestion of sickled red cells, which remain in and engorge the sinusoids, with masses of elongated sickled cells visible histologically (Plate 2, shown in colour between pp. 54 and 55). Macrophages lining the sinuses phagocytose the abnormally shaped red cells; this haemophagocytosis promotes hyperplasia of the macrophages. Over time, repeated episodes of sickling in the arterioles (which become progressively sclerosed) and sinusoids causes ischaemic necrosis of segments of spleen tissue. These resolve by fibrosis (the spleen does not regenerate) and scarring, and the spleen progressively shrinks. Eventually the state of 'autosplenectomy' is reached where the spleen is a small nubbin of tissue, < 20 g in weight, comprising scar tissue and deposits of crystalline iron and calcium-rich material that includes haemosiderin (the Gandy–Gamna nodules). Some patients suffer a more acute regional infarction of parts of the spleen as part of a sickle crisis or multi-organ failure. It is more frequent in those with HbSC and sickle thalassaemia than with HbSS [1]. Such infarction is also the probable basis of splenic abscesses which, like osteomyelitis, are usually due to non-typhoid *Salmonella* infection.

Consequences of asplenia

The lack of a spleen in many patients with sickle cell disease is well known to predispose to bacteraemia, particularly pneumococcal, through complex immunological abnormalities [24]. Bacterial infections are notably more frequent in the blood and all organs of SCD patients than in HbAS and normal populations [1].

HIV and SCD

One possible benefit from autosplenectomy, of unclear epidemiological significance, is the effect on the progression of HIV disease in HbSS or HbSC individuals. The chronic lack of the T-cell pool in the spleen appears to be associated with a slower progression to AIDS – i.e. higher CD4+ T-cell count and lower HIV load – than in non-SCD controls [25]. On the other hand, pneumococcal sepsis and meningitis are significantly more common in HIV-positive SCD patients than the HIV-negative majority [26].

Acute sequestration crisis in the spleen

This mainly occurs in children and is a significant cause of mortality [1], although it is occasionally fatal in adults [27]. Obviously it can only occur in patients who have retained their spleen. Clinically, the spleen is palpable well below the left costal margin, and there is severe anaemia. An underlying precipitating factor is usually not evident. The pathological finding is a large dark red spleen, with the sinusoids dilated and packed with sickled red cells. In non-malaria regions, splenectomy may be performed as treatment for recurrent episodes when the patient has attained the age of 2 years.

Hypersplenism

There is an unusual syndrome of chronic enlarged spleen with consequent depletion of the circulating blood cells. It appears to be more frequent in HbSC disease [28]. Pathological studies are limited, but erythrocyte sickling, sinusoidal dilatation and haemophagocytosis by macrophages are seen.

Hyperhaemolysis syndrome

A few patients – adults and children – undergo an abnormal reaction to apparently matched blood transfusion that results in severe protracted haemolysis and splenomegaly. There is destruction of both transfused and autologous red cells; serological studies might reveal multiple red cell allo-antibodies, but usually the serology is negative [29]. Pathologically, there is erythroid hyperplasia in the marrow and splenomegaly [30], indicating peripheral destruction of red cells. The spleen shows congestion and hyperactive macrophages with erythrophagocytosis. Intravenous immunoglobulin therapy may arrest the haemolysis (by blocking adhesion of sickled red cells and reticulocytes to macrophages), but death may occur from severe anaemia. The syndrome is most common in HbSS patients but has also been seen in sickle thalassaemia [31].

Intestines

The intestines are rarely critically affected in SCD [1], and there is no chronic malabsorption syndrome. The clinical syndrome of abdominal painful crisis appears to relate mainly to rib bone pain, spleen and liver sequestration, possibly to mesenteric lymph node, and to small bowel ileus. A single case report documents ischaemic mucosal necrosis of the colon during a crisis, due to microvascular sickling [32]. Occlusion of the major intra-abdominal vessels is uncommon, in line with the lack of deep vein thrombosis in SCD [33]. Portal vein thrombosis, and associated occlusion of hepatic, mesenteric and splenic veins, has occasionally been documented as a cause of abdominal crisis [34] and following laparoscopic surgery [35].

Kidney

Overview

The renal lesions found in sickle patients are the most variable and complex that affect any organ [36, 37]. This is because the vascular microanatomy of the kidney is highly organized, and red cell–endothelial cell interactions are critical. Good overviews are presented by Bhathena [38] and Wesson [39]. The main pathologies are:
- papillary necrosis and interstitial nephritis
- hypercellularity and enlargement of glomeruli
- focal segmental glomerulosclerosis and nephrotic syndrome
- membranoproliferative and other glomerulonephritides
- end-stage chronic renal failure
- acute renal cortical necrosis
- carcinoma of the kidney.

The kidneys of chronically ill SCD patients typically are smaller than normal, with cortical scarring from glomerular and interstitial disease. In earlier more acute presentations, they are engorged and the individual glomeruli are visible through congestion and enlargement.

Papillary necrosis

Papillary necrosis is common in SCD, and is caused by vaso-occlusion within the vasa rectae vessels of the medulla – associated with hypertonicity and acidity [40]. The necrotic slough may occasionally block the ureters to cause acute renal failure; otherwise, it is associated with reduced concentrating ability. Morphologically the pyramids are missing, with secondary hydronephrosis.

Glomerular disease

Hypercellularity

A universal finding in SCD patients is enlarged glomeruli due to hyperplasia. Ultrastructural studies show capillaries with double contours, associated with mesangial interposition [41]. Epithelial podocytes are also abnormal with stretch lesions and eventual loss, as they cannot replicate [42], leading to impairment of the filtration barrier. These lesions are associated with hyperfiltration, and are the result of interaction between sickle cells and glomerular endothelial cells, and endothelial injury. It is presumed that they are the precursor lesions to focal segmental glomerulosclerosis in SCD. Although immune complexes may be found in glomeruli, they are secondary phenomena, not the cause of the abnormality [38].

Focal segmental glomerulosclerosis (FSGS)

End-stage renal failure (ESRF) occurs in up to 20% of SCD patients who survive to adulthood [43] and at a significantly earlier age than in the general population. The cause of this ESRF is predominantly focal segmental glomerulosclerosis (FSGS) (Plate 3, shown in colour between pp. 54 and 55). This is the 'classic' form of FSGS (not the 'collapsing' variant as typified by HIV nephropathy) [39]. The pathogenesis of FSGS is unclear and there are

several hypotheses concerning the initial lesion: local capillary thrombosis, raised intracapillary pressure, capillary disruption, mesangial interposition are all posited – the result of sickle and endothelial cell interactions. The consequent progressive inflammatory mediator damage leads to tuft adhesion between glomerular capillary and Bowman's capsule [38, 39]. The capillary wall hyalinizes and the lumen becomes obliterated. Mesangial cell matrix production contributes to the sclerosis. The parietal epithelium ruptures, enabling leakage of filtrate in the renal interstitium, and contributing to the interstitial chronic inflammation that accompanies FSGS. There is secondary atrophy and dilatation of the renal tubules. It is becoming evident that genetic variations in response to injury are important in determining which SCD patients are more likely to develop FSGS.

Membranoproliferative and other glomerulonephritides

The other patterns of glomerulonephritis encountered, apart from that associated with parvovirus (see below) are not so specific to SCD patients. They are not as frequent or significant as FSGS. Membranoproliferative glomerulonephritis is similar morphologically to the usual form in general patients, but immune complexes are not so frequently seen [39]. The usual causes of acute immune complex-mediated glomerulonephritis, e.g. post-streptococcal, can occur in SCD patients. One notable association is with parvovirus B19 infection. Nephrotic syndrome with segmental proliferative glomerulonephritis was found in SCD patients within days of aplastic crisis due to parvovirus B19 infection. The outcomes included complete recovery, death from chronic renal failure and chronic impaired renal function [44].

Acute cortical necrosis

Focal infarction of the superficial cortex is due to microvascular sickling and obstruction of the small arteries (arcuate) in the kidney (Plate 4, shown in colour between pp. 54 and 55). It is found in conjunction with generalized vaso-occlusion in many organs, part of the multi-organ failure syndrome, and thus diagnosed mainly at autopsy.

Carcinoma of the kidney

An unusual renal tumour has been specifically associated with SCD. Renal medullary carcinoma – clinically, genetically and pathologically distinct from collecting duct carcinoma – is described in children and adults with HbSS, HbSC or HbAS genotype. It presents with haematuria, or suspected renal and urinary tract infection, and metastases. The mortality rate is high with a mean survival of 4 months [45]. At the time of presentation, there are usually distant metastases (e.g. lung, brain) and lymphatic involvement [46]. The diagnosis has been made by fine-needle aspiration [47]. The pathogenesis is postulated to involve chronic hypoxia of the renal medulla.

Lung

Pulmonary involvement in SCD is a major cause of morbidity and mortality; its aetio-pathogenesis is not completely understood. The main clinico-pathological syndromes can be divided into acute and chronic.

Acute syndromes

1 Pulmonary sequestration and acute chest syndrome (ACS).
2 Bacterial pneumonia – which is not pathologically different from usual patterns.

Acute chest syndrome

Acute chest syndrome has a clinical rather than a patho-morphological case definition. There is chest pain, fever, hypoxia, dyspnoea, new infiltrates on chest X-ray and declining haemoglobin level. It is important because it may develop rapidly, is a major cause of mortality in SCD, and yet is treatable with good prognosis if managed in time. Acute chest syndrome is precipitated by many often overlapping factors [19, 48–50]:
• community-acquired pulmonary and systemic infections
• rib fracture

• bone sickle crisis (infarction)
• fat or bone marrow embolism
• surgical operations.

The pulmonary infections associated with acute chest syndrome include *Chlamydia pneumoniae*, *Streptococcus pneumoniae* and *Haemophilus influenzae* [1, 51]; however, in up to half of acute chest syndrome cases, no identifiable precipitating factor is found [52]. The pathology is characteristic (Plate 5, shown in colour between pp. 54 and 55). Grossly the lungs are dark red and heavy, without macroscopically evident pulmonary embolism. Histologically, the small arterioles, capillaries and venules of the pulmonary circulation are dilated and stuffed with sickled red cells. In the arterioles in many cases – especially where a bone vaso-occlusive crisis has been the precursor of acute chest syndrome – fat emboli and sometimes bone marrow emboli are found [53]. These originate in the bone marrow, following infarction there, and may be seen embedded in fibrin within the vessel. Infarction of the lung tissue may be seen: this may be regional or, more frequently, focal and evident only microscopically [54, 55]. Essentially, acute chest syndrome is an intravascular sickling crisis occurring in the small vessels of the lung, seizing up the blood flow, inducing cardio-pulmonary failure with acute right heart strain, and sometimes causing local lung infarction. Pathogenetically, the lung is predisposed to such sickling: the mixed venous oxygen tension in the pulmonary capillary bed is low, as is the pH; there may be shunting of blood within the pulmonary circulation; and uniquely, the pulmonary vascular bed constricts with hypoxia [55, 56]. Diagnostically, in cases of fat embolism, broncho-alveolar lavage (BAL) frequently reveals fat globules in alveolar macrophages [50].

Chronic

1 Pulmonary thromboembolism.
2 Pulmonary hypertension.

As is generally agreed, there is no predilection in SCD patients to develop deep leg vein thrombosis, and autopsy studies do not commonly find gross pulmonary emboli in the pulmonary vasculature [57]. However, there is a syndrome of chronic lung disease with progressive vascular thrombotic obstruction, pulmonary hypertension and cor pulmonale [58, 59]. The lungs of these patients may show old (grey) and recent (reddish) obliteration of the lumens of small pulmonary arteries on careful gross examination. Microscopically, there is mild to severe muscular hypertrophy of the arteries, the mark of pulmonary hypertension (Plate 6, shown in colour between pp. 54 and 55). Using the standard histological grading scheme for this disease, intimal fibro-elastosis, dilatation lesions and plexiform (aneurysmal) lesions may also be found, but the most advanced angiomatoid lesions and fibrinoid necrosis of arteries are not seen [58]. The second group of arterial lesions are recanalization of thrombi [58, 59]. Their pathogenesis is not well understood, but if thrombus is present it is probably formed locally, not embolic. In some cases, previous fat or marrow embolism may have precipitated the process. The complex interactions of sickled red cells with endothelial cells in an environment of hypoxia are also critical. Shear stress, inflammatory cytokines, altered adhesion properties of endothelial cells, local prothrombotic factors and altered local nitric oxide synthase production are among the factors proposed as relevant [58, 60].

Heart

There is no SCD-specific cardiomyopathy [61, 62] but a range of changes are encountered in people who have this haemoglobinopathy. These include work hypertrophy and the sequelae of ischaemic damage with fibrosis. A challenge for the pathologist is to identify (or exclude) subtle cardiac lesions in people with SCD and sickle cell trait who have suddenly and unexpectedly died, and assess their contribution to death. Because of the anaemia and increased cardiac work, left ventricular hypertrophy is usual in children as well as in long-term survivors [63]. Right ventricular hypertrophy accompanies pulmonary hypertension (see above), but is also regularly seen in milder form in those without clinical hypertension. Fibrosis, irregularly distributed through the left myocardium, is a persistently noted feature

of the heart in SCD [1], without myocardial disarray.

Myocardial infarction

Acute myocardial infarction is uncommon in SCD [64]. A US autopsy series from 1950 to 1982 documented 10% of patients as having old or recent infarction in the absence of classical coronary atherosclerosis and superimposed occlusive thrombosis [65, 66]. Instead, microthrombi were seen in intramyocardial arterioles; this is very similar to the phenomena encountered in the lungs with *in situ* thrombosis in the more distal pulmonary arteries, and the pathogenetic mechanisms are probably similar (see above). Other series have not found evidence of infarction, and conclude that heart failure results from chronic anaemia reducing the heart muscle reserve with superimposed pulmonary disease or acquired valvular disease [62]. Much evidently depends on case selection. Circumstances that predispose to regional myocardial infarction in SCD include anaesthesia, cor pulmonale and sepsis [67, 68]. Personal experience of hearts from sickle patients who have died unexpectedly notes an increased prevalence of micro-scars in the left ventricular myocardium which are presumably the result of episodes of microvascular sickling, obstruction and local ischaemia. Ultrastructural observations of sickle heart myofibres, through endomyocardial biopsy, find degenerative cellular changes and local oedema that are consistent with microvascular occlusion [69]. Patients who died from multi-organ failure frequently show micro-infarction in the left ventricle muscle on microscopic examination. The presence of an acute inflammatory reaction helps to establish that these lesions are pre-terminal. If there are only contraction band necroses, then the possible pathogenetic contribution of inotropic agents during attempted resuscitation may be impossible to distinguish from pre-mortem microvascular obstruction and ischaemia. Patients who had acute chest syndrome, with effective cessation of pulmonary blood flow, may show acute contraction band necrosis of the right ventricular muscle; this is presumably due to acute pulmonary hypertensive stress.

Autonomic dysfunction and arterial dysplasia

Physiological studies on sickle cell patients show differences from control subjects that suggest autonomic dysfunction [70] and, because autonomic nervous dysfunction is associated with sudden cardiac death in other disease, it has been proposed that this might explain such deaths that occur in people with SCD and sickle cell trait where gross changes (e.g. infarction) are not evident. The morphological bases for this proposal have not been systematically studied, and with few normal controls, but a detailed and thoughtful paper [71] provides some clues. Fibrosis of the atrioventricular (AV) node, the bundle of His and upper septal muscle are documented and, throughout the heart and particularly near the conducting system, fibromuscular dysplasia (FMD) of arterioles (Plate 7, shown in colour between pp. 54 and 55). This includes some medial thickening and prominent intimal thickening that comprises fibroblasts, smooth muscle cells and some elastic reduplication. The FMD induces local ischaemic damage and fibrosis. The cause of FMD is proposed to be the cumulative physical effect of sickled cells damaging endothelium.

Brain

Overview

The brain is frequently affected by SCD, particularly in children who are not under optimal management, and the major pathologies are due to cerebrovascular disease. Bacterial meningitis is also common, but is a manifestation of the general predilection to sepsis in SCD. In order of frequency, the major abnormalities encountered, over all age groups, are:

1 cerebral infarction
2 subarachnoid haemorrhage
3 intracerebral haemorrhage
4 fat embolism
5 dural venous sinus thrombosis.

Cerebral infarction

The incidence of cerebral infarction peaks in children (< 15 years) and adults > 30 years. Intracranial haemorrhage is uncommon in children and occurs mainly in adults [72]. Cerebral infarction in sickle syndromes predominantly affects the internal capsule and the boundary zones between the main cerebral arteries, particularly the anterior-middle artery territories [73]. The grey and white matter pathology of old and recent infarcts is similar to that in non-SCD subjects, but the underlying arterial pathology differs. The vascular pathology is better documented in the literature by angiography than morbid anatomy. The circle of Willis, the main cerebral arteries and their proximal main branches show intimal hyperplasia, thrombi, and organization and recanalization of these thrombi [74, 75]. Less frequently the internal carotid artery is thrombosed, with intimal hyperplasia [76]. Exactly how SCD leads to thrombosis and intimal damage in these relatively large arteries is still unclear. Suggestions that occlusion of the vasa vasorum of the cerebral arteries is the initial lesion are controversial, and unlikely given the rarity of such intra-arterial vessels in the cerebral circulation. Complex prothrombotic tendencies, secondary to red cell–endothelial cell interactions, are postulated [77], but their importance is not yet clear. An association of inherited thrombophilic states with cerebrovascular disease in sickle patients is not yet supported [78].

Haemorrhage

Infarction and intracerebral haemorrhage can occur simultaneously [75]. The pathogenesis of the intracranial haemorrhage syndromes is not so well understood. Intracerebral haemorrhage is less common than subarachnoid haemorrhage (SAH), and the presence of an identifiable arterial aneurysm associated with SAH increases with age, being uncommon in children [79]. Aneurysms are multiple in more than half of the patients with SAH, in different locations from the non-SCD-related berry aneurysms [80]. A unifying hypothesis to account for both intracerebral and SAH has been proposed [81]: adherent sickled red cells damage the endothelium; the resulting injury reaction fragments the elastic lamina of the media and causes smooth muscle degeneration (analogous to atherosclerotic processes and aneurysm formation);

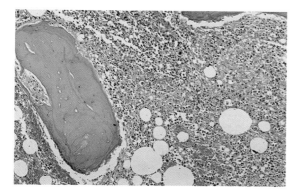

Plate 1 Sickle cell crisis with bone infarction; the necrotic (anuclear) bone trabeculum sits in necrotic haemopoietic marrow. H&E × 200.

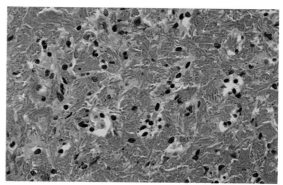

Plate 2 Spleen in sickle crisis; the sinusoids are dilated and packed with elongated sickled red cells. H&E ×400.

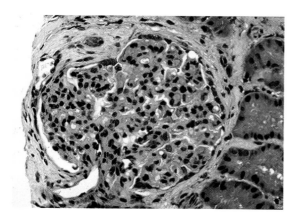

Plate 3 Focal segmental glomerulosclerosis (FSGS) with nephritic syndrome; the glomerular capillary loops are becoming thickened as is the mesangium. H&E ×200.

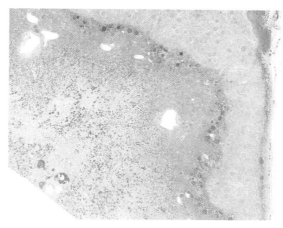

Plate 4 Kidney with regional cortical infarction in SCD; the lower congested zone is viable and the upper anuclear zone is infarcted. H&E ×100.

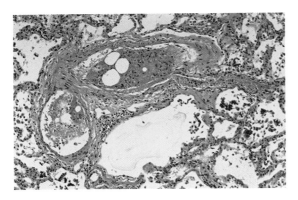

Plate 5 Lung in acute chest syndrome; the small arteriole has embolic fat droplets (the round clear spaces) and the alveolar capillaries are dilated with sickled red cells. H&E ×100.

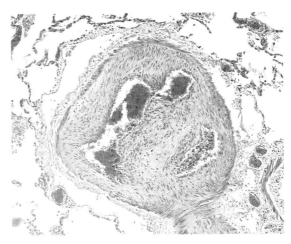

Plate 6 Lung in SCD patient with pulmonary hypertension; the small arteriole has intimal and muscular hyperplasia and the lumen shows recanalization. H&E ×100.

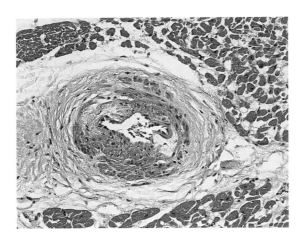

Plate 7 Heart in SCD: intramyocardial arteriole in the septum showing fibromuscular dysplasia. H&E ×100.

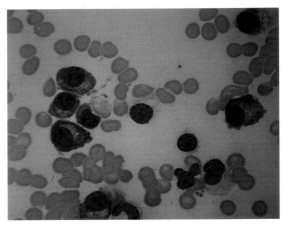

Plate 8 Multiple myeloma presenting with generalised acute bone pains, and mimicking sickle cell crisis. This diagnostic bone marrow aspirate shows plasmacytosis and erythrocyte rouleaux formation.

haemodynamic stress results in aneurysm formation and rupture. Ruptured (and hence invisible) aneurysms on small intracerebral arteries could account for the haemorrhages there. In a rare case of spinal cord involvement, the dorsal cervical cord was infarcted in association with recanalized thrombi in the vertebral artery and smaller arachnoid arterioles [82].

Fat embolism

Fat embolism to the brain causes multiple white matter lesions with focally limited perivascular necroses and ring haemorrhages [83]. This is no different from fat embolism encountered following fractures and orthopaedic surgical procedures in non-SCD patients, and has pathophysiological similarities to the small vessel obstruction seen in falciparum malaria. It is likely that fat embolism underlies some of the reported cases of demyelinating leukoencephalopathy associated with the acute chest syndrome [84, 85], as marrow embolism is a frequent precipitator of acute chest syndrome.

Venous thrombosis

Venous thrombosis is generally uncommon in SCD. Rare fatal cases of dural venous sinus thrombosis with coma and cerebral haemorrhage are reported [86]; dehydration is a factor, and a similar syndrome may rarely occur in sickle cell trait [87].

Pethidine-induced seizures

When pethidine was more frequently used for pain control in sickle crisis, fatalities occurred, because pethidine can induce seizures [1]. There are no specific morphological features in addition to the standard changes of hypoxic encephalopathy if the patient has survived more than a day or so, and of sickled cells within congested cerebral vessels.

Multi-organ failure

Individual organ failure and pathology has been considered separately up to this point. However, in reality, it has long been recognized that in many acute clinical syndromes in SCD patients more than one organ may be significantly damaged. In several accounts of painful sickle cell crisis, combinations of acute lung, liver and renal failure were noted [1, 88]. In series which document painful crises, autopsies find sequestration crisis (in liver and spleen), marrow and fat embolism to the lung, and infection (pneumonia and septicaemia) [89]. However, the deaths of a significant proportion of such patients remain unexplained in terms of gross pathology. From other published and personal observations it is likely that many result from microvascular sickling and ischaemic damage in critical organs such as the heart and lungs. This occurs in all phenotypic types of SCD. Multiple small foci of acute infarctive necrosis are seen in the heart (similar geographically to that found in acute cocaine and inotrope toxicity, where microvascular spasm is the accepted pathophysiology), in the pituitary [55], and in the peripheral renal cortex. The lungs may also show multiple areas of infarction, not necessarily related to small arterial thrombi [55]. Colonic infarction during sickle cell crisis is discussed above. A useful analogy of severe multi-organ failure in SCD has been made with thrombotic thrombocytopenic purpura (TTP) [90]. Although the aetio-pathogenesis of the two syndromes is different, the microvascular ischaemic effect on many of the organs is similar.

Maternal mortality

In the UK, with a generally low maternal mortality rate, HbSS and HbSC diseases are still disproportionately associated with death related to pregnancy [91, 92]. In countries with markedly higher overall rates of maternal mortality, SCD patients have even higher death rates [93]. The precise pathological causes of these deaths, which mostly occur around the time of delivery, are not well documented, but they include both direct causes (obstetric disease) and indirect causes (other conditions exacerbated by pregnancy, such as SCD). They include:
• genital tract haemorrhage
• pulmonary thromboembolism and chronic sickle lung disease [94, 95]
• acute chest syndrome

- septicaemia
- hypertensive disorder with chronic renal disease
- multi-organ failure with disseminated intravascular coagulation [91]
- acquired cardiac disease including myocardial fibrosis
- ischaemic necrotizing colitis with sickling in arterioles [96]
- aorto-caval compression [97].

Maternal mortality and sickle cell trait

Sickle cell trait is also reported in association with maternal morbidity and mortality, although there are no epidemiological series to support a true causal relationship. The exertion associated with delivery could induce red cell sickling and blood vessel occlusion in some people with sickle cell trait; a situation similar to vaso-occlusive crisis in SCD. The documented abnormalities encountered include:

- post-partum hypopituitism [98]
- fatal peripartum cardiomyopathy exacerbated by intravascular sickling [99].

Pathology of sickle cell trait

Severe pathology from sickling in HbAS individuals is very uncommon, as disease caused by sickling-related processes is fortunately rare. However, under certain circumstances, the red cells will sickle in small vessels and induce the related pathology. It is now agreed that a limited number of clinical syndromes are epidemiologically more frequent among HbAS persons compared with HbAA controls [1, 100]. These include:

- haematuria
- hyposthenuria
- renal medullary carcinoma
- bacteriuria in pregnant and non-pregnant women
- splenic infarction at reduced oxygen levels (e.g. altitude)
- pulmonary embolism
- sudden unexplained death.

The renal abnormalities of haematuria and hyposthenuria are generally explained as following

disruption of the vasa recta vascular system, although the aetiology of the carcinoma is unknown. Splenic infarction can also occasionally occur in sickle cell trait without altitude or similar hypoxic stress [101]. Many of the other abnormalities encountered in SCD occur occasionally in sickle cell trait. These include:

- subcortical cerebral infarction with arteriolar sickling but not thrombosis [102]
- sagittal sinus thrombosis [87]
- avascular necrosis of the femoral head [103]
- pulmonary infarction and acute chest syndrome [54, 104].

Exertional rhabdomyolysis and sudden death in sickle cell trait

The most important aspect of the pathology of sickle cell trait revolves around sudden death. The literature contains numerous case reports of HbAS persons who have collapsed and died unexpectedly, nearly always under conditions of extreme exertion. They include athletes and military personnel, and co-risk factors include heat stress, viral illness, poor physical conditioning and dehydration [105]. In the landmark epidemiological study of US army recruits, Kark *et al.* [106] found an odds ratio of x27.6 for HbAS soldiers to die of unexplained causes compared with HbAA soldiers. The majority of these unexplained deaths occurred through cardio-respiratory failure, co-morbidities having been excluded. Two clinico-pathological patterns emerge from the case reports:

1 Many of the patients had developed exertional rhabdomyolysis. They present in collapse with profound metabolic acidosis, lactic acidaemia, myoglobinuria, renal failure and disseminated intravascular coagulation (DIC). At autopsy, widespread multi-organ small vessel sickling is seen and the lungs often have the typical histopathology of acute chest syndrome [107–110].

2 Other patients, also having exerted themselves, do not have rhabdomyolysis. They collapse and show the widespread sickling, often with small infarcts in many organs, and are presumed to have died of multi-organ failure of which the most important aspect is cardio-pulmonary arrest [106, 111, 112].

One unfortunate aspect of this exertion–collapse syndrome, albeit uncommon, is death in custody with body restraint or following police pursuit. Agitation is sometimes a precursor factor. This is best documented in the USA [113, 114] but also happens in the UK (personal observations). Again, not all the patients have had rhabdomyolysis. Finally, there may be an association between fatal multi-organ sickling of red blood cells in sickle cell trait and dehydration from hyperosmolar diabetic coma (personal observations).

Causes of death in SCD

As indicated, there is significant variation over time and place in when and why SCD patients die. In developed countries, the majority of patients now live beyond 50 years [115], but previously undiagnosed HbSS and HbSC individuals may still present with fatal, acute SCD-related illness [49, 116]. Universal screening at birth cannot prevent this, because some of the affected individuals might have moved to the area of screening later in life. Two decades ago in Jamaica [117], the main causes of SCD-related death were:
- acute chest syndrome
- bacterial infections
- acute splenic sequestration
- chronic renal failure
- cerebrovascular accident.

A recent European survey found the following main causes of death [118]:
- multi-organ failure with intravascular sickling
- acute chest syndrome
- bacterial infections
- chronic organ disease – mainly liver cirrhosis.

Of practical significance is the fact that over one-third of those dying of multi-organ failure and acute chest syndrome had had only mild disease before the final events [118].

Appendix

The autopsy in SCD and sickle cell trait

The following guidelines are adapted from the Royal College of Pathologists 'Guidelines for Autopsy Practice' on the website www.rcpath.org (2003).

The role of the autopsy

To determine the pathologies that led to death and the contribution of SCD or sickle cell trait.

A significant proportion of deaths occur perioperatively and require careful examination to determine what took place.

Abnormalities and causes of death encountered at autopsy

The main causes of death in HbSS and HbSC individuals include:
1 Acute chest syndrome (ACS).
2 Pulmonary vascular thrombosis and cor pulmonale.
3 Sudden cardiac failure from fibrosis in adults.
4 Multi-organ failure following sickle cell crisis.
5 Bacterial infections: pneumonia, meningitis, bacteraemia, osteomyelitis.
6 Acute splenic sequestration (in children).
7 Chronic renal failure.
8 Cerebrovascular accident.
9 Pregnancy-related: with multi-organ failure and pulmonary disease.
10 Hyperhaemolysis (post-transfusion) syndrome in adults.
11 Aplastic crisis (in children).
12 Seizures induced by pethidine.
13 Respiratory depression from fentanyl patches and other opiates.

In patients with HbAS (sickle cell trait), unexplained death from acute cardio-respiratory arrest is ~28 times more frequent than among normal HbAA persons; this usually occurs after severe exertion [106].

Clinical information relevant to the autopsy

- All the present relevant and past medical history details: particularly the mode of death, recent operation records, drug and pain relief therapy, current radiology; laboratory results such as blood cultures must be gathered.
- Discussion with the clinicians is always helpful

to understand the complex patho-physiological processes taking place.

The autopsy procedure

Standard full autopsy should be done, with careful attention to the coronary, pulmonary and cerebral arteries. Include vertebral bone marrow sampling. If agreement is obtained (and stress its importance), remove one femur and split it longitudinally; this enables examination of marrow hyperplasia and sampling of old and recent sites of bone infarction. It can be replaced to strut the leg during reconstruction.

Minimum blocks for histological examination

Histological studies are essential in all cases of SCD-related death. Gross observation and pathological guesswork only will fail to provide the correct cause of death within the complex of sickle cell disorders, will not satisfy the clinicians or help them with clinical governance issues, and will certainly not satisfy the relatives of the deceased. The following represents recommended practice:
• Heart: if cardiac malfunction is the likely significant event, take at least three blocks of the left ventricle and one of the right ventricle. Ideally, also take the right AV septal block for fixation and serial slicing to examine the AV node and the bundle of His area.
• Lungs: multiple samples (at least one per lobe) to identify acute chest syndrome, pneumonia, or small pulmonary arterial thrombosis.
• Vertebra, femoral bone and marrow (proximal, mid and distal).
• Both kidneys.
• Spleen.
• Liver.
• Skeletal muscle (particularly if crush injury is suspected).
• Any recent operation sites.
• Brain if a CVA was clinically suspected or is pathologically evident.
  Fix the samples in buffered formalin, to reduce artefactual post-mortem sickling of red cells.

Other samples required

1 Urine, blood, meninges and lung cultures for sepsis.
2 Peripheral blood, urine and vitreous humour if opiates were administered during the final medical management. (Note: fentanyl is not detected by routine screening for drugs of abuse, it must be specified.)
3 Centrifuged blood for serology, e.g. parvovirus B19 infection; for mast cell tryptase analysis if acute anaphylaxis is suspected.
4 Whole blood for haemoglobinopathy screening if the Hb genotype had not been determined pre-autopsy but is suspected clinically or morbid anatomically.

The clinico-pathological summary

• Determine whether SCD is the underlying factor in the cause of death sequence, played a contributory role, or was irrelevant to the cause of death.
• Consider whether drug overdose caused fatal respiratory depression or seizures.
• Lay out the pathological sequence logically; the clinicians and relatives are going to study the autopsy report closely.
• Consult a more experienced pathologist to review the case and histology, etc. if the pathology and cause of death are not clear.

Specimen cause of death opinions/statements

1a. Acute cardio-respiratory failure
1b. Acute chest syndrome following painful crisis
1c. Sickle cell disease
1a. Anaemia
1b. Hyperhaemolysis syndrome
1c. Sickle cell disease
1a. Septicaemia
1b. Cholecystitis (laparoscopic cholecystectomy on dd/mm/yy)
1c. Sickle cell disease
1a. Acute cardio-respiratory failure
1b. Exertion and sickle cell trait (HbAS)

References

1. Serjeant GR, Serjeant BE. *Sickle Cell Disease*. Oxford: Oxford University Press, 2001.

2. Narla M. New views of sickle cell disease, pathophysiology and treatment: sickle cell adhesion. *Hematology* 2000; (1): 2.

3. Steinberg MH, Rodgers GP. Pathophysiology of sickle cell disease: role of cellular and genetic modifiers. *Semin Hematol* 2001; **38**: 299–306.

4. Cheung AT, Chen PC, Larkin EC *et al*. Microvascular abnormalities in sickle cell disease: a computer-assisted intravital microscopic study. *Blood* 2002; **99**: 3999–4005.

5. Serjeant GR, Lethbridge R, Morris J, Singhal A, Thomas PW. The painful crisis of homozygous sickle cell disease: clinical features. *Br J Haematol* 1994; **87**: 586–91.

6. Lowe SH, Prins JM, van der Lelie J, Lange JMA. Does HAART induce sickle cell crises? *AIDS* 2002; **16**: 1572–4.

7. Serjeant GR, Serjeant BE, Thomas PW *et al*. Human parvovirus infection in homozygous sickle cell disease. *Lancet* 1993; **341**: 1237–40.

8. Anderson MJ, Davies LR, Hodgson J *et al*. Occurrence of infection with a paravovirus-like agent in children with sickle cell anemia during a 2-year period. *J Clin Pathol* 1982; **35**: 744–9.

9. Godeau P, Galacteros F, Schaeffer A *et al*. Aplastic crisis due to extensive bone marrow necrosis and human parvovirus infection in sickle cell disease. *Am J Med* 1991; **91**: 557–8.

10. Ataga KI, Orringer EP. Bone marrow necrosis in sickle cell disease: a description of three cases and a review of the literature. *Am J Med Sci* 2000; **320**: 342–7.

11. Wright J, Thomas P, Serjeant GR. Septicemia caused by Salmonella infection: an overlooked complication of sickle cell disese. *J Pediatr* 1997; **130**: 394–9.

12. Rennels MB, Tenney JH, Luddy RE, Dunne MG. Intestinal *Salmonella* carriage in patients with major sickle cell hemoglobinopathies. *South Med J* 1985; **78**: 310–11.

13. Ballas SK. Iron overload is a determinant of morbidity and mortality in adult patients with sickle cell disease. *Semin Hematol* 2001; **38** (1 Suppl 1): 30–6.

14. Mills LR, Mwakyusa D, Milner PF. Histopathologic features of liver biopsy specimens in sickle cell disease. *Arch Pathol Lab Med* 1988; **112**: 290–4.

15. Teixeira AL, Viana MB, Roquette ML, Toppa NH. Sickle cell disease: a clinical and histopathologic study of the liver in living children. *J Pediatr Hematol Oncol* 2002; **24**: 125–9.

16. Akinyanju O, Ladapo F. Cholelithiasis and biliary tract disease in sickle cell disease in Nigerians. *Postgrad Med J* 1979; **55**: 400–2.

17. Meshikhes AN, al-Dhurais SA, al-Jama A *et al*. Laparoscopic cholecystectomy in patients with sickle cell disease. *J R Coll Surg Edinb* 1995; **40**: 383–5.

18. Koshy M, Weiner SJ, Miller ST *et al*. Surgery and anesthesia in sickle cell disease. Cooperative Study of Sickle Cell Diseases. *Blood* 1995; **86**: 3676–84.

19. Delatte SJ, Hebra A, Tagge EP *et al*. Acute chest syndrome in the postoperative sickle cell patient. *J Pediatr Surg* 1999; **34**: 188–92.

20. Charlotte F, Bachir D, Nenert M *et al*. Vascular lesions of the liver in sickle cell disease. A clinicopathological study in 26 living patients. *Arch Pathol Lab Med* 1995; **119**: 46–52.

21. Sty JR. Ultrasonography: hepatic vein thrombosis in sickle cell anemia. *Am J Pediatr Hematol Oncol* 1982; **4**: 213–15.

22. Zakaria N, Knisely A, Portmann B *et al*. Acute sickle cell hepatopathy represents a potential contraindication for percutaneous liver biopsy. *Blood* 2003; **101**: 101–3.

23. Diggs LW. Siderofibrosis of the spleen in sickle cell anemia. *JAMA* 1935; **104**: 538–41.

24. Wong WY, Overturf GD, Powars DR. Infection caused by *Streptococcus pneumoniae* in children with sickle cell disease: epidemiology, immunologic mechanisms, prophylaxis, and vaccination. *Clin Infect Dis* 1992; **14**: 1124–36.

25. Bagasra O, Steiner RM, Ballas SK *et al*. Viral burden and disease progression in HIV-1 infected patients with sickle cell anemia. *Am J Hematol* 1998; **59**: 199–207.

26. Godeau P, Bachir D, Schaeffer A *et al*. Severe pneumococcal sepsis and meningitis in HIV infected adults with sickle cell disease. *Clin Infect Dis* 1992; **15**: 327–9.

27. Hutchins KD, Ballas SK, Phatak D, Natarajan GA. Sudden unexpected death in a patient with splenic sequestration and sickle beta thalassaemia syndrome. *J Forensic Sci* 2001; **46**: 412–14.

28. Zimmerman SA, Ware RE. Palpable splenomegaly in children with haemoglobin SC disease: haematological and clinical manifestations. *Clin Lab Haematol* 2000; **22**: 150.

29. Petz LD. Hemolytic transfusion reactions in patients with sickle cell anaemia. *Hematology* 2000; (1): 2.

30. Win N, Doughty H, Telfer P, Wild BJ, Pearson TC. Hyperhemolytic transfusion reaction in sickle cell disease. *Transfusion* 2001; **41**: 323–8.

31. Grainger JD, Makar Y, McManus A, Wynn R. Refractory hyperhaemolysis in a patient with beta-thalassaemia major. *Transfus Med* 2001; **11**: 55–7.

32. Karim A, Ahmed S, Rossoff LJ *et al*. Fulminant ischaemic colitis with atypical clinical features compli-

cating sickle cell disease. *Postgrad Med J* 2002; **78**: 370–2.

33. Humphries JE, Wheby MS. Case report: sickle cell trait and recurrent deep venous thrombosis. *Am J Med Sci* 1992; **303**: 112–14.

34. Arnold KE, Char G, Serjeant GR. Portal vein thrombosis in a child with homozygous sickle cell disease. *West Indian Med J* 1993; **42**: 27–8.

35. Ng PC, Ashari L. Portal vein thrombosis following laparoscopic surgery in a patient with sickle cell disease. *Surg Endosc* 2003; **17**: 831.

36. Ataga KI, Orringer EP. Renal abnormalities in sickle cell disease. *Am J Hematol* 2000; **63**: 205–11.

37. Morgan AG, Shah DJ, Williams W. Renal pathology in adults over age 40 with sickle cell disease. *West Indian Med J* 1987; **36**: 241–50.

38. Bhathena DB. Sickling disorders. In: Jennette JC, Olson JL, Schwartz MM, Silva FG, eds. *Heptinstall's Pathology of the Kidney*. Philadelphia: Lippincott-Raven, 1998: 1231–46.

39. Wesson DE. The initiation and progression of sickle cell nephropathy. *Kidney Int* 2002; **61**: 2277–86.

40. Vaamonde CA. Renal papillary necrosis in sickle cell hemoglobinopathies. *Semin Nephrol* 1984; **4**: 48–64.

41. Vogler C, Wood E, Lane P *et al*. Microangiopathic glomerulopathy in children with sickle cell anemia. *Pediatr Pathol Lab Med* 1996; **16**: 275–84.

42. Schmitt F, Martinez F, Brillet G *et al*. Early glomerular dysfunction in patients with sickle cell anemia. *Am J Kidney Dis* 1998; **32**: 208–14.

43. Powars DR, Elliot-Mills DD, Chan L. Chronic renal failure in sickle cell disease: risk factors, course, and mortality. *Ann Intern Med* 1991; **115**: 614–20.

44. Wierenga KJ, Pattison JR, Brink N *et al*. Glomerulonephritis after parvovirus infection in homozygous sickle cell disease. *Lancet* 1995; **346**: 475–6.

45. Swartz MA, Karth J, Schneider DT *et al*. Renal medullary carcinoma: clinical, pathologic, immunohistochemical, and genetic analysis with pathogenetic implications. *Urology* 2002; **60**: 1083–9.

46. Dimashkieh H, Choe J, Mutema G. Renal medullary carcinoma: a report of 2 cases and review of the literature. *Arch Pathol Lab Med* 2003; **127**: 135–8.

47. Qi J, Shen PU, Rezuke WN *et al*. Fine needle aspiration cytology diagnosis of renal medullary carcinoma: a case report. *Acta Cytol* 2001; **45**: 735–9.

48. Davies SC, Win AA, Luce PJ, Riordan JF, Brozovic M. Acute chest syndrome in sickle cell disease. *Lancet* 1984; **i**: 36–8.

49. Ballas SK. Sickle cell disease: clinical management. *Baillieres Clin Haematol* 1998; **11**: 185–214.

50. Maitre B, Habibi A, Roulot-Thoraval F *et al*. Acute chest syndrome in adults with sickle cell disease. *Chest* 2000; **117**: 1386–92.

51. Dean D, Neumayr LD, Kelly DM *et al*. *Chlamydia pneumoniae* and acute chest syndrome in patients with sickle cell disease. *J Pediatr Hematol Oncol* 2003; **25**: 46–55.

52. Vichinsky EP, Neumayr LD, Earles AN *et al*. Causes and outcomes of the acute chest syndrome in sickle cell disease. National Acute Chest Syndrome Study Group. *N Engl J Med* 2000; **342**: 1855–65.

53. McMahon LEC, Shepard J-AO, Mark EJ. Sickle lung disease: case presentation of the Massachusetts General Hospital. *N Engl J Med* 1997; **337**: 1293–301.

54. Hasleton PS, Orr K, Webster A, Lawson RAM. Evolution of acute chest syndrome in sickle cell trait: an ultrastructural and light microscope study. *Thorax* 1989; **44**: 1057–8.

55. Athanasou NA, Hatton C, McGee J'OD, Weatherall DJ. Vascular occlusion and infarction in sickle cell crisis and the sickle chest syndrome. *J Clin Pathol* 1985; **38**: 659–64.

56. Stuart MJ, Setty BN. Acute chest syndrome of sickle cell disease: new light on an old problem. *Curr Opin Hematol* 2001; **8**: 111–22.

57. Zaidi Y, Sivakumaran M, Graham C, Hutchinson RM. Fatal bone marrow embolism in a patient with sickle cell beta thalassemia. *J Clin Pathol* 1996; **49**: 774–5.

58. Haque AK, Gokhale S, Rampy BA *et al*. Pulmonary hypertension in sickle cell hemoglobinopathy: a clinicopathologic study of 20 cases. *Hum Pathol* 2002; **33**: 1037–43.

59. Collins FS, Orringer EP. Pulmonary hypertension and cor pulmonale in the sickle hemoglobinopathies. *Am J Med* 1982; **73**: 814–21.

60. Belhassen L, Pelle G, Sediame S *et al*. Endothelial dysfunction in patients with sickle cell disease is related to selective impairment of shear stress-mediated vasodilatation. *Blood* 2001; **97**: 1584–9.

61. Covitz W, Espeland M, Gallagher D *et al*. The heart in sickle cell anemia. The Cooperative Study of Sickle Cell Disease (CSSCD). *Chest* 1995; **108**: 1214–9.

62. Gerry JL, Bulkley BH, Hutchins GM. Clinicopathologic analysis of cardiac dysfunction in 52 patients with sickle cell anemia. *Am J Cardiol* 1978; **42**: 211–16.

63. Batra AS, Acherman RJ, Wong WY *et al*. Cardiac abnormalities in children with sickle cell anemia. *Am J Hematol* 2002; **70**: 306–12.

64. Saad ST, Arruda VR, Junqueira OO, Schelini FA, Coelho OB. Acute myocardial infarction in sickle cell anaemia associated with severe hypoxia. *Postgrad Med J* 1990; **66**: 1068–70.

65. Martin CR, Johnson CS, Cobb C, Tatter D, Haywood LJ. Myocardial infarction in sickle cell disease. *J Natl Med Assoc* 1996; **88**: 428–32.

66. McCormick WF. Massive nonatherosclerotic myocardial infarction in sickle cell anemia. *Am J Forensic Med Pathol* 1988; **9**: 151–4.

67. Mansi IA, Rosner F. Myocardial infarction in sickle cell disease. *J Natl Med Assoc* 2002; **94**: 448–52.

68. Rockoff AS, Christy D, Zeldis N, Tsai DJ, Kramer RA. Myocardial necrosis following general anesthesia in hemoglobin SC disease. *Pediatrics* 1978; **61**: 73–6.

69. Tap San M, Mete UO, Kaya M. Ultrastructural alterations in the myocardium of patients with sickle cell anemia. *J Submicrosc Cytol Pathol* 2001; **33**: 156.

70. Romero Mestre JC, Hernaandez A, Agramonte O, Hernandez P. Cardiovascular autonomic dysfunction in sickle cell anemia: a possible risk factor for sudden death. *Clin Auton Res* 1997; **7**: 121–5.

71. James TN, Riddick L, Massing GK. Sickle cells and sudden death: morphologic abnormalities of the cardiac conducting system. *J Lab Clin Med* 1994; **124**: 507–20.

72. Ohene-Frempong K, Weiner SJ, Sleeper LA *et al*. Cerebrovascular accidents in sickle cell disease: rates and risk factors. *Blood* 1998; **91**: 288–94.

73. Rothman SM, Fulling KH, Nelson JS. Sickle cell anemia and central nervous system infarction: a neuropathological study. *Ann Neurol* 1986; **20**: 684–90.

74. Merkel KH, Ginsberg PL, Parker JC, Post MJ. Cerebrovascular disease in sickle cell anemia: a clinical, pathological and radiological correlation. *Stroke* 1978; **9**: 45–52.

75. Koshy M, Thomas C, Goodwin J. Vascular lesions in the central nervous system in sickle cell disease (neuropathology). *J Assoc Minor Phys* 1990; **1**: 71–8.

76. Tuohy AM, McVie V, Manci EA, Adams RJ. Internal carotid artery occlusion in a child with sickle cell disease: case report and immunohistochemical study. *J Pediatr Hematol Oncol* 1997; **19**: 455–8.

77. Bayazit AK, Kilinc Y. Natural coagulation inhibitors in patients with sickle cell anemia in a steady state. *Pediatr Int* 2001; **43**: 592–6.

78. Andrade FL, Annichino-Bizzacchi JM, Saad ST, Costa FF, Arruda VR. Prothrombin mutant, factor V Leiden, and thermolabile variant of methylenetetrahydrofolate reductase among patients with sickle cell disease in Brazil. *Am J Hematol* 1998; **59**: 46–50.

79. Van Hoff J, Ritchey AK, Shayawitz BA. Intracranial hemorrhage in children with sickle cell disease. *Am J Dis Child* 1985; **139**: 1120–3.

80. Preul MC, Cendes F, Just N, Mohr G. Intracranial aneurysms and sickle cell anemia: multiplicity and propensity for the vertebrobasilar territory. *Neurosurgery* 1998; **42**: 977–8.

81. Oyesiku NM, Barrow DL, Eckman JR, Tindall SC, Colohan AR. Intracranial aneurysms in sickle cell anaemia: clinical features and pathogenesis. *J Neurosurg* 1991; **75**: 356–63.

82. Rothman SM, Nelson JS. Spinal cord infarction in a patient with sickle cell anemia. *Neurology* 1980; **30**: 1072–6.

83. Kolquist KA, Vnencak-Jones CL, Swift L *et al*. Fatal fat embolism syndrome in a child with undiagnosed hemoglobin S/beta-thalassemia: a complication of acute parvovirus B19 infection. *Pediatr Pathol Lab Med* 1996; **16**: 71–82.

84. Henderson JN, Noetzel MJ, McKinstry RC *et al*. Reversible posterior leukoencephalopathy syndrome and silent cerebral infarcts are associated with severe acute chest syndrome in children with sickle cell disease. *Blood* 2003; **101**: 415–19.

85. Lee KH, McKie VC, Sekul EA, Adams RJ, Nichols FT. Unusual encephalopathy after acute chest syndrome in sickle cell disease: acute necrotizing encephalitis. *J Pediatr Hematol Oncol* 2002; **24**: 585–8.

86. Di Roio C, Jourdan C, Yilmaz H, Artu F. Cerebral deep vein thrombosis: 3 cases. *Rev Neurol* 1999; **155**: 583–7.

87. Feldenzer JA, Bueche MJ, Venes JL, Gebarski SS. Superior sagittal sinus thrombosis with infarction in sickle cell trait. *Stroke* 1987; **18**: 656–60.

88. Hassell KL, Eckman JR, Lane PA. Acute multiorgan failure syndrome: a potentially catastrophic complication of severe sickle cell pain episodes. *Am J Med* 1994; **96**: 155–62.

89. Parfrey NA, Moore GW, Hutchins GM. Is pain crisis a cause of death in sickle cell disease? *Am J Clin Pathol* 1985; **84**: 209–12.

90. Chehal A, Taher A, Shamseddine A. Sicklemia with multi-organ failure syndrome and thrombotic thrombocytopenic purpura. *Hemoglobin* 2002; **26**: 345–51.

91. NICE. *Why Mothers Die: 1997–1999*. London: RCOG Press, 2001.

92. Howard RJ, Tuck SM, Pearson TC. Pregnancy in sickle cell disease in the UK: results of a multicentre survey of the effect of prophylactic blood tranfusion on maternal and fetal outcome. *Br J Obstet Gynaecol* 1995; **102**: 947–51.

93. Odum CU, Anorlu RI, Dim SI, Oyekan TO. Pregnancy outcome in HbSS sickle cell disease in Lagos, Nigeria. *West Afr Med J* 2002; **21**: 19–23.

94. el-Shafei AM, Sandhu AK, Dhaliwal JK. Maternal mortality in Bahrain with special reference to sickle cell disease. *Aust N Z J Obstet Gynaecol* 1988; **28**: 41–4.

95. van Enk A, Visschers G, Jansen W, Statius van Eps LW. Maternal death due to sickle cell chronic lung disease. *Br J Obstet Gynaecol* 1992; **99**: 162–3.

96. van der Neut FW, Statius van Eps LW, van Enk A, van de Sandt MN. Maternal death due to acute necrotizing colitis in homozygous sickle cell disease. *Neth J Med* 1993; **42**: 132–3.

97. Anaesthesia Advisory Committee to Chief Coroner of Ontario. Intraoperative death during Caesarian section in a patient with sickle cell trait. *Can J Anaesth* 1987; **34**: 67–70.

98. Tollin SR, Seely EW. Case report: postpartum hypopi-

tuitism in a patient with sickle cell trait. *Am J Med Sci* 1994; **308**: 36–7.

99. Pastorek KG, Seiler B. Maternal death associated with sickle cell trait. *Am J Obstet Gynecol* 1985; **151**: 295–7.

100. Sears DA. The morbidity of sickle cell trait. A review of the literature. *Am J Med* 1978; **64**: 1021–6.

101. Gitlin SD, Thompson CB. Non-altitude related splenic infarction in a patient with sickle cell trait. *Am J Med* 1989; **87**: 697–8.

102. Reyes MG. Subcortical cerebral infarctions in sickle cell trait. *J Neurol Neurosurg Psychiatry* 1989; **52**: 516–18.

103. Taylor PW, Thorpe WP, Trueblood MC. Osteonecrosis in sickle cell trait. *J Rheumatol* 1986; **13**: 643–6.

104. Israel RH, Salipante JS. Pulmonary infarction in sickle cell trait. *Am J Med* 1979; **66**: 867–9.

105. Wirthwein DP, Spotswood SD, Barnard JJ, Prahlow JA. Death due to microvascular occlusion in sickle cell trait following physical exertion. *J Forensic Sci* 2001; **46**: 399–401.

106. Kark JA, Posey DM, Schumacher HR, Ruehle CJ. Sickle cell trait as a risk factor for sudden death in physical training. *N Engl J Med* 1987; **317**: 781–7.

107. Hynd RF, Bharadwaja K, Mitas JA, Lord JT. Rhabdomyolysis, acute renal failure, and disseminated intravascular coagulation in a man with sickle cell trait. *South Med J* 1985; **78**: 890–1.

108. Le Gallais D, Bile A, Mercier I. Exercise-induced death in sickle cell trait: role of aging, training and deconditioning. *Med Sci Sports Exerc* 1995; **28**: 541–4.

109. Murray MJ. Sudden exertional death in a soldier with sickle cell trait. *Milit Med* 1996; **161**: 303–5.

110. Kerle KK, Nishimura KD. Exertional collapse and sudden death associated with sickle cell trait. *Am Fam Physician* 1996; **54**: 237–40.

111. Charache S. Sudden death in sickle cell trait. *Am J Med* 1988; **84**: 459–61.

112. Dudley AW, Waddell CC. Crisis in sickle cell trait. *Hum Pathol* 1991; **22**: 616–18.

113. Thogmartin JR. Sudden death in police pursuit. *J Forensic Sci* 1998; **43**: 1228–31.

114. Mercy JA, Heath CW, Rosenberg I. Mortality associated with the use of upper-body control holds by police. *Violence Vict* 1990; **5**: 215–22.

115. Platt OS, Brambilla DJ, Rosse WF *et al*. Mortality in sickle cell disease. Life expectancy and risk factors for early death. *N Engl J Med* 1994; **330**: 1639–44.

116. de la Grandmaison GL, Paraire F. Postmortem relevation of sickle cell disease following fatal episode of acute bronchial asthma. *Forensic Sci Int* 2002; **126**: 48–52.

117. Thomas AN, Pattison C, Serjeant GR. Causes of death in sickle cell disease in Jamaica. *BMJ* 1982; **285**: 633–7.

118. Perronne V, Roberts-Harewood M, Bachir D *et al*. Patterns of mortality in sickle cell disease in adults in France and England. *Hematol J* 2002; **3**: 56–60.

Chapter 7
Sickle cell crisis

Iheanyi E Okpala

Definition

Occlusion of blood vessels in various parts of the body occurs continually in sickle cell disease (SCD). If the resultant ischaemic or infarctive pain is considered negligible or mild, it could be ignored or treated with analgesics without the attention of health professionals. Episodes of such negligible or mild pain occur in 'steady-state' SCD and are not regarded as crises by affected persons or health-care staff. People with SCD on hydroxyurea report a decrease in the frequency of these 'niggling' pains distinct from acute painful crises. There is evidence of inflammatory reaction to the ischaemic tissue damage caused by such subclinical vaso-occlusive painful episodes in the form of increased levels of acute phase proteins during steady-state [1]. They indicate that recurrent inflammation occurs even during steady-state SCD. It is apparently when the pains are of greater severity, generalized, or affecting some vital organ that medical attention is sought. Sickle cell crisis is therefore an increase in the intensity of what usually happens during steady-state SCD. It can be defined as an acute illness characterized by exacerbation of the clinical features of SCD, such as pain, anaemia or jaundice. Sickle cell crisis is a sudden change in the individual's state of health defined on clinical grounds. This sometimes makes it difficult to differentiate crisis from steady-state disease.

What brings on sickle cell crisis?

A number of conditions within or external to the in-dividual precipitate sickle cell crisis, although in a considerable proportion of people no precipitating factor is identified. Infection stands out as the predominant precipitant of sickle cell crisis. Hypoxia, exposure to cold, dehydration, physical exertion, acidosis, extensive trauma or injury, and psychological stress can also bring on crisis. Improved understanding of the importance of interaction between vascular endothelium, blood cells and plasma proteins in the pathogenesis of small vessel occlusion has shed some light on how different conditions could lead to sickle cell crisis [2]. Acute inflammatory reaction to infection or tissue injury increases the local and circulating levels of tumour necrosis factor-alpha (TNF-α) and interleukin-1β, which activate leucocytes to express more adhesion molecules on their surfaces, and vascular endothelial cells to express more ligands (receptors) for the adhesion molecules on blood cells. This increases aggregation of blood cells to each other and their adhesion to the vessel wall, reducing the size of the lumen. Erythrocytes adhere more to the activated endothelium and leucocytes, leading to microvascular occlusion and sickle cell crisis. Dehydration causes loss of water from erythrocytes. This increases the concentration of HbS inside red cells, and encourages crystallization of HbS and sickling. Sickled erythrocytes are more rigid than their normal counterparts, and attach more readily to vascular endothelium and leucocytes. This facilitates vaso-occlusion. Acidosis causes an increase in the plasma concentration of hydrogen ions, which displace oxygen from HbS. It is deoxy-HbS, and not oxy-HbS, that crystallizes and causes sickling. Hypoxia has a similar effect. Exposure to cold causes vasoconstriction and narrows the lumen of blood vessels. The hormonal and neuronal interactions of the limbic and endocrine systems with each other and the blood vessel wall might be the basis of observations that psychological stress predisposes to sickle cell crisis.

Management of sickle cell crisis

Specific therapy for sickle cell crisis depends on the type. However, irrespective of whether it is vaso-occlusive, aplastic or sequestration crisis, some broad guidelines are helpful in clinical management.
- Make the patient comfortable.
- Give effective analgesia.
- Administer oxygen if there is hypoxia ($SaO_2 <$ 92%).
- Ensure optimal hydration.
- Antimicrobial therapy for infections.
- Blood transfusion if indicated.
- Treat specific clinical problems, e.g. priapism.

Acute chest syndrome and stroke are special forms of sickle cell crisis discussed in Chapters 10 and 15, respectively. If the patient is in pain, it is advisable to conduct a quick clinical evaluation within minutes and administer an appropriate dose of an analgesic before going on to detailed medical history, physical examination and investigations. This approach helps to keep the patient comfortable and to win the co-operation required for the other management measures. Attempts to take a full clinical history, examine or take samples for investigations from a patient in crisis pain may be met with poor co-operation and lack of confidence in the healthcare professional. Once pain is adequately controlled, one could proceed to full clinical evaluation and the following investigations that may facilitate diagnosis of the specific type of sickle cell crisis, and guide medical treatment.
- Full blood count with reticulocyte count.
- Examination of the blood film.
- Plasma levels of total and conjugated bilirubin.
- Serum urea, electrolytes and creatinine levels.
- Infection screen on blood or other specimens.
- X-rays or other imaging of relevant parts of the body.

- Pulse oximetry or measurement of arterial blood gases.

Vaso-occlusive crisis

Vaso-occlusive crisis is the hallmark of clinical presentation of SCD. It is characterized by skeletal or soft tissue pain of sudden onset; the result of ischaemia or infarction caused by obstruction of blood vessels [2]. Signs and symptoms of a precipitating factor such as infection may be present; or the patient might give suggestive history, such as having been out in cold weather. The importance of efficacious therapy for the acute pain of sickle cell crisis (and chronic pain in SCD) is such that a separate chapter (Chapter 8) has been devoted to pain management. Sickle cell crisis tends to reduce the patient's appetite for food and water. Dehydration should be sought for and treated, or prevented if not yet present. Oral hydration is preferred; however, if the patient is unable to take fluid orally, parenteral fluid administration is advised. With the common feature of inability to concentrate urine (hyposthenuria), patients in sickle cell crisis who are not receiving sufficient fluid input may become dehydrated and run the risk of complications such as acute renal shutdown. Optimal hydration is required. Too much fluid may lead to pulmonary oedema and increase the risk of the life-threatening acute chest syndrome.

A total daily fluid intake (oral and parenteral) of $1.5 \, L/m^2$ is advised; equivalent to about 3 L/day for most adults. The type of parenteral fluid given is important. Hyposthenuric patients cannot excrete the sodium in normal saline as well as normal individuals [3]. If normal saline (0.09% NaCl solution) is infused continuously, plasma osmolality may build up, with intracellular dehydration of erythrocytes, increasing the concentration of HbS inside the cells. This facilitates crystallization of HbS and sickling of red blood cells. Therefore, 5% dextrose solution or 5% dextrose in 25% saline (dextrose in saline) is preferred.

Oxygen therapy is only needed if there is hypoxaemia (blood oxygen saturation < 92%). Humidified oxygen is given, so as not to facilitate dehydration. Different methods of oxygen delivery are used; techniques like continuous positive airways pressure (CPAP) may be appropriate for patients with acute chest syndrome being ventilated in the High Dependency or Intensive Care Units. Although sickling of red blood cells is caused by hypoxia and pathophysiological considerations might lead one to administer oxygen to all patients in sickle cell crisis, there is no evidence from large clinical trials on which to base such practice. Hypoxaemia is not a common feature of uncomplicated sickle cell crisis, and its presence should alert one to look out for acute chest syndrome. Two small clinical trials that were randomized and controlled showed no benefit from routine oxygen therapy [4, 5]. People with chronic sickle lung disease may have blood oxygen saturation < 92% even in steady-state, and this ought to be taken into account if they are in sickle cell crisis. Pulse oximetry readings will suffice in the majority of SCD patients, although the readings do not correlate with arterial blood gas measurements as well as in HbAA individuals. This is because HbS has a lower oxygen affinity than HbA, and a different oxygen dissociation curve. If in doubt, pulse oximetry readings should be confirmed with arterial blood gas measurement. However, this is not often necessary.

In the presence of fever suggestive of infection (temperature ≥ 38 °C) broad-spectrum antibiotics should be started after taking specimens for infection screen. Mortality in SCD patients is most frequently caused by infections, which are also the most common precipitating factors for sickle cell crisis. Therapy for infections should therefore be prompt and vigorous, more so because people with SCD have various immunological abnormalities that reduce their ability to kill microbes [6–9]. Common pathogens in SCD include staphylococcus, salmonella organisms and atypical microbes. An example of effective combination chemotherapy would be flucloxacillin for staphylococcus, ciprofloxacin for salmonella and clarithromycin for atypical pneumonia. In cases of tooth infection or osteomyelitis of the jawbones, anaerobic cover with metronidazole is required. Clinical experience shows that long-term antibiotic therapy for 2–3 months is usually necessary in SCD patients with acute osteomyelitis or septic arthritis to avoid chronicity of the infection.

The most reliable indication for blood transfusion is the presence of acute symptoms or signs of anaemia, such as getting tired more easily than usual, weakness, unexplained breathlessness or tachycardia. These imply that oxygen delivery to the tissues is not sufficient. The body has had time to adjust to the chronic anaemia in steady-state SCD, and affected individuals are usually haemodynamically stable. Therefore they do not need blood transfusion just because the Hb level is lower than normal. Rather, the aim of blood transfusion is to abolish the acute clinical features of anaemia that may develop during sickle cell crisis as a result of increased sickling and haemolysis with further reduction in Hb level. In most people simple (top-up) transfusion to restore the Hb level to the steady-state value will suffice. If the individual's steady-state Hb level is not known, a threshold value of 6 g/dL could be used as a guide below which transfusion may be given, especially if the reticulocyte count is below 100×10^9/L. Very high reticulocyte counts (e.g. $> 200 \times 10^9$/L) indicate good bone marrow response to the symptomatic anaemia. In such situations, if the Hb level is 5–6 g/dL, blood transfusion could safely be withheld because spontaneous recovery to the usual steady-state value may occur. Acute signs and symptoms of anaemia may be expected to develop when the Hb level falls by > 2 g/dL below the steady-state value; which ranges from 7 to 9 g/dL in the majority of HbSS individuals. Such a patient whose steady-state Hb level is known should be considered for blood transfusion if it drops by > 2g/dL during sickle cell crisis. Exchange blood transfusion may be indicated for special forms of crisis such as cerebrovascular accidents and acute chest syndrome (discussed in Chapters 10, 11 and 15). SCD patients develop antibodies against blood group antigens more frequently than HbAA controls and, in all cases, should be transfused with blood matched for the six red cell antigens that most frequently cause alloimmunization: K, C, E, S, Fy and Jk [10].

Vaso-occlusive crisis involving abdominal organs could be difficult to distinguish from acute surgical abdomen. Affected patients benefit from review by the surgeons. If the differential diagnosis is not clear and the patient is improving clinically on conservative medical treatment, this should be continued and surgery deferred. Clinical deterioration despite conservative management calls for surgical intervention.

Splenic/hepatic sequestration crisis

Splenic/hepatic sequestration crisis is acute pooling of a large proportion of circulating erythrocytes in the spleen or liver. The spleen is more frequently involved than the liver, and HbSS children are affected more often than adults, who are likely to have undergone autosplenectomy. However, adults with Hb genotype SC or Sβ thalassaemia may have sequestration crises because infarction of the spleen is less extensive in these two conditions. The symptoms and signs of acute splenic or hepatic sequestration include extreme weakness or irritability in children, abdominal pain, tenderness and distension, very severe pallor, progressive enlargement of the spleen and/or the liver, tachycardia, low volume or weak pulses, with cold and clammy extremities. As a large proportion of the circulating blood is trapped in the spleen, the patient has clinical features of circulatory collapse or hypovolaemic shock. The degree of pallor worsens very rapidly as the haemoglobin level falls precipitously; it may drop below 3 g/dL in < 5 hours. A good bone marrow response (manifesting as reticulocytosis and/or numerous nucleated red cells in the blood film) helps to differentiate sequestration from aplastic crisis, the latter is characterized by a low reticulocyte count. This is useful in differential diagnosis when aplastic crisis occurs in a person with pre-existing (chronic) enlargement of the spleen or liver, as could be found in malaria-endemic regions of the world.

Timely transfusion of red blood cell concentrate revives the patient. Top-up transfusion is more feasible in the emergency situation than exchange transfusion. Following transfusion of normal red cells containing HbA, the patient's HbS-containing red cells trapped in the spleen/liver gradually return to the circulation, and the total haemoglobin level rises more than would be expected from the number of units of blood given. In attempt to reduce high childhood mortality from splenic sequestration, which can recur in up to half of affected individuals, splenectomy has been done in those older than 2 years who have one severe episode or recurrent mild/moderate episodes [11, 12]. This improved survival in Jamaica [13], and can be safely done in other malaria-free countries. Where malaria exists, removal of the spleen in young children may increase the risk of death from cerebral malaria. An effective alternative in that situation is regular exchange blood transfusions (EBT) or a hypertransfusion programme. EBT is less likely to cause iron overload than hypertransfusion, although both increase body iron. In both malaria-endemic and malaria-free regions, educating parents and those who look after affected children on how to examine the abdomen for hepato-splenomegaly facilitates early diagnosis of sequestration crisis, with reduction in associated loss of lives.

Aplastic crisis

Aplastic crisis is caused by infection of immature blood cells in the bone marrow by parvovirus B19 [14]. Although other microbial infections have been reported in association with transient erythroid hypoplasia in SCD [15], this is uncommon. The virus gains entry into haemopoietic cells by attaching to the P blood group antigen (globoside) in the cell membrane [16]. As this antigen is well expressed by erythroid cells relative to other haemopoietic cells, and fully mature red cells that have the antigen lack nuclei and the protein synthetic machinery required by parvovirus B19 for its replication, nucleated erythroid precursor cells bear the brunt of the infection. As a result, only a minority of bone marrow erythroid cells mature beyond the normoblast stage; and the number of young red cells or reticulocytes is markedly reduced in the peripheral blood. Whereas reticulocytopenia (< 2%) is the main diagnostic feature of aplastic crisis caused by parvovirus B19, reduction in the platelet or white blood cell count also occurs [12]. This suggests that the virus may also infect nucleated haemopoietic cells that have the capacity to differentiate into white blood cells or megakaryocytes. Consistent with this possibility is the finding that intrauterine infection of the fetus by parvovirus B19 leads to anaemia, leukopenia, and thrombocytopenia [14]. Other features of aplastic crisis include fever, easy tiredness of insidious onset because the

Hb level falls gradually over a number of days rather than hours (unlike in sequestration crisis), marked pallor, skin rash in the cheeks, circulating IgM antibodies to parvovirus B19, and the presence of the viral DNA in plasma and nucleated erythroid cells in the blood/bone marrow. IgM antibodies are used for diagnosis because IgG antibodies may be the result of a previous infection. Aplastic crisis is more common in children than adults, who are more likely to have had contact with parvovirus B19 in childhood, usually with lifelong immunity.

The first step in the practical management of aplastic crisis is to isolate the patient. In particular, contact with expectant mothers should be avoided because, as noted above, parvovirus B19 infection of the fetus causes long-term aplastic anaemia lasting well beyond birth [14]. With the objective of bringing the Hb level up to the patient's steady-state value, blood transfusion is given when necessary. Intravenous immunoglobulin therapy may be required in patients with immunodeficiency. In most people with SCD, no specific antiviral treatment is required and the infection runs its natural course, with recovery in 1–2 weeks. In normal individuals parvovirus B19 infection does not lead to as much reduction in haemoglobin level as in people with haemolytic states such as SCD, hereditary spherocytosis or thalassaemia. This is because the lifespan of red blood cells in the circulation is about 120 days, and arrest of erythropoiesis during the comparatively short viral infection of 2 weeks is not likely to make the Hb level drop to values at which symptoms of anaemia occur.

Hyperbilirubinaemia

The three types of sickle cell crisis may be associated with increased destruction of red blood cells and increased plasma bilirubin level. Other causes of hyperbilirubinaemia may need to be considered in differential diagnosis. Malaria causes haemolysis and, in the main, a rise in the level of unconjugated bilirubin. Diagnosis is based on detection of plasmodium in red blood cells. This task, which could sometimes be tricky, is made a lot easier by the use of quinacrine buffy coat (QBC) stain; rather than the more traditional examination of stained peripheral blood films. Red blood cells infected by the

malaria parasite are less dense than normal uninfected erythrocytes. After centrifugation of a blood sample stained with quinacrine, red blood cells containing the parasite are found in the buffy coat layer with white blood cells, which are also less dense than uninfected erythrocytes. Plasmodium DNA stained with quinacrine fluoresces under ultraviolet light. As the mature red blood cell has no nucleus, the test can detect as few as one infected red cell out of a million non-infected cells. This degree of sensitivity approaches that of DNA analytic procedures and is clearly a quantum leap from that of examination of blood films which require a critical level of parasitaemia to give positive results. It is also pertinent to bear in mind that, as a major systemic infection, malaria often precipitates and can therefore co-exist with sickle cell crisis.

Blood transfusion reactions also cause haemolysis and increased levels of unconjugated bilirubin. The diagnosis is made from a positive direct antiglobulin test. Delayed reactions manifesting as hyperbilirubinaemia 1–2 weeks after the blood transfusion are less likely to be detected than immediate reactions. As they are more likely to need a blood transfusion than healthy individuals, people with SCD are at increased risk of infection by hepatitis viruses, which are blood-borne pathogens. Viral hepatitis is another cause of predominantly unconjugated hyperbilirubinaemia, and is diagnosed by positive viral serology and detection of specific viral RNA or DNA. By contrast, gall bladder stones, a common complication of SCD, cause a rise in the level of conjugated bilirubin. Ultrasonography is the mainstay of diagnosis.

Priapism

Priapism is a form of vaso-occlusive crisis affecting the penile circulation. This causes prolonged painful erection with or without prior sexual stimulation. It is a common manifestation of SCD. Various studies found that 42–89% of affected males have experienced priapism by the age of 20 years [17, 18]. Rarely, priapism occurs in people who have sickle cell trait [19]. The exact magnitude of the problem in SCD or sickle cell trait is difficult to determine because affected persons may be reluctant to give the information even when it is specifically requested, and even less likely to give the history voluntarily. This is more so when seeing a female health professional. As a result, priapism may be under-reported, under-recognized, and so under-treated. It is more likely that a positive history will be obtained if male staff attend to the affected person. Clinical experience and research findings show that priapism usually starts at night and early morning, and less often in the afternoon [17, 20]. There are two types of priapism.

The more severe variety is called major or fulminant priapism. It can last from 1 hour to several days and can lead to infarction and fibrosis of the erectile tissue of the phallus, loss of the ability to have erection and psycho-social problems [21]. Stuttering priapsm is the more frequent, less severe, form that lasts < 1 hour and resolves on its own without medical treatment.

Over 67% of episodes of major priapism are preceded by repeated occurrence of the stuttering variety. A person with frequently recurring stuttering priapism could therefore be regarded as being at increased risk of developing a fulminant attack, and offered preventive therapy.

Assessment of the patient with priapism includes medical history to ascertain when the episode began, if the major or stuttering variety had occurred in the past, and whether the person is able to pass urine. A general clinical examination is carried out before the specifics to detect the presence of bladder distension, urinary retention, tenderness and turgidity confined to the corpora cavernosa or also involving the corpus spongiosum. A soft glans penis and ability to pass urine imply that the corpus spongiosum is not involved, and that a glans–cavernosa shunt operation may confer clinical benefit if considered necessary. On the other hand, urinary retention and engorgement of the glans suggest that the corpus spongiosum is involved and possibly infarcted. In such situations, a glans–cavernosa shunt may not be effective in relieving the priapism [22]. When the spongiosum is affected, a shunt between the corpus cavernosum and the dorsal vein of the penis may lead to detumescence. The urology surgeons may also consider shunting blood from the cavernosa to the great saphenous vein in the thigh.

Before blood shunting procedures are initiated, conservative medical treatment should be given.

The first essential step is to provide effective analgesia for the pain of major priapism while taking measures to achieve detumescence. The urology surgeons have a major role in the management of major priapism in SCD, and should be involved at an early stage for optimal results. Even with timely treatment, the results are not always satisfactory, and the search continues for an effective way of bringing about detumescence. Various studies have found the alpha-adrenergic agonist, etilefrine, to be effective in the prevention and treatment of priapism caused by SCD in 50–100% of patients [17, 20, 23, 24]. In St Thomas' Hospital, London, UK, the following protocol is used for specific management of priapism in SCD. People with normal erectile function who have recurrent stuttering priapism or have had one previous major attack are given prophylactic treatment with slow-release etilefrine tablet 25–100 mg daily. Prophylaxis is started with 25 mg of the tablet, which has a duration of action of 8–9 hours, taken at bedtime. The rationale is to achieve effective blood concentrations of the drug during the critical hours of the night and early morning when the onset of priapism is most likely. The dose is increased by 25 mg every fortnight until the patient has good clinical response: absence of major priapism, with stuttering episodes not more than once in 2 weeks and not longer than 10 minutes in duration. The maximum daily dose is 100 mg, as recommended by the manufacturers. Daily doses > 50 mg are divided into 25–50 mg taken by 4–5 pm, and 50 mg at bedtime. The blood pressure and erectile function are closely monitored. People who have hypertension, cerebral vascular disease, transient ischaemic attacks or other contraindications to the use of etilefrine are not treated with the drug. Although there is no evidence from its use to date that etilefrine reduces penile erectile function, the drug is not given to patients with erectile dysfunction based on theoretical consideration that a drug that prevents and relieves priapism might affect normal penile erection. Individuals with erectile dysfunction are referred to urosurgeons for expert management, including consideration for the implantation of penile prosthesis. People with recurrent priapism not preventable with etilefrine 100 mg/day are given, in addition, the oestrogen analogue stiboesterol, or the anti-androgen cyproterone, or hydroxyurea [20]. If recurrent priapism is unresponsive to any of the above combinations, a programme of regular exchange blood transfusion (EBT) is usually effective in preventing further attacks [20].

Treatment of major attacks of priapism in our centre depends on whether or not the affected individual was previously on prophylactic etilefrine. People on prophylactic etilefrine are advised to take 50 mg orally and to attend the Accident and Emergency Department of the hospital if they have priapism that lasts up to 1 hour (major episode). On arrival at the hospital, the patient is kept comfortable and assessed, given analgesics, hydrated and observed while the urosurgeon is called. A bladder catheter is inserted in cases of urinary retention. If the priapism does not resolve satisfactorily 1 hour after the 50 mg etilefrine was taken, the urosurgeons irrigate the corpora cavernosa with 6–10 mg of etilefrine diluted in 5% dextrose solution. This is repeated after 1 hour if no clinical benefit is observed. Surgical operation to shunt blood from the corpora cavernosa is performed if a second irrigation with dilute etilefrine does not lead to resolution of the priapism. Individuals not previously on prophylactic etilefrine who develop major priapism are given 50 mg of oral etilefrine in the Accident and Emergency Department, and observed for 1 hour as above. If there is no satisfactory detumescence after this period, they are treated with intracavernous irrigation using dilute etilefrine. In contrast to the efficacy of regular EBT for preventing priapism, the procedure does not usually reverse an already established major episode. It could be that a sufficient amount of transfused normal blood does not flow into the penile blood vessels once fulminant priapism is fully established. Following a single episode of major priapism, prophylactic etilefrine is commenced if the patient has no contraindications. The person is also advised to empty the bladder before going to bed, avoid conditions that precipitate sickle cell crisis such as dehydration, and minimize intake of alcohol, a potent diuretic that can cause dehydration.

The mechanism of action of etilefrine in priapism is not known. Other alpha-adrenergic agonists such as phenylephrine have similar but less potent effects. It is paradoxical that a drug that causes vessel constriction prevents and ameliorates priapism, which is thought to result from vaso-occlusion in SCD. Elucidation of its mode of action may shed light on why etilefrine does not work in some patients [20]. It is intriguing that a small proportion of people with sickle cell trait (HbAS) experience priapism [19, 20]. A number of biological and environmental variables influence the manifestation and severity of SCD. These include the number of alpha globin genes inherited by the individual and proportion of HbF in the blood [25], leucocyte count [8, 26], and the expression of adhesion molecules on white blood cells [27]. It is also conceivable that the likelihood of vaso-occlusion in an HbAS individual is affected by these variables and the percentage of HbS in the blood, which ranges from 25% to 45%. Thus an HbAS person who has five alpha globin genes ($\alpha\alpha/\alpha\alpha\alpha$), %HbS, leucocyte count and adhesion molecule expression in the upper limits of normal, and a low HbF level, might be predisposed to develop vessel occlusion during an episode of infection or dehydration. Such a combination of inherited and acquired factors may also account for the occurrence in some HbAS individuals of renal papillary necrosis, haematuria and hyposthenuria [28, 29], or red cell sickling, rhabdomyolysis and sudden death after strenuous exercise or exposure to extreme cold [30].

Is it sickle cell crisis?

Case no. 1

A 40-year-old black man presented at night to the Accident and Emergency Department with a history of fever and severe bone pains in the hips, shoulders and knees for the previous 3 days. He had a temperature of 38.1°C, pallor with Hb of 9.7g/dL, leucocyte count 6.7×10^9/L, platelet count 96×10^9/L, jaundice with a bilirubin level of 38µmol/L (reference range 0–22), normal levels of liver enzymes and creatinine, total protein level 95g/L (ref. 64–86), albumin 28g/L (ref. 35–46), bilateral crepitations in the lung fields, and no abnormality on abdominal examination. High-performance liquid chromatography (HPLC) could not be done to determine the Hb genotype because it was outside normal working hours, but the sickle solubility test gave a positive result. The clinical impression was of sickle cell crisis precipitated by respiratory tract infection. Myeloma and lymphoma were noted as differential diagnoses. He was started on broad-spectrum antibiotics for the infection, diamorphine injections to relieve the severe bone pains, and admitted into the hospital ward.

On review the following morning the patient was feeling much better, his pains were well controlled on the opiate injections, and the temperature was down to normal. Further history taking revealed that (at the age of 40 years) he had no previous episode of generalized severe bone pains, had never had a blood transfusion and no member of his nuclear or extended family had SCD. The working diagnosis of sickle cell crisis was re-considered. HPLC on his blood sample was expedited. It showed his Hb genotype as AS. To find out the basis of his anaemia and jaundice, investigations for the causes of haemolytic anaemia were done. The direct anti-globulin test was positive. In the absence of any previous blood transfusion, the diagnosis was autoimmune haemolytic anaemia. A bone marrow aspiration and biopsy were done the same day, in search of the cause of his severe bone pains, hyper-proteinaemia and borderline thrombocytopenia. The reference range for platelet count in black people is $100-300 \times 10^9/L$ [31]. The marrow aspirate showed numerous immature plasma cells (Plate 8, shown in colour between pp. 54 and 55). Final diagnosis: multiple myeloma complicated by auto-immune haemolytic anaemia. Among the unusual aspects of this patient's illness is that auto-immune haemolytic anaemia is uncommon as a complication of myeloma, although it is more usual in other lymphoproliferative disorders such as chronic lymphocytic leukaemia and lymphoma. On the whole, the mode of presentation was an interesting reminder to keep an open mind when dealing with a clinical problem.

Case no. 2

A young woman known to have HbSS disease sought urgent medical attention because in the previous 48 hours she had fever, abdominal distension, constipation and lower abdominal pain not relieved by combination of paracetamol with codeine. On clinical examination she was pale, jaundiced and febrile. There was fullness in the lower abdomen, tenderness on deep palpation of the suprapubic region and both iliac fossae, and reduced bowel sounds. She had no dysuria, abnormalities in the chest or skeletal tenderness. Urinalysis gave normal results. The differential diagnoses included sepsis with no identified focus of infection, vaso-occlusive crisis involving the bowels and surgical acute abdomen. Samples of blood and mid-stream urine were sent for microbiology and broad-spectrum antibiotics were started. Urgent ultrasound scan of the abdomen and pelvis was requested. Ultrasono-graphy detected 33 mm of fluid in the pouch of Douglas and adhesions between the adnexae, suggestive of pelvic inflammatory disease. The patient was referred to gynaecologists for further management.

References

1. Hedo CC, Aken'Ova AY, Okpala IE, Durojaiye AO, Salimonu LS. Acute phase reactants and the severity of homozygous sickle cell disease. *J Intern Med* 1993; **233**: 467–70.
2. Frenette PS. Sickle cell vaso-occlusion: multistep and multicellular paradigm. *Curr Opin Hematol* 2002; **9**: 101–6.
3. Addae SK, Konotey-Ahulu FID. Lack of diurnal variation in sodium, potassium and osmolal excretion in the sickle cell patient. *Afr J Med Sci* 1971; **2**: 349–59.
4. Robieux IC, Kellner JD, Coppes MJ. Analgesia in children with sickle cell crisis: comparison of intermittent opioids vs continous infusion of morphine and placebo controlled study of oxygen inhalation. *Pediatr Hematol Oncol* 1992; **9**: 317–26.
5. Zipursky A, Robieux IC, Brown EJ *et al.* Oxygen therapy in sickle cell disease. *Am J Pediatr Hematol Oncol* 1992; **14**: 222–8.
6. Johnston RB Jr, Hewman SL, Struth AC. An abnormality of the alternative pathway of complement activation in sickle cell disease. *N Engl J Med* 1973; **288**: 803–5.
7. Anyaegbu CC, Okpala IE, Aken'Ova AY, Salimonu LS. Complement haemolytic activity, circulating immune complexes and the morbidity of sickle cell anaemia. *Acta Pathol Microbiol Scand* 1999; **107**: 699–702.
8. Anyaegbu CC, Okpala IE, Aken'Ova AY, Salimonu LS. Peripheral blood neutrophil count and candidacidal activity correlate with the clinical severity of sickle cell anaemia. *Eur J Haematol* 1998; **60**: 267–8.

9. Mollapour E, Porter JB, Kacmarski R, Linch D, Roberts PJ. Raised neutrophil phospholipase A2 activity and defective priming of NADPH oxidase and phospholipase A2 in sickle cell disease. *Blood* 1998; **91**: 3423–9.

10. Davies SC, Olatunji PO. Blood transfusion in sickle cell disease. *Vox Sang* 1995; **68**: 145–51.

11. Emond AM, Morias P, Venugopal S, Carpenter RG, Serjeant GR. Role of splenectomy in homozygous sickle cell disease in childhood. *Lancet* 1984; i: 88–90.

12. Serjeant GR. *Sickle Cell Disease*. Oxford: Oxford University Press, 1992.

13. Rogers DW, Clarke JM, Cepidore L *et al*. Early deaths in Jamaican children with sickle cell disease. *BMJ* 1978; **1**: 1515–16.

14. Brown KE, Young NS. Parvovirus B19 infection and haematopoiesis. *Blood Rev* 1995; **9**: 176–82.

15. Megas H, Papdaki E, Constantinides B. Salmonella septicaemia and aplastic crisis in a patient with sickle cell anaemia. *Acta Pediatr* 1961; **50**: 517–21.

16. Brown KE, Anderson SM, Young NS. Erythrocyte P antigen: cellular receptor for B19 parvovirus. *Science* 1993; **262**: 114–17.

17. Virag R, Bachir D, Lee K, Galacteros F. Preventive treatment of priapism in sickle cell disease with oral and self-administered intracavernous injection of etilefrine. *Urology* 1996; **47**: 777–81.

18. Mantadakis E, Ewalt DH, Cavender JD *et al*. Outpatient penile aspiration and epinephrine irrigation for young patients with sickle cell anaemia and prolonged priapism. *Blood* 2000; **95**: 78–82.

19. Fowler JE Jr, Koshy M, Strub M, Chin SK. Priapism associated with the sickle haemoglobinopathies: prevalence, natural history and sequelae. *J Urol* 1991; **145**: 65–8.

20. Okpala IE, Westerdale N, Jegede T, Cheung B. Etilefrine for the prevention of priapism in adult sickle cell disease. *Br J Haematol* 2002; **118**: 918–21.

21. Ihekwaba FN. Priapism in sickle cell anaemia. *J R Coll Surg Edinb* 1980; **25**: 133.

22. Winter CC. Priapism cured by creation of fistulas between glans penis and corpora cavernosa. *J Urol* 1978; **119**: 227–8.

23. Gbadoe AD, Atakouma Y, Kusiaku K, Assimadi JK. Management of sickle cell priapism with etilefrine. *Arch Dis Child* 2001; **85**: 52–3.

24. Bachir D, Galacteros E, Lee K, Virag R. Two years experience in management of priapism and impotence in sickle cell disease. *Blood* 1996; **88** (Suppl): 14a.

25. Steinberg MH, Rodgers GP. Pathophysiology of sickle cell disease: role of genetic and cellular modifiers. *Semin Hematol* 2001; **38**: 229–306.

26. Platt OS, Brambilla DJ, Rosse WF *et al*. Mortality in sickle cell disease – life expectancy and risk factors for early death. *N Engl J Med* 1994; **330**: 1639–43.

27. Okpala IE, Daniel Y, Haynes R, Odoemene D, Goldman JM. Relationship between the clinical manifestations of sickle cell disease and the expression of adhesion molecules on white blood cells. *Eur J Haematol* 2002; **69**: 135–44.

28. Herard A, Colin J, Youinou Y, Drancourt E, Brandt B. Massive hematuria in a sickle cell trait patient with renal papillary necrosis. *Eur Urol* 1998; **34**: 161–2.

29. Ataga KI, Orringer EU. Renal abnormalities in sickle cell disease. *Am J Hematol* 2000; **63**: 205–11.

30. Kark JA, Posey DM, Schumacher HR Jr, Ruehle CJ. Sickle cell trait as a risk factor for sudden death in physical training. *N Engl J Med* 1987; **317**: 781–7.

31. Essien EM. Platelets and platelet disorders in Africa (review). *Baillieres Clin Haematol* 1992; **5**: 441–56.

Chapter 8
Treatment modalities for pain in sickle cell disease

Iheanyi E Okpala

Introduction

From the point of view of affected persons, pain is the most distressing symptom of sickle cell disease (SCD). Its intensity in sickle cell crisis could be so much that the patient is deeply frightened and concerned about surviving the painful episode. This psychological distress adds to the feeling of pain, which is subjective in essence. Pain is an emotional and unpleasant experience associated with actual or potential damage to the body. The subjective nature of pain and lack of an objective method of measuring its intensity mean that clinical assessment depends on the feeling of the patient and the opinion of the health-care giver. Therefore, the field of pain management is a fertile ground for differences in opinion between individuals, and practice between health-care centres. In recognition of this, the treatment regimens and modalities described in this chapter reflect the practice in the author's institution. Whatever the place or the method of treatment, pain control is crucial in relieving suffering from SCD. Failure to achieve adequate analgesia creates problems in the relationship between patients and health-care professionals.

A very common and characteristic feature of SCD, pain was given due prominence in the history of this illness passed by word of mouth down generations in Africa [1], and in the first written description of the condition [2]. Considering the geographical distribution of the haemoglobinopathy and the total number of people affected worldwide, pain caused by SCD is a major public health problem on a global scale [3]. Two types of pain that may co-exist in the same person are direct results of tissue damage in SCD. Acute pain, typical of vaso-occlusive crisis, is caused by a recent tissue infarction. It is usually of sudden and unpredictable onset, intense, affects bony or soft tissues, and stops when the sickle cell crisis has resolved. Chronic pain is usually due to avascular necrosis of bone in the joints; leg ulceration is another cause. The femoral head is most commonly involved, the shoulder less frequently, the ankle seldom. The spine is usually affected by avascular necrosis. This shows on radiographs as 'fish-mouth' vertebrae. The knee is rarely affected. Chronic pain caused by SCD is not simply a continuation of acute pain from sickle cell crisis. Acute and chronic pain due to SCD can occur simultaneously in the same person; for example, a patient who has previous avascular joint necrosis with acute exacerbation of pain in the same joint as a result of new injury induced by movement or recent vaso-occlusive event. Similarly, generalized painful crisis could develop in an individual who had chronic pain in one or more sites. Pain control measures that produced satisfactory analgesia for the chronic pain caused by avascular necrosis may become inadequate when acute pain supervenes. In such situations, it is appropriate to discontinue medications such as parenteral opiates when the crisis resolves. The cause of pain in SCD patients may be unrelated to the haemoglobinopathy, e.g. a surgical acute abdomen or rheumatoid arthritis.

Case no. 1

A 35-year-old HbSS female with avascular necrosis of the left femoral head developed very severe pain of increasing intensity in the right hip. The pain was not relieved with doses of opiates that produced analgesia in the left hip. Pelvic radiographs and magnetic resonance imaging (MRI) scan showed no abnormalities. Over the following 2 weeks she became anorexic, more anaemic and lost about 5 kg in weight. A repeat MRI detected excess fluid in the right hip joint. Recalling that she was treated for tuberculosis 5 years previously, the joint fluid was aspirated and sent for bacteriology. Initial Ziehl–Neelsen (Z–N) staining showed no tubercle bacilli. After 6 weeks culture of her joint aspirate, the mycobacterium was isolated. Anti-tuberculosis treatment was started, and the right hip pain subsequently resolved.

Acute pain

With respect to pain control, people with SCD may be regarded as either opiate-naive or -tolerant. The regime and modality of pain treatment in SCD depend on degree of tolerance to opioid analgesics, and the type of pain. It is advisable to use analgesics in a stepwise manner, similar to methods for treating high blood pressure or hyperglycaemia. Patients who are not known to the health-care staff can be asked what doses and types of painkillers have been effective previously; these are used for the current painful episode so long as there are no contraindications. This approach generally saves the patient a lot of distress; although the few individuals with opiate-seeking behaviour may exaggerate the degree of their pain or the effective doses so as to receive more medication. Analgesics are administered at regular intervals for acute pain. In opiate-naive individuals, mild to moderate pain can be treated with dihydrocodeine tablets 30 mg 4-hourly combined with paracetamol 1 g 6-hourly. As an alternative, two tablets of co-codamol or co-proxamol could be given every 4 hours. Even opiate-naive patients may require small doses of these drugs for effective control of severe crisis pain, e.g. subcutaneous (s.c.) diamorphine injection 3–5 mg given 4–6-hourly. By contrast, opiate-tolerant people would normally require such drugs for satisfactory treatment of mild to moderate pain. Examples are immediate-release morphine sulphate (tablet or suspension) 10–20 mg or hydromorphone tablets

1.3–3.9 mg, both given 4-hourly. Adequate control of severe pain in opiate-tolerant patients invariably requires administration of parenteral preparations of these analgesics, such as diamorphine s.c. 10–20 mg given 4-hourly.

Although diamorphine is usually given at intervals of 4–6 hours, some people become so opiate-tolerant that more frequent doses every 2 hours are needed to maintain effective pain control. Such high degrees of tolerance create difficulties in pain control because there is a limited number of parenteral opioids available suitable for severe acute pain. To minimize the chances of developing high levels of tolerance, analgesics with different modes of action (such as paracetamol and non-steroidal anti-inflammatory drugs, NSAIDs) are used in conjunction with diamorphine, to reduce the dose of the opiate. Another beneficial effect of NSAIDs is reduction of the inflammatory component of the pain caused by ischaemia or infarction in vaso-occlusive events. SCD patients without contraindications to NSAIDs (kidney dysfunction, asthma, peptic ulcer) have a cyclo-oxygenase 2 (Cox-2) inhibitor such as rofecoxib added to the analgesic regime for acute pain. NSAIDs that are not specific Cox-2 inhibitors, such as ibuprofen and diclofenac, are less preferable. However, a diclofenac suppository has two advantages: it can be given to patients who are vomiting or otherwise unable to intake orally, and rectal administration bypasses the stomach and reduces the risk of peptic ulceration. Another side-effect of NSAIDs that is relevant in the context of SCD is nephrotoxocity, because it can worsen sickle nephropathy. Therefore, NSAIDs tend not to be used for more than 10 days for the treatment of pain in people with the haemoglobinopathy.

If the acute pain is not relieved by intermittent injections of the initial opiate dose, small increments (e.g. diamorphine 2–3 mg) are made every 4–6 hours to reduce the risk of respiratory depression. The dose is reduced by similar amounts as the sickle cell crisis and pain resolve. This strategy prevents development of opiate withdrawal syndrome. Clinical features of opiate withdrawal include dysphoria, tremors, seizures, nasal congestion, nausea, diarrhoea, vomiting and a feeling of increased pain. Therefore, opiate withdrawal can mimic sickle cell crisis. Diarrhoea and vomiting may cause dehydration and exacerbate an already resolving sickle cell crisis or precipitate a new one. The patient may repeatedly return to hospital with apparently 'recurrent crises' if opiates are stopped abruptly after administration for a few days when the crisis and pain have resolved. If intermittent injection of diamorphine is started with a dose > 10 mg, oral immediate-release morphine sulphate is given instead when the dose has been reduced to < 10 mg per injection. In patients started on < 10 mg per injection, oral morphine equivalent to the last dose of injection is given for about 3 days before stopping opiate therapy. The equivalent dose of oral immediate-release morphine sulphate is twice the dose of diamorphine injection. For example, 10 mg of oral morphine is equivalent to 5 mg of diamorphine injection, because 1 mole of diamorphine is metabolized to 2 moles of morphine in the body. The amount of oral morphine given should depend on how sensitive the individual is to opiates, and not solely on the theoretical equivalent doses. In people who are very sensitive to opiates, there is a risk of overdosage with depression of the central nervous system if the dose of oral morphine is based exclusively on the theoretical equivalent amounts.

Patient-controlled analgesia (PCA) is an alternative method of administering parenteral opiates. It is effective, safe, and preferred by some patients [4]. Continuous subcutaneous infusion of an opioid provides background analgesia that is supplemented by intermittent bolus doses when the patient feels the need for more pain relief. The total amount of opiate that can be delivered is set within safe limits and according to the intensity of pain.

Diamorphine is used in preference to pethidine in treatment of acute pain because it has several advantages. Norpethidine, a metabolite of pethidine, is neuro-excitatory. It may accumulate in the body and cause convulsions. Diamorphine is a more potent analgesic than pethidine. Unlike the latter, it is sufficiently soluble to be given as subcutaneous injections. Pethidine, on the contrary, needs to be given intramuscularly. The muscles are damaged by repeated injections, heal by fibrosis, and may develop contractures. This limits movement around the joints served by the damaged muscles. Moreover, as fibrotic tissue does not have as many blood vessels as skeletal muscles, absorption of subsequent injec-

tions of pethidine from the site is impaired. As a result, the analgesic effect is reduced, and larger doses are needed, causing more fibrosis. Of greater concern, it also increases the risk of opiate dependence or addiction (discussed further in Chapter 21).

Other side-effects of opiates more often experienced during therapy are constipation, nausea, vomiting and respiratory depression. Constipation is treated with laxatives such as lactulose, senna, sodium docussate, glycerol suppository or phosphate enema. Nausea or vomiting can be relieved with metoclopramide or cylizine. Pruritus does not imply allergy to an opiate and it does not often warrant switching to another drug. To avoid further sedation of the patient on opiates, non-sedative antihistamines (such as desloratadine) are preferred for its treatment. Opiate-induced pruritus appears to be more common in black people than in other ethnic groups, suggesting a genetic basis for its occurrence. By far the most serious side-effect of opiate therapy is respiratory depression because it is a life-threatening emergency that calls for urgent treatment with opiate antagonists such as naloxone.

Chronic pain

Multidisciplinary treatment is given to people who have chronic pain due to SCD. Management involves the use of analgesic medications, adjuvant therapy, physiotherapy, psychological support that includes cognitive behaviour therapy (CBT), and orthopaedic intervention or surgery. A combination of paracetamol and dihydrocodeine or the compound formulation co-proxamol is used for mild chronic pain. If the pain is of such intensity that it is not relieved by maximum doses of the above drugs, it is regarded as moderate/severe, and morphine is given. Long-term, background analgesia is provided with slow-release tablets of morphine sulphate or hydromorphone, taken 12-hourly. For breakthrough pain, immediate-release tablets of morphine sulphate or hydromorphone are taken. When tolerance develops to one drug, a switch is made to the other. Clinical experience shows that after a long time of not taking a particular opiate to which tolerance had developed, it may be used again with significant benefit. Other morphine-based drugs such as oxycodone and fentanyl can be used. NSAIDs are used for short periods not exceeding 10 days in the management of chronic pain, usually in combination with other analgesics.

Patients who need opioids for relief of chronic pain are considered for other modalities of therapy. Psychotherapy, especially CBT, enhances the person's coping strategies for dealing with the emotional aspects of chronic pain and other types of psychological stress associated with SCD [5]. Physiotherapy helps to prevent muscle contractures and reduces joint pain and stiffness, as well as overall physical disability. People who have avascular necrosis of joints with chronic pain uncontrolled by medications are reviewed jointly by orthopaedic surgeons and haematologists in the Sickle/Orthopaedic component of the Comprehensive Clinic as discussed in Chapter 1. Appliances that provide back support and make up for the difference in length between the legs ameliorate chronic pain in the back and hips. Some patients have avascular necrosis with chronic pain that can only be effectively relieved by orthopaedic surgery. For such people, early surgery is preferred. In others, surgery is deferred for as long as the individual can cope on other modalities of pain treatment. This policy is adopted because certain procedures such as hip replacement confer clinical benefit for a limited period [6, 7], usually not longer than 10 years. Thereafter, repeat surgery may be required. Adjuvant therapy, with medications that enhance pain relief although they are strictly not regarded as analgesics, helps in chronic pain control. For example, gabapentin and amitryptiline have been found to be beneficial by some patients who have neuropathic pain. Similarly, transcutaneous electrical nerve stimulation (TENS) machines are regularly used by some people to enhance analgesia. Chronic pain from avascular necrosis of the femoral heads, intervertebral joints or shoulders can be ameliorated for periods up to 3 months following local nerve block by the anaesthetists. This procedure helps to reduce the doses of opiates required by the individual, and so reduces the risk of side-effects.

Case no. 2

A young man with homozygous (HbSS) SCD and avascular necrosis of the left femoral head underwent osteotomy in the left hip to relieve chronic pain. The surgery was complicated by infection with methicillin-resistant *Staphylococcus aureus* (MRSA). Healing of the surgical wound was delayed. The chronic pain in the left hip persisted, uncontrollable with opiate analgesics. The probability of reactivating MRSA infection made it inadvisable to perform further orthopaedic surgery. The anaesthetists carried out left hip nerve block, which reduced the chronic pain to such an extent that it was subsequently controllable with hydromorphone 16 mg 12-hourly. Repeat nerve blocks were needed about every 4 months to maintain satisfactory analgesia.

References

1. Konotey-Ahulu FID. Hereditary qualitative and quantitative erythrocyte defects in Ghana: an historical and geographical survey. *Ghana Med J* 1968; 7: 118–19.
2. Africanus Horton JB. *The Diseases of Tropical Climates and their Treatment*. London: Churchill, 1874.
3. Weatherall DJ, Clegg JB. Inherited haemoglobin disorders: an increasing global health problem. *Bull World Health Organ* 2001; 79: 704–12.
4. Gonzales ER, Bahal N, Hansen LA *et al*. Intermittent injection vs patient controlled analgesia for sickle cell crisis pain. Comparison in patients in the emergency department. *Arch Intern Med* 1991; 51: 1373–6.
5. Thomas VJ. Cognitive behavioural therapy in pain management for sickle cell disease. *Int J Palliat Nurs* 2000; 6: 434–42.
6. Iwegbu CG, Fleming AF. Avascular necrosis of the femoral head in sickle cell disease. *J Bone Joint Surg* 1985; 67: 29–32.
7. Moran MC. Osteonecrosis of the hip in sickle cell haemoglobinopathy. *Am J Orthoped* 1995; 24: 18–24.

Chapter 9
Management of sickle cell disease in childhood

Moira Dick

Introduction

The outcome in childhood sickle cell disease (SCD) has improved greatly over the past two decades since the introduction of neonatal screening. Early diagnosis allows the introduction of penicillin prophylaxis by 3 months of age to prevent invasive pneumococcal infection, and the education of parents to recognize significant signs such as sudden enlargement of the spleen in acute splenic sequestration. Mortality in the first few years of life can be reduced to < 1% [1] but there is still an increased risk of death in the first 18 years of life due to complications such as acute chest syndrome and stroke. Because of the variability of the disorder there are children who may have few symptoms and can be managed in primary care or in the outpatient setting. Over two-thirds, however, will have a hospital admission at some point in their lives and many school days are lost due to repeated episodes of painful crisis or ill health. Most vaso-occlusive episodes can be managed safely at home. A small minority of children will have frequent hospital admissions but even this number is less than previously due to the introduction of hydroxyurea. Attention should therefore be paid to improving quality of life and allowing children to participate fully in all activities according to their tolerance. In addition, inclusion and access to education is important, as there has been a growing awareness of the impact that silent stroke can have on a child's learning and self-esteem and ability to cope with their illness. An estimated 20% will have evidence of infarction on magnetic resonance (MR) scanning by the time they are 20 years old [2].

This chapter sets out a guide to the management of children with sickle cell disorders, recognizing that not all units will necessarily have as much expertise and resources as others. The key to successful paediatric management is:

1 having a neonatal screening programme
2 engaging the family early (during the antenatal period if possible) and the child as soon as they are able to understand simple aspects of their condition
3 having a multidisciplinary team that can provide holistic care to the child and family
4 having recourse to specialist services as and when they are needed.

Neonatal screening

Neonatal screening for haemoglobinopathies will be universal throughout England from 2004 [3]. Similar programmes are implemented or planned in several countries. There is no benefit from screening without counselling and good paediatric and haematology follow-up. In the UK, there are currently no national guidelines for follow-up arrangements or clinical management of SCD in childhood.

Children will still be diagnosed after the neonatal period either because they were born before the universal screening programme was introduced or they moved to the area where neonatal screening is done. Therefore, health professionals will need to be alert to the diagnosis. Dactylitis is pathognomic of SCD and overwhelming pneumococcal sepsis or acute splenic sequestration may be the first indication that a child has the condition.

Types of sickle cell disorders

The most commonly encountered forms of SCD are:
- Sickle cell anaemia (HbSS)
- HbSC disease
- HbS β^0 thalassaemia
- HbS β^+ thalassaemia
- HbSD Punjab.

Haemoglobin HbS/HPFH (sickle with hereditary persistence of haemoglobin) is not considered to be a significant sickle cell disorder. It should not be confused with the more common HbSS with a high HbF level. Unless both parental phenotypes are known it is impossible to distinguish HbSS from HbS β^0 thalassaemia and HbS/HPFH at birth. HbSC and HbS β^+ thalassaemia are more likely to run a milder course than HbSS, HbS/HbD or HbS β^0 thalassaemia. Although these conditions vary in presentation and prognosis, routine outpatient management should be identical, at least in the early years. However, clinicians should be aware of the particular phenotype, especially on admission, as steady-state Hb levels vary greatly and certain complications, e.g. stroke, are much less frequent in HbSC disease or HbS/β^+ thalassaemia.

Multidisciplinary team

The multidisciplinary team will vary depending on the stage of the child's life. The following is a guide to the optimal team.
- Antenatal period: GPs, midwives, genetic counsellors, and/or specialist nurse counsellors for haemoglobinopathies, haematologists.
- Neonatal period: specialist nurse counsellors, health visitors, GPs, paediatricians, paediatric haematologists.
- Paediatric care: as above for neonatal period, clinical psychologists, school nurses, community paediatricians, teachers, educational psychologists, specialist nurses, Accident and Emergency staff.
- Joint clinics/protocols: paediatric neurologists, orthopaedic surgeons, ophthalmologists.
- Transition: haematology team for adults with SCD.

Recourse to specialist services

A paediatrician, or a paediatric haematologist with experience of general paediatrics, should lead the multidisciplinary team. SCD can affect all aspects of a child's growth and development. It is important to have good links with specialist paediatric services such as neurology for investigation of stroke and other neurological problems, orthopaedic surgeons for the management of avascular necrosis and endocrinologists for those children who may be severely growth delayed or iron overloaded as a result of regular transfusion therapy. Children will need to be referred to a specialist unit if bone marrow transplantation is being considered.

An approach to outpatient care

The care of a child who has SCD is mostly carried out in the outpatient setting. The rationale for regular follow-up is to prevent or anticipate some of the complications of the condition and for parents to feel confident in managing most of the straightforward episodes themselves. Regular follow-up from birth can reduce hospital admissions significantly. The aims of the clinic should be explicit and communicated with parents, as otherwise the value of attending clinic will not be apparent and, as with many chronic conditions, attendance will decline. Usual practice is to register the child in the paediatric clinic at about 2 months of age, assuming that the child was picked up by the neonatal screening programme and that the diagnosis has already been disclosed to the parents. In high prevalence areas, the diagnosis is usually imparted at home by specialist nurses, but if not, this should be done by another professional with knowledge and expertise.

Prevention strategies

- Primary: penicillin prophylaxis, pneumococcal and other immunization.
- Secondary: education of parents to manage simple complications and to recognize and anticipate serious illness; education of children and care plans for transition to adult clinic.

• Tertiary: screening for cerebral vasculopathy, chronic lung disease, renal disease.

Primary prevention

Children with SCD are liable to develop splenic hypofunction in the first 6 months of life as their fetal haemoglobin declines and episodes of infarction occur in the spleen. Splenic hypofunction and the absence of type-specific antibody means that young children are at great risk of infection by organisms containing polysaccharide-coated antigen such as *Pneumococcus* or *Haemophilus influenzae*.

Penicillin prophylaxis

This works if taken regularly [4]. Resistance has not become a major problem in the UK, currently being found in about 6% of infections.

Penicillin V dosage:

• 62.5 mg orally twice daily at < 1 year (or < 10 kg)
• 125 mg orally twice daily at 1–5 years
• 250 mg orally twice daily at > 5 years.

If there is a genuine allergy to penicillin, erythromycin can be substituted. In the UK it is recommended that penicillin is continued throughout life and certainly throughout childhood. The incidence of pneumococcal infection in the general population falls dramatically after the age of 5 years and it may be possible with the introduction of conjugate pneumococcal vaccination to discontinue penicillin much earlier.

Immunization

See Table 9.1 for a proposed vaccine schedule.

Pneumococcal infection

The heptavalent conjugate pneumococcal vaccine (Prevenar®) has been licensed for use in under 2-year-olds since January 2002 [5]. Infectious disease specialists also recommend its use in at-risk children over the age of 2 years [6]. As the polysaccharide vaccine, Pneumovax®, is 23 valent, it should also be given at 2 years and 5-yearly thereafter.

The recommended scheme comprises 7 valent Prevenar®, three doses of 0.5 mL intramuscularly (i.m.) at 2, 3 and 4 months (with DPT, Hib, MenC

Table 9.1 Proposed vaccine schedule

Vaccine	Age
DPT, Hib, polio, MenC, Prevenar®	2 months
DPT, Hib, polio, MenC, Prevenar®	3 months
DPT, Hib, polio, MenC, Prevenar®	4 months
MMR	13 months
HepB	12 months
Hep B	15 months
Hep B	18 months
Prevenar	6, 8 and 14 months or twice in second year of life if no Prevenar® in primary course
Pneumovax®	2 years
Pneumovax®	7 years
Pneumovax®	12 years
Pneumovax®	17 years
Influenza	Annually from 2 years of age

and polio). If a child misses the primary course, the catch-up scheme comprises two doses of 0.5 mL i.m. at > 6 < 12 months at least 1 month apart and a third dose at 12–16 months *or* two doses of 0.5 mL i.m. at > 12 < 23 months at least 1 month apart *and* 23 valent Pneumovax, one dose of 0.5 mL i.m. at 24 months and 5-yearly thereafter.

Haemophilus influenzae

The conjugate Hib vaccine is part of the primary course of immunization together with diphtheria, tetanus, pertussis, meningitis C and polio and should be given at the same time as the Prevenar® at 2, 3 and 4 months.

Hepatitis B

Children with SCD are likely to receive one or more blood transfusions in their life and it is good practice to safeguard them from hepatitis B. Many antenatal clinics screen for hepatitis B and neonates will automatically be offered immunization in positive cases. In the rest a course of hepatitis B vaccination should be given at the beginning of the second year of life.

Influenza

There is no impaired immune response to viral infections such as influenza but it is considered good practice to offer influenza vaccination annually in order to prevent chest complications.

Secondary prevention

1 Written information, e.g. parent handbook [7] or pages in parent handbook or child passport
2 Haemoglobinopathy card with diagnosis, steady-state haemoglobin and blood group
3 Verbal reinforcement at every clinic visit or other contact, e.g. by specialist nurse.

The areas that should be covered and continually reinforced are:
• Simple understanding of condition
• Crucial importance of penicillin prophylaxis and pneumococcal vaccination
• Recognition of pallor (very important in aplastic crisis, acute splenic sequestration)
• Palpation of spleen
• Knowledge of steady-state haemoglobin level
• Temperature measurement and management
• Recognition of dactylitis
• Pain relief
• When to come to hospital
• The importance of visual disturbance particularly in HbSC disease
• Genetic counselling
• Information for future pregnancies.

Children who have parents who manage their condition grow up to be adults who can cope with their condition [8]. It is therefore important to communicate effectively with parents as they will be the role models for their children, but children must also be actively engaged from an early age. Mishandling of a sickle cell admission early on can lead to loss of trust by the parent and poor adjustment by the child. A good transition plan will stop adolescents falling out of clinic follow-up and help to ensure that they are able to manage their condition satisfactorily.

The sickle cell team should address the following:
1 An understanding of a child's view of illness and pain at different ages by all staff
2 Education and training of all staff to assess and manage the condition effectively
3 Continuity of care
4 Children's and teenage workshops
5 Videos and leaflets for children
6 Teenage handbook
7 Transition clinics and a different model for adolescent care.

Tertiary prevention

1 Monitoring of cerebral blood flow velocities to anticipate stroke
2 Measuring lung function, steady-state oxygen saturation levels by pulse oximetry
3 Monitoring blood pressure
4 Monitoring urine for microalbuminuria.

What should take place in the clinic?

The first visit will be important in going over the likely diagnosis, exploring the parents' understanding, answering any questions and taking a confirmatory blood sample. Follow-up visits should address the following topics.

General examination

Children should be examined on most clinic visits. Presence of pallor, jaundice and splenomegaly should be noted. Height and weight measurements should be recorded on appropriate centile charts. The spleen should be palpated and measured. In children under 5 years the parents should be taught how to feel the spleen. Most children who are anaemic have a short ejection systolic murmur heard loudest at the left sternal edge. This does not need further investigation if the rest of the cardiac system is normal.

Monitoring steady-state values

The value of monitoring haematological, biochemical or other steady-state values is to be able to compare if the child becomes unwell and requires admission to hospital. If the child is well, blood tests should only be done on an annual or possibly 2-yearly basis. The added advantage of this approach is that the child is less likely to become phobic of needles and the outpatient visit can be a relaxed event. A suggested plan for steady-state investigations is set out in Table 9.2.

Blood pressure, urinalysis and an oxygen saturation level when well should be recorded annually. Blood pressure levels are lower in patients with sickle cell anaemia and this should be

Birth	HPLC on Guthrie spot
3 months	Confirmation HPLC, FBC, G6PD level
1 year	FBC and reticulocyte count, %HbF, HbA2 (if no parental phenotype), blood group, extended RBC genotype, electrolytes and urea, liver function tests
2 years	FBC and reticulocyte count, %HbF, electrolytes and urea, liver function tests
3 years	As above
4–17 years	As above + consider ultrasound abdomen and transcranial Doppler scan; repeat annually

Table 9.2 Suggested plan for steady-state investigations

HPLC, high-performance liquid chromatography; FBC, full blood count; G6PD, glucose-6-phosphate dehydrogenase; RBC, red blood cell.

taken into account when deciding on intervention [9].

An outpatient guide to pain relief

Most young children with pain will find relief from paracetamol (12 mg/kg/dose) 4-hourly and ibuprofen (10 mg/kg/dose) 8-hourly for mild to moderate pain. Codeine phosphate (0.5–1 mg/kg/dose) can be added in for severe pain. If there is no improvement and/or there are other factors such as a high temperature, the parent should seek medical advice.

Monitoring growth

Children typically are thin, although they grow steadily along the standard centiles despite an almost universal complaint by parents that they eat hardly anything. However, compared with ethnically matched controls, children are both shorter and thinner [10]. Chronic haemolytic anaemia and an increased metabolic rate are the accepted reasons for poor growth, and folate supplementation is often prescribed. However, specific nutritional deficiencies have not been described except for possible zinc deficiency [11]. The reason for the relative anorexia is not well understood although most children will drink large volumes of fluid because of functional hyposthenuria, due to sickling within the renal medulla affecting the concentrating mechanism.

Many children have pica for a range of substances, paper, foam and plaster being the commonest. Managing pica is difficult in the absence of an obvious nutritional deficiency and behavioural management techniques may only result in the pica

becoming secretive. Children start puberty on average 2 years later than their peers [12] and growth will slow in the early teenage years. Measurement of bone age reveals a bone age 2–3 years behind chronological age, and reassurance that they will go into puberty is normally sufficient. It is rare that a referral has to be made to a paediatric endocrinologist although some children, particularly boys, may have psychological difficulties due to their short height and a discussion with a specialist may be helpful.

Monitoring neurodevelopment

Most children will have surveillance by a health visitor in the pre-school years, although neurodevelopmental screening has become more targeted [13]. Because children with sickle cell anaemia are at risk of silent cerebral infarcts it is important to monitor their development not only during the pre-school years but also once they have started in school. Many children with SCD are not properly evaluated, as lack of progress is put down to their condition and time lost through illness. There should be good links with community services and school health teams to ensure that this does not happen. It is not infrequently found that children are missing school not because of illness but because they find the schoolwork difficult. Ideally all children should have a detailed neurodevelopmental assessment before starting school and at any other time if there are concerns about lack of academic progress.

Prevention of stroke

Between 5% and 10% of children with sickle cell

anaemia (HbSS) will have an overt stroke, usually between 18 months and 9 years, with a median age of 7 years [14]. MR scanning has shown that there is a generalized cerebral vasculopathy with narrowing or stenosis occurring most frequently in the middle cerebral arteries, but may include anterior and posterior cerebral arteries. This narrowing can be demonstrated by an increase in cerebral blood flow on transcranial Doppler imaging and this provides a quick and non-invasive technique of picking children up who may be at risk of developing stroke. Research in the USA has shown that transfusing children when the cerebral velocities are > 220 cm/s will prevent stroke in 60% [15]. It has therefore been recommended that regular transcranial Doppler flow measurements should be offered routinely from an early age. MR scan of the brain including MR angiography should be also carried out if the cerebral flows are consistently high.

Monitoring severity

A satisfactory measure of severity has never been established. As pain experience is a subjective phenomenon, the number of admissions to hospital with painful vaso-occlusive episodes is not necessarily a good measure, as some children may have low tolerance to pain or their parents may feel unable to cope. Conversely, with education and community support many parents manage quite severe painful episodes at home. It is useful to try and keep some record of the frequency of problems either by asking about school attendance or by asking the child to keep a pain diary, particularly if a trial of hydroxyurea is planned. A HbF > 7% is associated with less clinical symptoms and a better prognosis [16]. Dactylitis, severe anaemia (Hb < 7 g/dL), HbF < 13%, platelet count > 450×10^9/L and leucocytosis (> 8×10^9/L) by 2 years of age are associated with a worse prognosis [17].

Nocturnal enuresis

There is an increased rate of nocturnal enuresis in children, particularly boys, with sickle cell anaemia. The reason for this is not entirely clear.

Children pass large quantities of dilute urine and have nocturia but this should not necessarily lead to incontinence. A high ratio of overnight urinary volumes compared to maximum functional bladder capacity has been posed as a possible cause [18]. Parents report that their children are heavy sleepers. It has been shown that children with adenoidal hypertrophy and obstructive apnoea are more likely to have nocturnal enuresis [19] and it is possible that hypoxaemia plays a role in the aetiology of nocturnal enuresis. On the whole, sickle cell children do not respond to behavioural management techniques such as star charts or mattress alarms but can be 'trained' by intermittent alarms and parental waking to achieve continence. Many children respond to oral or nasal desmopressin and this is a useful adjunct, particularly for school trips.

Other medical complications

Gallstones occur in > 50% of children over the age of 10 years [20] but may not be the cause of intermittent abdominal pain, which is a relatively common symptom in all children. Laparoscopic cholecystectomy is advised in symptomatic biliary disease.

Avascular necrosis of the femoral head can be treated conservatively with partial weight-bearing on crutches and physiotherapy support.

Leg ulcers are relatively uncommon in the UK and should be treated with frequent dressing, support bandages and antibiotics if infected.

Stuttering priapism may affect adolescents in particular and may go unreported. Oral etilefrine may reduce the frequency of attacks and in a prolonged episode aspiration and irrigation of the corpora cavernosa with epinephrine or etilefrine is now the treatment of choice [21].

Children should be advised to seek treatment early.

Psychosocial support

Clinical nurse specialists play an important role in supporting the family but in an ideal service children should have access to a clinical psychologist with an interest in the condition. Sickle cell is a potentially fatal condition in childhood or early adulthood; it is a chronic illness, characterized by pain which may be severe enough to require opiate analgesia; silent strokes may affect cognitive development and behaviour. Psychologists are important for management of all these aspects, including the use of cognitive behavioural techniques and neuropsychometric assessments [22].

Travel information

It is important that families have good information about the risk of travelling abroad, particularly to malarious areas. Additional vaccinations should be given depending on the destination and should include meningitis A and C. Malaria prophylaxis is essential and advice about avoiding mosquito bites should be given. Many families assume that children with SCD are protected because of having sickle haemoglobin and this misinformation should be corrected. Advice to keep warm in the air-conditioned environment of an aeroplane, drink sufficient fluids and move around regularly are the only precautions that need to be taken when flying.

Managing transition

As neonatal screening becomes the norm, many children with SCD will have been managed all their life by the same paediatric team when they are required to transfer to the adult team. There is a case for not making this transfer until about 21 years of age, although individual young people will differ in their readiness for transition. Children are often physically immature at 16 years and the holistic approach of the paediatric clinic should perhaps support them through college and further education. In the absence of inpatient adolescent units in most hospitals, the reality is that once their 16th birthday is reached the child has to be admitted to an adult ward. Preparation for this event is therefore crucially important, as the experience of being in an adult ward with elderly sick patients can be extremely distressing.

The key components of good transition include:
1 Information about the condition and possible complications as they reach adolescence (e.g. pri-

apism, gallstones) and the adult services and the people involved.
2 An introduction to the adult team and facilities.
3 Comprehensive handover between the two teams, usually in a joint clinic with a chance for the teenager to express their current needs.
4 A gradual disengaging from the paediatric clinic if this is wished, even if the child might be admitted to the adult ward.
5 Genetic counselling.
6 Contraceptive advice.

An approach to inpatient management

The commonest causes of admission are acute chest syndrome, acute splenic sequestration in the under 5's, parvovirus-related aplasia, vaso-occlusive episodes and stroke. Osteomyelitis is relatively uncommon but is sometimes difficult to distinguish from a vaso-occlusive episode. Management of these acute complications is described elsewhere in this book. The Accident and Emergency Department is usually the first place parents take their child, often bypassing the general practitioner. This is perhaps not surprising given the potentially lethal nature of the condition and the anxiety that many parents feel. Potentially serious complications of SCD can present without pain, e.g. stroke, aplastic crisis. Guidelines are helpful but should always be used in conjunction with clinical acumen. It does not make sense to admit every febrile child as a potential pneumococcal sepsis or to take blood from every child in case they have an aplastic crisis. It should also be remembered that a child might present with a problem not related to their SCD. There should be an immediate triage system to assess the severity of the problem. Pain assessment should be carried out using a pain tool for children such as PATCh [23] that takes into account the child's perception and nursing and/or medical judgement. Algorithms for a sick child who is not necessarily in pain and for pain relief are given in Figs 9.1 and 9.2.

Some units recommend fast track admission to the children's ward, the rationale being that the child is more likely to be assessed quickly and by the paediatric team that knows them. This system can

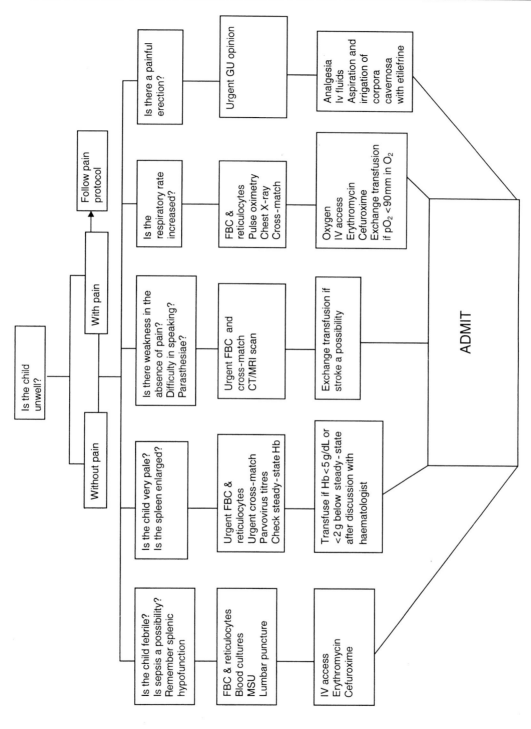

Fig. 9.1 Assessment of an unwell child in the Accident and Emergency Department.

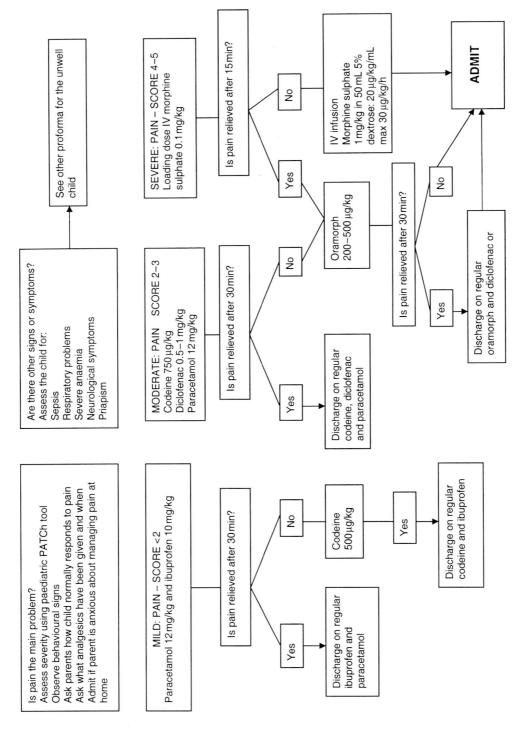

Fig. 9.2 Management of pain in children with sickle cell disease in the Accident and Emergency Department.

work well in a unit that is not very busy and with a moderate number of children on the sickle cell register, but may lead to unnecessary admission. It is difficult and potentially dangerous to attempt this in a very busy unit. Ideally the child should be assessed as far as possible by an experienced team, there should be an observation unit where the child's response to analgesia can be judged and the child should be sent home on an appropriate dose of medication.

Treatment

Treatment in an acute episode should consider the following factors.

Hydration

Most clinical guidelines stress the need for hydration in the management of an uncomplicated painful episode (usually 1.5 times the normal daily requirement). Certainly dehydration may worsen the sickling episode but there is no evidence that the painful episode is shortened by overhydration and attention should be paid to fluid balance, as inappropriate ADH secretion may complicate matters in a sick child. Where possible the child should be encouraged to drink rather than having intravenous (i.v.) fluids, particularly if afebrile. The less veins need to be cannulated the better it is for long-term management.

Pain relief

Pain experience is very subjective and there may be a degree of anxiety depending on previous experience of a painful episode. It is important to monitor pain relief in the same ways that pulse, blood pressure and temperature are monitored to be able to assess the efficacy of analgesia. A pain tool and guidelines for step increase of analgesics should be used as in the British Society of Haematology guidelines for the management of acute sickle cell crisis [24]. Most paediatric units favour the use of oral analgesia rather than parenteral unless the pain is very severe, in which case patient- or nurse-controlled analgesia using intravenous morphine is recommended. Laxatives should be prescribed with

codeine or morphine. It is important to make sure that paediatric and adult guidelines for pain relief agree to prevent a sudden increase in analgesic dosage at transition.

Antibiotics

Most children are mildly febrile with a painful crisis and antibiotics need not be given if there is no evidence of sepsis, although penicillin prophylaxis should continue. Some units advocate one dose of i.v. ceftriaxone in the Accident and Emergency Department, which can either be continued on review after 24 hours or discontinued if blood cultures are negative. If a child is unwell and febrile (> 38.5 °C) a broad-spectrum antibiotic should be used, such as augmentin or cefuroxime. If osteomyelitis is suspected an MR scan in the first 24 hours can help to distinguish from a vaso-occlusive episode. If there are chest signs, erythromycin should be added.

Blood transfusion

A simple top-up transfusion to bring the haemoglobin back to steady-state values is indicated for the treatment of acute splenic sequestration and parvovirus-related aplasia. Care should be taken not to increase the haemoglobin level too much in acute splenic sequestration, as the spleen returns to normal size after a few days, returning blood to the circulation. Exchange transfusion should be carried out as a matter of urgency in a child thought to have had a stroke and in acute chest syndrome. Regular monthly blood transfusions to maintain the haemoglobin S at about 30% are indicated for the management of stroke and should be considered if transcranial Doppler scans show elevated cerebral velocities > 220 cm/s on more than one occasion in the absence of an overt stroke. Hydroxyurea rather than chronic transfusion therapy is now the treatment of choice in frequent severe painful episodes or repeated acute chest syndrome. Once a child has been started on a long-term transfusion programme, education about the implications of iron overload should start. Subcutaneous desferrioxamine (35 mg/kg/night) administered either by an infusion or balloon pump should be started once the ferritin level is > 1000 µg/L, together with oral vitamin C to enhance iron excretion. Children receiving desferrioxamine should have annual ophthalmology and audiology reviews, regular ferritin levels and an annual MRI assessment of liver iron in children over 7 years.

Incentive spirometry

Acute chest syndrome is more likely to occur in those children with severe pain affecting particularly trunk and limb girdles. Incentive spirometry has been shown to improve ventilation and reduce the risk of chest crisis [25].

Oxygen

There is no evidence that oxygen therapy is beneficial in the acute painful crisis. It should be used if oxygen saturation levels measured by pulse oximetry are lower than steady-state levels. There is some evidence that lower nocturnal oxygen saturation levels are associated with a higher rate of painful crisis in childhood [26].

Other treatments

Hydroxyurea

Hydroxyurea is being used increasingly in managing not only frequent severe painful episodes requiring hospital admission but also less severe episodes leading to school loss and poor quality of life [27]. The starting dose is 15 mg/kg/day increasing after 3 months by 5 mg/kg/day. Initially, a blood test should be carried out every 2 weeks to monitor for myelotoxicitiy. It is usually not necessary to increase the dose to the maximum tolerated before seeing a positive effect.

Bone marrow transplantation

Hydroxyurea has not been shown to prevent the incidence of stroke [28] and bone marrow transplantation remains the only possible treatment other than regular blood transfusion once a stroke has occurred. However, it is possible that children will remain at risk from cerebral haemorrhage following the transplantation, depending on the extent of their cerebral vasculopathy. Bone marrow transplantation is currently the only cure for SCD. This is discussed in Chapter 19.

Pre-operative management

Children with SCD commonly have grommet insertion and/or adenotonsillectomy for adenoidal hypertrophy and serous otitis media. Other paediatric operations include orchidopexy and hernia repair. Children with repeated episodes of acute splenic sequestration need splenectomy and those with symptomatic gall bladder disease will need cholecystectomy. Pre-operative management varies according to the type of operation and previous complications experienced by the child. There is evidence that exchange transfusion confers no extra benefit over top-up transfusion pre-operatively [29] and omission of transfusion has been shown to be safe in short procedures [30]. The following guidelines are currently in use at King's College Hospital London, UK.

Group 1

Short procedure, e.g. grommet insertion, herniotomy in a child with no special risk factors.
   Action – discuss top-up transfusion if Hb < 7 g/dL.

Group 2

Intermediate risk surgery such as adenoidectomy for moderate obstructive sleep apnoea or cholecystectomy in a child with no special risk factors.
   Action – top-up transfusion to Hb 9–10 g/dL.

Group 3

Major surgery, e.g. thoracotomy or children who have had chest crises and/or severe vaso-occlusive crises.
   Action – plan exchange transfusion or sequential top-up transfusions to achieve HbS level of 30% and Hb not greater than 12 g/dL.

References

1. Center for Diseases Control, USA. Mortality among children with sickle cell disease identified by newborn screening during 1990–4 – California, Illinois, and New York. *MMWR* 1998; **47**: 169–72.

2. Pegelow CH, Macklin EA, Moser FG *et al*. Longitudinal changes in brain magnetic resonance imaging findings in children with sickle cell disease. *Blood* 2002; **99**: 3014–18.

3. *NHS Plan. A Plan for Investment a Plan for Reform.* www.nhs.uk/nhsplan

4. Gaston MH, Verter JI, Woods G *et al*. Prophylaxis with oral penicillin in children with sickle cell anemia. *N Engl J Med* 1986; **314**: 1593–9.

5. Chief Medical Officer guidance (2002) Pneumococcal vaccine for at risk under 2 year olds. http://www.doh.gov.uk/co/cmo0201

6. Finn A, Booy R, Moxon R, Sharland M, Heath P. Should the new pneumococcal vaccine be used in high risk children? *Arch Dis Child* 2002; **87**: 18–21.

7. Oni L, Dick M, Smalling B, Walters J. *Care and Management of Your Child – Sickle Cell Disease, A Parents' Guide.* Brent Sickle Cell & Thalassaemia Centre, 1997.

8. Maxwell K, Streetly A. Living with sickle cell pain. *Nurs Stand* 1998; **13**: 33.

9. Pegelow CH, Colangelo L, Steinberg M *et al*. Natural history of blood pressure in sickle cell disease: risks for stroke and death associated with relative hypertension in sickle cell anaemia. *Am J Med* 1997; **102**: 171–7.

10. Patey RA, Sylvester KP, Rafferty GF, Dick M, Greenough A. The importance of using ethnically appropriate reference ranges for growth assessment in sickle cell disease. *Arch Dis Child* 2002; **87**: 352–3.

11. Reed JD, Redding-Lallinger R, Orringer EP. Nutrition and sickle cell disease. *Am J Haematol* 1987; **24**: 441–55.

12. Serjeant GR, Singhal A, Hambleton IR. Sickle cell disease and age at menarche in Jamaican girls: observations from a cohort study. *Arch Dis Child* 2001; **85**: 375–8.

13. Hall DMB, Elliman D. *Health for All Children*, 4th edn. Oxford: Oxford University Press, 2003.

14. Ohene-Frempong K, Weiner SJ, Sleeper LA *et al*. Cerebrovascular accidents in sickle cell disease and risk factors. *Blood* 1998; **91**: 288–94.

15. Adams RJ, McKie VC, Hsu L *et al*. Prevention of first stroke by transfusions in children with sickle cell anaemia and abnormal results on transcranial Doppler ultrasonography. *N Engl J Med* 1998; **339**: 5–11.

16. Platt OS, Brambilla DJ, Rosse WF *et al*. Mortality in sickle cell diease. Life expectancy and risk factors for early death. *N Engl J Med* 1994; **330**: 1639–44.

17. Miller ST, Sleeper LA, Pegelow CH *et al*. Prediction of adverse outcomes in children with sickle cell disease. *N Engl J Med* 2000; **342**: 1612–31.

18. Readett DR, Morris J, Serjeant GR. Determinants of nocturnal enuresis in homozygous sickle cell disease. *Arch Dis Child* 1990; **65**: 615–81.

19. Brooks LJ, Topol HI. Enuresis in children with sleep apnoea. *J Pediatr* 2003; **142**: 515–18.

20. Bond LR, Hatty SR, Horn ME *et al*. Gall stones in sickle cell disease in the United Kingdom. *BMJ* 1987; **295**: 234–6.

21. Mantadakis E, Ewalt DH, Cavender JD, Rogers ZR, Buchanan GR. Outpatient penile aspiration and epinephrine irrigation for young patients with sickle cell anaemia and prolonged priapism. *Blood* 2000; **95**: 78–82.

22. Helps S, Fuggle P, Udwin O, Dick M. Psychosocial and neurocognitive aspects of sickle cell disease. *Child and Adolescent Mental Health* 2003; **8**: 11–17.

23. Qureshi J, Buckingham S. A pain assessment tool for all children. *Paediatr Nurs* 1994; **6**: 11–13.

24. Rees DC, Olujohungbe AD, Parker NE *et al*. Guidelines for the management of the acute painful crisis in sickle cell disease. *Br J Haematol* 2003; **120**: 744–52.

25. Bellett PS, Kalinyak KA, Shukla R, Gelland MJ, Rucknagel DL. Incentive spirometry to prevent acute pulmonary complications in sickle cell disease. *N Engl J Med* 1995; **333**: 699–703.

26. Hargrave DR, Wade A, Evans JP, Hewes DK, Kirkham FJ. Nocturnal oxygen saturation and painful sickle cell crises in children. *Blood* 2003; **101**: 846–8.

27. Roberts I. The role of hydroxyurea in sickle cell disease. *Br J Haematol* 2003; **120**: 177–86.

28. Vichinsky EP, Lubin BH. A cautionary note regarding hydroxyurea in sickle cell disease. *Blood* 1994; **83**: 1124–8.

29. Vichinsky EP, Haberkern CM, Neumayr L *et al*. A comparison of conservative and aggressive transfusion regimens in the peri-operative management of sickle cell disease. *N Engl J Med* 1995; **333**: 251–2.

30. Griffin TC, Buchanan GR. Elective surgery in children with sickle cell disease without pre-operative blood transfusion. *J Pediatr Surg* 1993; **28**: 681–5.

Chapter 10

Acute chest syndrome in sickle cell disease

J Wright

Introduction

Under normal circumstances, oxygen loading of HbS-containing red cells occurs in a well-ventilated lung, making this the major site of sickle depolymerization. Normal gas exchange offers protection against excessive sickle polymerization and vaso-occlusion. Therefore it is not surprising that lung dysfunction can have severe consequences for the patient with sickle cell disease (SCD). When exposed to low oxygen tension, most organs respond by vasodilation to increase blood flow and hence oxygen delivery. The lung is unique in that in the presence of regional hypoxia vasoconstriction occurs to reduce shunting of blood through non-ventilated lung. In the non-sickle patient this mechanism will reduce ventilation–perfusion mismatch and improve oxygenation of blood passing through the pulmonary microcirculation. In the sickle patient it may also slow capillary transit times and increase erythrocyte–endothelial interaction, exacerbating vaso-occlusion and contributing to tissue infarction.

The lungs of patients with SCD can be affected by either acute or chronic forms of lung injury. The acute chest syndrome of SCD is the second most frequent cause of hospital admission for this group of patients [1]. More importantly it is a common cause of death in all age groups, accounting for 25% of deaths in SCD, and a leading cause of morbidity [2–4]. Chronic lung disease is increasingly recognized in older patients and is probably under-diagnosed. The final stages of sickle-mediated lung damage result in a severe restrictive lung defect with impaired gas transfer and pulmonary hypertension [1].

Definition

The acute chest syndrome represents a spectrum of lung injury with several underlying pathological processes. An appropriate clinical definition of acute chest syndrome would be a syndrome consisting of chest pain, dyspnoea, fever and pulmonary infiltrates on chest X-ray. A strict interpretation of this definition means that straightforward pneumonia (which of course presents with dyspnoea, fever and infiltrates) cannot be diagnosed in SCD. Although this is probably not entirely true it demonstrates the complex nature of acute chest syndrome; treatment of acute chest syndrome as infection alone is unlikely to be successful.

Incidence and risk factors

In the USA the Co-operative Study of Sickle Cell Disease [5] followed several thousand patients with a variety of sickling disorders, and identified 2100 episodes of acute chest syndrome in 1085 patients of all ages. The incidence was higher in the phenotypically more severe disorders (HbSS disease and HbS β^0 thalassaemia). Risk factors for the development of acute chest syndrome were younger age, low HbF, higher steady-state Hb and higher steady-state white cell count [5].

Pathophysiology

Several pathophysiological processes including fat emboli from infarcted bone marrow, infection, atelectasis and splinting from rib infarction, *in situ* thrombus formation and vessel occlusion, and red cell sequestration in the pulmonary microvasculature have been implicated in acute chest syndrome. An individual episode is likely to represent a combination of pathological processes accounting for the wide clinical spectrum.

Pulmonary fat embolism

The presence of embolic fragments of infarcted bone marrow in the pulmonary vasculature was first noted as an autopsy finding of uncertain significance [6]. Subsequently broncho-alveolar lavage has suggested that the presence of fat embolism is a common occurrence in acute chest syndrome [7]. Fat-containing macrophages are seen in both children and adults with acute chest syndrome in 40–60% of cases [7, 8]. Indeed there are many similarities between acute chest syndrome and the clinical syndrome of fat embolism that may follow trauma. Recently Vichinsky and the National Acute Chest Syndrome Study Group [9] published details of a prospective multicentre series of 671 episodes and again fat embolism featured prominently as a causative factor. They also noted that a typical skeletal painful crisis was effectively the prodrome for acute chest syndrome, occurring 2–3 days before the onset of acute chest syndrome in almost half the cases. It is likely that the fat emboli arise from areas of infarcted bone marrow. This is supported by the temporal relationship between pain and acute chest syndrome and the occasional autopsy finding of infarcted bone marrow even including bony spicules in the pulmonary vasculature.

Elevated levels of secretory phospholipase A2 (PLA2) have also been demonstrated in acute chest syndrome. This enzyme is an important inflammatory mediator that liberates free fatty acids. These free fatty acids are felt to be at least partially responsible for the lung injury following fat embolism. Elevated levels of secretory PLA2 may precede and predict the development of an episode of acute chest syndrome [10].

Infection

The poor response of acute chest syndrome to an-

Table 10.1 Infectious pathogens implicated in acute chest syndrome

Mycoplasma pneumoniae
Chlamydia pneumoniae
Respiratory syncytial virus
Streptococcus pneumoniae
Haemophilus influenzae
Escherichia coli
Legionella pneumophila
Influenza and parainflunenza viruses
Staphylococcus aureus

tibiotics alone and the impressively rapid response to transfusion support a non-infective cause for the majority of cases. However, the presence of an immune defect not wholly explained by hyposplenism along with areas of infarcted lung tissue provide an excellent environment for infection even if this was not the primary event. The organisms implicated in acute chest syndrome vary. An aggressive search for organisms by the National Acute Chest Syndrome Study Group detected evidence of infection in just over one-third of their 671 cases; 27 different organisms were implicated, including viruses, typical and atypical organisms [9] (Table 10.1). Although widespread use of penicillin prophylaxis and vaccination against *Pneumococcus* and *Haemophilus influenzae* B may have reduced the frequency, these organisms may still be isolated from patients with acute chest syndrome. Atypical organisms such as mycoplasma and chlamydia also occur and were the most common organisms isolated by the National Acute Chest Syndrome Study Group.

Recently parvovirus B19 has also been associated with acute chest syndrome, possibly by causing marrow necrosis and embolization [11].

Hypoventilation and splinting

The hypothesis that pain and hypoventilation may contribute to the development of acute chest syndrome was based on the observation that rib infarction was temporally related to the development of acute chest syndrome [12]. A recent study looking at breathing patterns in patients with thoracic and non-thoracic sickle pain has confirmed that thoracic pain leads to acute chest syndrome in part due to shallow breathing [13]. Other studies have convincingly demonstrated the link between rib infarction and radiographic changes of acute chest syndrome. The low tidal volume–high respiratory rate associated with splinting probably leads to regional hypoxia and atelectasis, providing a good environment for a vicious cycle of further vaso-occlusion, further hypoxia, etc. Supporting this concept, a randomized trial of incentive spirometry to improve ventilation reduced the incidence of pulmonary complications [14]. Over-narcotization and consequent hypoventilation may also contribute [15]. Although pain control is important in acute chest syndrome, care should be taken that this is not at the expense of oxygenation.

Thrombus formation/endothelial dysfunction

There is ample evidence of a biochemical hyper-coagulable state in SCD [16, 17]. The endothelium is also activated [18], with increased levels of vaso-constrictors and decreased production of nitric oxide [19], which further exacerbates this tendency to constriction. Increased expression of endothelial adhesion molecules (such as VCAM-1) induced by hypoxia and cytokines further exacerbates pulmonary vascular occlusion [20]. In this setting microvascular thrombus formation and tissue infarction is likely to be secondary to *in situ* phenomena rather than representing embolism from distant sites.

Red cell sequestration

The phenomenon of trapping or sequestration of sickle red cells in vascular beds is a recurrent theme in several complications of SCD, for example, acute splenic or hepatic sequestration. Patients showing rapid clinical deterioration, hypoxia and a progressive 'white out' on chest X-ray associated with a rapid decline in Hb demonstrate the most extreme form of pulmonary sequestration and, if caught early enough, can respond dramatically to transfusion [21]. A rapid decrease in Hb of approximately 1 g/dL is a common finding in many patients with acute chest syndrome and may represent a more moderate form of sequestration.

Other contributory factors

Based upon a questionnaire study, smoking may increase the risk of acute chest syndrome [22] and common sense would dictate that prolonged and regular consumption may contribute to the development of chronic lung disease.

Reversible airway obstruction is likely to be a contributory factor; 20% of patients treated with bronchodilators in the National Acute Chest Syndrome Study Group showed a significant improvement in FEV1 [9]. There are occasional reports of mucinous casts occluding the bronchial tree; once removed at bronchoscopy there is a rapid improvement in oxygenation [23]. Figure 10.1 gives a diagrammatic illustration of the pathogenesis of acute chest syndrome [24].

Clinical features and diagnosis

By definition, patients will present with cough, fever, dyspnoea and chest pain. However, there is variation in the frequency of these symptoms with age, fever and cough with evidence of reversible airways obstruction being more common in the under-10s and chest pain and breathlessness predominating in the older patient. A seasonal predilection is present in young children, with an increase in the winter months suggesting an infective component [25]. A prodrome of skeletal painful crisis becomes an increasingly common finding in the over-20s [25]. Presenting symptoms observed during a first episode of acute chest syndrome are predictive of symptoms during subsequent events (Table 10.2).

Examination

The most common findings are crepitations and dullness to percussion [25]. Clinical signs suggestive of pleural effusion may be present more frequently in adults than in children, but this does not predict an infective aetiology. It is important to remember that about a third of patients may have a normal chest examination [25].

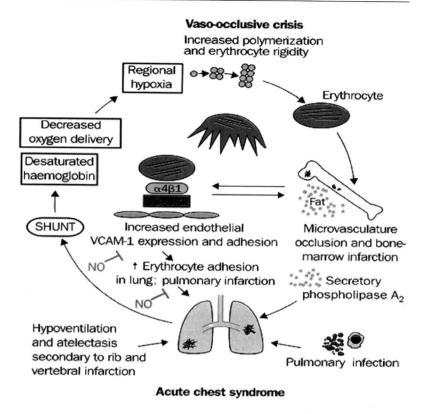

Fig. 10.1 The pathogenesis of acute chest (taken from Gladwin and Rodgers [24]).

Table 10.2 Differences in presentation of acute chest syndrome in children and adults

Children	Adults
Seasonal predilection (winter > summer)	High rates of morbidity and mortality
Commonly present with fever, cough and wheeze	Present with chest pain, dyspnoea and painful crisis
Radiographs show more frequent upper and middle lobe changes	Radiographs show lower and multilobe changes
Bacteraemia and viraemia more common	Organisms rarely isolated
Fewer transfusions necessary	High rate of transfusion

Radiology

A chest X-ray should always be performed in patients with SCD and respiratory symptoms. Although lower lobe involvement is the most common finding in all ages, radiographic findings vary with age; young children have more frequent isolated involvement of the upper and middle lobes [25]. Adults, on the other hand, present more commonly with multilobe involvement and pleural effusion. Clinical signs often lag behind radiological findings.

Isotope bone scans can demonstrate the presence of rib infarction, although usually the diagnosis of rib pain is clear on clinical grounds alone [12].

The diagnosis of pulmonary embolus (PE) represents a challenge in SCD. VQ scanning is difficult to interpret under normal circumstances, and many non-sickle patients have indeterminate scans. Add to this the complicating factor of SCD with possible previous lung damage, *in situ* vaso-occlusion, and scans become even harder to interpret. The availability of previous scans for comparison may be helpful but the VQ scan can be abnormal even in the absence of an acute pulmonary event [26]. Pulmonary angiography is rarely performed because of the interventional nature of the procedure and the theoretical risks of contrast media, but even this test can be difficult to interpret because of abnormalities in the pulmonary vascular tree. The confident diagnosis of a PE is therefore a difficult one to make.

'Common things occur commonly' is a phrase much used in medical education and in general the sickle patient with chest pain fever and dyspnoea should be treated as having acute chest syndrome rather than PE. Although infarction may feature in the pathogenesis of this disorder it is likely to be secondary to *in situ* changes and bone marrow/fat embolus rather than a clot migrating from the deep veins of the leg or pelvis. Postoperative and postpartum periods are both known to be associated with an increased risk of vascular thromboembolism (VTE) (as well as acute chest syndrome) and if a PE is suspected in these situations imaging of deep veins to look for deep vein thrombosis (DVT) may be helpful as supporting evidence for a PE. However, a brisk response to transfusion is more suggestive of an episode of acute chest syndrome rather than VTE.

Laboratory investigations

The development of acute chest syndrome is almost invariably associated with a drop in haemoglobin (generally 0.7–1 g/dL but occasionally more) from steady-state values [9]. Reticulocytes may be either increased as an appropriate response to anaemia or decreased suggesting a temporary erythroid hypoplasia. The white cell count will increase with a prominent neutrophilia [25]. Platelet counts may be relatively decreased in some patients at the time of diagnosis, but thrombocytosis is common in the recovery period [27]. A platelet count of $< 200 \times 10^9$ is a predictor of morbidity and mortality. Inflammatory markers such as C-reactive protein (CRP) are raised even in steady-state [28] but are likely to increase further during acute chest syndrome.

Oxygen saturation and blood gases

Several studies have assessed the optimal approach to monitoring of oxygenation in SCD. Many patients with SCD have low baseline oxygen saturation. There are several potential mechanisms for this. The right-shifted oxygen dissociation curve (HbS being a low affinity haemoglobin) may contribute and some patients with previous episodes may have early undiagnosed changes of chronic sickle lung disease. In the Jamaican cohort study mean oxygen saturation by pulse oximetry was 92.5% in a population of patients with homozygous SCD in steady-state [29]. Almost a quarter of this group had saturations below 90%. Other studies have established that pulse oximetry is a reliable method for monitoring these patients, although values calculated from blood gas analysis tend to underestimate saturation even in steady-state [30–32]. Monitoring of trends in pulse oximetry supplemented by blood gas analysis as required is therefore indicated.

Management

Periods of increased risk

As discussed above the presence of painful crisis and rib/sternal/thoracic spine infarction may contribute to the pathogenesis of acute chest syndrome. Other clinical scenarios are also associated with an increased risk (Table 10.3). Postoperatively, especially following abdominal surgery, the sickle patient maybe immobile and in pain with diaphragmatic splinting. The acute phase response that follows surgery constitutes a further component increasing the likelihood of acute chest syndrome, which may occur in 10% of patients [33]. Optimal peri-operative management is discussed elsewhere in this book, but this increased risk of acute chest syndrome is one of the reasons transfusion is recommended by many as pre-operative preparation. Similarly, the sickle patient who is in the final trimester of pregnancy or postpartum

Table 10.3 Periods of increased risk for the development of acute chest syndrome

Risk period	Contributory factors
Postoperative (particularly after abdominal surgery)	Splinting, dehydration, infection
During painful crisis	Fat embolus, dehydration
Patient with rib pain	Fat embolus, splinting
Postpartum	Unknown
Final trimester of pregnancy	Unknown
Post general anaesthetic	

appears to be at increased risk [34, 35]. These groups of patients should therefore be monitored closely for evidence of hypoxia, fever and consolidation.

Prevention

The risks of acute chest syndrome maybe reduced for patients in the above high risk situations by the use of incentive spirometry [14]. Encouraging the patient to take 10 maximal inspirations every 2 hours while awake has been shown to significantly reduce the incidence of acute chest syndrome in patients with thoracic pain and is also likely to be useful in other high risk situations.

Hydroxyurea is a very useful agent in SCD, in addition to the reduction in frequency and intensity of pain seen in a multicentre, randomized, blinded trial of hydroxyurea, the patients on hydroxyurea have a 50% reduction in the frequency of acute chest syndrome [36]. This reduction in acute chest syndrome in adults on hydroxyurea may be a result of the reduced incidence of bone marrow infarction and hence fat embolism. As recurrent acute chest syndrome is likely to be a risk factor for the development of chronic lung disease, this agent can be used to reduce this risk and possibly slow progression in patients who have recurrent attacks of acute chest syndrome [37].

Chronic transfusion programmes will also reduce or abolish attacks of acute chest syndrome; however, this mode of treatment carries significant long-term side-effects relating particularly to iron overload and allo-immunization and should not be undertaken lightly [38].

Bone marrow transplantation has also been employed in patients with recurrent acute chest syndrome.

Treatment

In the absence of randomized trials many of the recommendations in this section are based on the large follow-up studies carried out in the USA. As in many of the complications of SCD the foundations for a proper evidence-based approach are lacking. In general the diagnosis of acute chest syndrome is not difficult and appropriate management will reduce the risks of morbidity and mortality. Problems arise when the diagnosis and the vascular nature of the event are not recognized. The key to correct treatment is therefore early and accurate diagnosis.

The mainstays of therapy for this condition are: monitoring, supplemental oxygen, antimicrobial agents, analgesia, hydration and transfusion.

Monitoring

Several studies have assessed the optimal approach to monitoring of oxygen saturation [30–32]. Continuous (or at least 6-hourly) pulse oximetry would seem to be the optimal approach, possibly supplemented by blood gas analysis at baseline and in the event of deterioration.

Patients also require monitoring of haemoglobin, as significant decreases may occur with the acute chest syndrome. Reticulocyte counts may either be appropriately increased in response to the anaemia or may fall, signalling erythroid hypoplasia as a non-specific response. Erythroid aplasia is unusual, although it is occasionally seen with severe bacterial infections as well as parvovirus B19 [39].

Antimicrobial agents

The presence or absence of infection is difficult to

establish by routine studies such as blood/sputum cultures. Empirical antibiotics should therefore be prescribed. The National ACS Study Group in the USA identified a variety of typical, atypical and viral organisms. A cephalosporin such as cefuroxime or ceftazidime will cover the appropriate bacterial culprits and the addition of a macrolide such as erythromycin will treat mycoplasma or chlamydial infections [9]. Bronchoscopy is not routinely indicated.

Analgesia

Many patients will require analgesia for chest pain or other sickle-related skeletal pain. Opiates supplemented by non-steroidal agents are appropriate. Care should be taken to avoid over-narcotization, which may exacerbate hypoxia.

Hydration

Hyposthenuria, an inability to concentrate urine, is a feature of SCD present almost from birth [40]. Patients with pain and under the influence of opiates may fail to drink and pyrexia increases insensible losses. Dehydration is thus a constant threat and will contribute to HbS polymerization. Fluid balance should be monitored carefully in all patients. Care should be taken to avoid fluid overload in the patient with acute chest syndrome, because pulmonary oedema will contribute to hypoxia. There is little evidence to direct the choice of intravenous fluids, although there are some theoretical problems associated with the overuse of normal saline. A sensible approach would be the use of 5% dextrose saline.

Supplemental oxygen

Patients will be hypoxic in association with acute chest syndrome and require supplemental O_2. Failure of saturation to rise in response to high concentrations of oxygen should prompt transfusion.

Bronchodilators

The acute phase of acute chest syndrome is associated with significant reductions in FEV1. Up to 20% of these patients demonstrate clinical improvement and increase in FEV1 when treated with bronchodilators [9]. The use of, for example, nebulized salbutamol should be encouraged, particularly in children.

Transfusion

Transfusion of packed cells is currently the mainstay of treatment and has a number of theoretical benefits:
• Correction of a more severe anaemia may improve oxygen delivery.
• It will decrease the fraction of HbS-containing cells.
• It will decrease viscosity in the case of exchange transfusion.

Many studies have demonstrated the benefits of transfusion in acute chest syndrome. Marked and rapid improvement in oxygenation, lysis of fever and improvement in the general clinical status are seen in many patients of all ages [9, 41–43]. However, there are no randomized controlled trials on which to base firm recommendations as to the extent, type (exchange or top-up) and timing of transfusion. Despite the lack of trials there is no doubt that transfusion is beneficial in curtailing the episode of acute chest syndrome, indeed failure to transfuse is an all too frequent cause of death in this condition.

The key to appropriate transfusion in acute chest syndrome is the timing rather than the volume of blood used or the target %HbS. In most cases an *early* top-up or partial exchange transfusion is the optimal approach. The National ACS Study Group showed that simple top-up transfusion was used in 68% of patients using an average of 3.2 units of packed cells. This appeared to be as effective as an exchange transfusion [9]. Many haematology departments now have access to automated cell separators that can reduce %HbS to very low levels. These have been demonstrated to be effective in several series [44, 45]. The problem with this approach is that frequently staff may be unavailable to perform such a time-consuming procedure on an urgent basis. In the hypoxic deteriorating patient with acute chest syndrome such delays can have severe consequences. The findings of Vichinsky *et al.* [9] are therefore very reassuring for those with limited access to automated pheresis facilities.

In the absence of a randomized controlled trial a sensible approach is to use simple top-up transfusion, aiming for a haemoglobin of no more than 9–10 g/dL, in patients with relatively mild episodes or those with severe anaemia (e.g. < 5 g/dL) and to use exchange transfusion in the more severe cases. Again the timing of exchange transfusion is crucial. It is preferable to perform a limited manual partial exchange urgently rather than wait for several hours or overnight until staff are available to perform an automated exchange. The procedure of partial manual exchange transfusion is detailed in Chapter 20. Transfused blood should be matched for Rhesus and Kell antigens, this precaution will reduce rates of allo-immunization, previously reported at up to 20% [46], to single figures. If extended red cell phenotype of the patient is unknown the patient should be given either R0 or rr blood. Most patients only require a single transfusion episode, with oxygenation and overall clinical status improving over 12 hours or so post-transfusion. Because of the high risk of line-related sepsis and thrombosis in this patient group central lines should be removed as soon as possible.

Role of critical care service

Depending upon ward staffing levels and nursing expertise it maybe appropriate to manage some patients on High Dependency Units or to involve Critical Care Outreach teams to optimize care. If this is felt to be appropriate early involvement of such teams is advised. Occasional patients may deteriorate rapidly and become severely hypoxic. Transfusion is still the top priority; however, ventilatory or CPAP support may become necessary. In the National ACS Study Group, 13% of patients required ventilatory support and the vast majority of these made a good recovery [9]. CPAP has been used with some success in small numbers of patients.

Other measures

The difficulty in diagnosing PE, the presence of biochemical evidence of coagulation and platelet activation with fibrin deposition in the pulmonary microcirculation prompt the question 'what is the role of anticoagulants in acute chest syndrome?'. There are certainly theoretical grounds for the use of anticoagulants, although there are no clinical data on which to base a reasoned answer to this question. It is the author's practice to use prophylactic subcutaneous low molecular weight heparin in patients with acute chest syndrome.

Outcome of acute chest syndrome

If managed correctly the vast majority of episodes will resolve without long-term sequelae. Acute chest syndrome in children tends to resolve more quickly; this is reflected in shorter average hospital stays (5–6 days) compared with adults (10–11 days) [9, 25]. Overall mortality rates are about 2%; however, there is a striking difference between adults and children, risk being significantly higher in adults [9, 25]. There appears to be an increase in the frequency of neurological events during acute chest syndrome, such as seizure and cerebrovascular accidents, presumably representing the effect of hypoxia or severe anaemia on an already compromised cerebral circulation [9]. Recurrent episodes of acute chest syndrome may contribute to the development of chronic sickle lung.

Say NO to acute chest syndrome

Much of the morbidity associated with acute chest syndrome arises from pulmonary vascular occlusion and ischaemia regardless of the aetiology. Reduction of hypoventilation/atelectasis can be achieved by the use of incentive spirometry, painful crisis frequency and hence incidence of bone marrow/fat embolism can be reduced by the use of hydroxyurea. However, to date, other than transfusion there are limited measures which may reduce the severity and duration of an established episode of acute chest syndrome. As this remains a major cause of morbidity and mortality in all age groups there is an urgent need for other treatments.

A novel approach would be to reduce the hypoxia and shunting which accompany acute chest syndrome and contribute to the maintenance of the vicious cycle of sickling–vascular occlusion–hypoxia–more sickling. If this potential therapeutic compound could also favourably influence the erythrocyte–endothelial interaction then it would hold great promise . . . enter nitric oxide (NO) [19, 47].

NO is generated from L-arginine by NO synthases. Among its functions is the maintenance of vascular tone [48]. NO is a potent vasodilator and cytoprotective agent with a high affinity for oxygenated haemoglobin. Subtle changes in the structure of haemoglobin in the presence of reduced oxygen tension favour the dissociation of NO, which may then mediate local vasodilation, via changes in subendothelial muscle tone, improving blood supply to the hypoxic area [49, 50]. This mechanism has particular relevance for the pulmonary microvasculature, which constricts with hypoxia unlike other vascular beds. As reduced capillary transit time is an important determinant of HbS polymerization [51], then there are theoretical advantages to reducing vasoconstriction. Furthermore, there is *in vitro* evidence that NO may inhibit erythrocyte adhesion to hypoxic endothelium [47]. Available data suggest that NO and its metabolites are reduced in acute chest syndrome [19]. There are therefore several potential pathways by which NO may positively influence the course of acute chest syndrome.

Limited experience in adult respiratory distress syndrome (ARDS) – which is also characterized by intrapulmonary shunting, hypoxaemia, vasoconstriction and widespread occlusion of the pulmonary vasculature – adds further support to the use of NO. In a small study of 10 patients with ARDS, inhalation of low concentrations of NO reduced pulmonary artery pressure and increased oxygenation by improving matching of ventilation and perfusion [52]. Using inhalation as the route of delivery means that the vasodilatory effect of NO should be limited to the ventilated regions of the lung. This is in contrast to systemically administered vasodilators, which may cause widespread vasodilation and worsen ventilation–perfusion mismatch. Interestingly, hydroxyurea has recently been shown to be a NO donor, possibly contributing to its protective effect on acute chest syndrome [53].

There are, however, potential risks to the use of therapeutic NO in the sick patient. Inhaled or endogenously produced NO may generate powerful oxidants which may contribute to lung injury [54]. Binding to haemoglobin may adversely alter oxygen affinity [55]. A phenomenon of rebound hypoxia and pulmonary hypertension has been seen in other conditions after the use of NO, with a possible recurrence of the original pathology on withdrawal of treatment [56].

Despite these caveats, NO is a potentially exciting development in the management of acute chest syndrome, although thus far experience is limited to occasional cases [57].

Other potential developments

As discussed above, a rise in serum PLA2 levels can predict the onset of acute chest syndrome even before clinical signs/symptoms. Ongoing studies are assessing the use of pre-emptive transfusion in patients with painful crisis and elevated PLA2.

Flocor, a non-ionic surfactant, appears to decrease red cell–endothelial interaction and has been shown to prevent lung injury in animal models [58]. Phase I studies in the treatment of acute chest syndrome have commenced.

References

1. Powars D, Weidman JA, Odom-Maryon T, Niland JC, Johnson C. Sickle cell chronic lung disease and the role of pulmonary failure. *Medicine* 1988; **67**: 66–76.
2. Platt OS, Brambilla DJ, Rosse WF *et al*. Mortality in sickle cell disease: life expectancy in sickle cell disease in the U.S. *N Engl J Med* 1994; **30**: 1639–44.
3. Thomas AN, Pattison C, Serjeant GR. Causes of death in sickle cell disease in Jamaica. *BMJ* 1982; **285**: 633–5.
4. Gray A, Anionwu EN, Davies SC, Brozovic M. Patterns of mortality in sickle cell disease in the UK. *J Clin Pathol* 1994; **44**: 459–63.
5. Castro O, Brambilla DJ, Thorington B *et al*. The acute chest syndrome of sickle cell disease: incidence and risk factors. The Co-operative Study of Sickle Cell Disease. *Blood* 1994; **84**: 643–9.
6. Haupt HM, Moor GW, Bauer TW. The lung in sickle cell disease. *Chest* 1982; **81**: 332–7.
7. Vichinsky E, Williams R, Das M *et al*. Pulmonary fat embolism: a distinct cause of severe acute chest syndrome in sickle cell anaemia. *Blood* 1994; **83**: 3107–12.
8. Godeau B, Schaeffer A, Bachir D *et al*. Bronchoalveolar lavage in adult sickle cell patients with acute chest syn-

drome: value for diagnostic assessment of fat embolism. *Am J Respir Crit Care Med* 1996; **153**: 1691–6.

9. Vichinsky E, Neumayr L, Earles AN *et al.* Causes and outcomes of the acute chest syndrome in sickle cell disease. *N Engl J Med* 2000; **342**: 1855–65.

10. Styles LA, Schalkwijk CG, Aarsmam AJ *et al.* Phospholipase A$_2$ levels in acute chest syndrome. *Blood* 1996; **87**: 2573–7.

11. Lowenthal EL, Wells A, Emanuel PD, Player R, Prehal JT. Sickle cell acute chest syndrome associated with parvovirus B19 infection. Case series and review. *Am J Hematol* 1996; **51**: 207–13.

12. Gelfand MJ, Daya SA, Rucknagel DL, Kalinyak KA, Paltiel HS. Simultaneous occurrence of rib infarction and pulmonary infiltrates in sickle cell disease patients with acute chest syndromes. *J Nucl Med* 1993; **34**: 614–18.

13. Needleman JP, Benjamin LJ, Sykes JA, Aldrich TK. Breathing patterns during vaso-occlusive crisis of sickle cell disease. *Chest* 2002; **122**: 43–6.

14. Bellet PS, Kalinyak KA, Shukla R, Gelfand M J, Rucknagel DL. Incentive spirometry to prevent acute pulmonary complications in sickle cell diseases. *N Engl J Med* 1995; **333**: 699–703.

15. Palmer J, Broderick KA, Naiman JL. Acute lung syndrome during painful sickle cell crisis: relation to site of pain and narcotic requirement. *Blood* 1983; **62**: 59a.

16. Wright JG, Malia R, Cooper P *et al.* Protein C and protein S in homozygous sickle cell disease: does hepatic dysfunction contribute to low levels. *Br J Haematol* 1997; **98**: 627–31.

17. Peters M, Plaat BE, Tencate H *et al.* Enhanced thrombin generation in children with sickle cell disease. *Thromb Haemost* 1994; **71**: 169–72.

18. Blann AD, Marwah S, Serjeant G, Bareford D, Wright J. Platelet activation and endothelial cell dysfunction in sickle cell disease is unrelated to reduced anti-oxident capacity. *Blood Coagul Fibrinolysis* 2003; **14**: 255–9.

19. Stuart MJ, Setty BNY. Sickle cell acute chest syndrome: pathogenesis and rationale for treatment. *Blood* 1999; **94**: 1555–60.

20. Setty BNY, Stuart MJ. Vascular cell adhesion molecule-1 is involved in mediating hypoxia induced sickle red blood cell adherence to the endothelium: potential role in sickle cell disease. *Blood* 1996; **88**: 2311–20.

21. Serjeant GR, Serjeant BE. *Sickle Cell Disease*, 3rd edn. Oxford: Oxford University Press, 2001.

22. Young RC, Rachal RE, Hackeney RL, Uy CG, Scott RB. Smoking is a factor in causing acute chest syndrome in sickle cell anaemia. *J Natl Med Assoc* 1992; **8**: 267–71.

23. Raghuram N, Pettignano R, Gal A, Horsch A, Adamkiewicz T. Plastic bronchitis: an unusual complication associated with sickle cell disease and the acute chest syndrome. *Pediatrics* 1997; **100**: 139–42.

24. Gladwin MT, Rodgers GP. Pathogenesis and treatment

of acute chest syndrome in sickle cell anaemia. *Lancet* 2000; **355**: 1476–8.

25. Vichinsky EP, Styles LA, Colangelo LH *et al.* Acute chest syndrome in sickle cell disease: clinical presentation and course. *Blood* 1997; **89**: 1787–92.

26. Walker BK, Ballas SK, Burka ER. The diagnosis of pulmonary thromboembolism in sickle cell disease. *Am J Hematol* 1979; **1**: 219–32.

27. Van Agfmael MA, Cheng JD, Nossent HC. Acute chest syndrome in adult Afro-Caribbean patients with sickle cell disease. *Arch Intern Med* 1994; **154**: 557–61.

28. Singhal A, Doherty JF, Raynes JG *et al.* Is there an acute phase response in steady state sickle cell disease? *Lancet* 1993; **341**: 651–3.

29. Homi J, Levec L, Higgs D, Thomas P, Serjeant G. Pulse oximetry in a cohort study of sickle cell disease. *Clin Lab Haematol* 1997; **19**: 17–22.

30. Rackoff WR, Kunkel N, Silber JH, Asakura T, Ohene-Frempong K. Pulse oximetry and factors associated with haemoglobin oxygen desaturation in children with sickle cell disease. *Blood* 1993; **81**: 3422–7.

31. Kress JP, Pahlman AS, Hall JB. Determination of haemoglobin saturation in patients with acute sickle chest syndrome: a comparison of arterial blood gases and pulse oximetry. *Chest* 1999; **115**: 1316–20.

32. Ortiz FO, Aldrich TK, Nagel RL, Benjamin LJ. Accuracy of pulse oximetry in sickle cell disease. *Am J Respir Crit Care Med* 1999; **159**: 447–51.

33. Vichinsky EP, Haberkern CM, Neumayr L *et al.* A comparison of conservative and aggressive transfusion regimens in the peri-operative management of sickle cell disease. *N Engl J Med* 1995; **333**: 206–13.

34. Poddar D, Maude GH, Plant MJ, Scorer H, Serjeant GR. Pregnancy in Jamaican women with homozygous sickle cell disease. Fetal and maternal outcome. *Br J Obstet Gynaecol* 1986; **6**: 727–32.

35. Smith JA, Espeland M, Bellvue R *et al.* Pregnancy in sickle cell disease: experience of the cooperative study of sickle cell disease. *Obstet Gynecol* 1996; **87**: 199–204.

36. Charache S, Terrin ML, Moore RD *et al.* Effect of hydroxyurea on the frequency of painful crisis in sickle cell anaemia. *N Engl J Med* 1995; **332**: 1317–22.

37. Koren A, Segal-Kupeshmit D, Lalman L *et al.* Effect of hydroxyurea in sickle cell anaemia: a clinical trial in teenagers with severe sickle cell anaemia and sickle β thalassaemia. *Pediatr Hematol Oncol* 1999; **16**: 221–32.

38. Serjeant GR. Chronic transfusions regimes in sickle cell disease. Problem or panacea. *Br J Haematol* 1997; **97**: 253–5.

39. Wright J, Thomas P, Serjeant GR. Septicaemia caused by salmonella infection; an overlooked complication of sickle cell disease. *J Pediatr* 1997; **130**: 394–9.

40. Keitel HG, Thompason D, Itario HA. Hyposthenuria in sickle cell anaemia: a reversible renal defect. *J Clin Invest* 1957; **39**: 998–1007.

41. Van de Pelte JEW, Pearson TC, Slater NGP. Exchange transfusion in life threatening sickling crisis. *J R Soc Med* 1982; **83**: 3107–12.

42. Mallouh AA, Asha M. Beneficial effects of blood transfusion in children with sickle chest syndrome. *Am J Dis Child* 1998; **142**: 178–82.

43. Emre U, Miller ST, Gutierez M *et al*. Effect of transfusion in acute chest syndrome of sickle cell disease. *J Pediatr* 1995; **127**: 901–4.

44. Jones SL, Pocock M, Bishop E, Bevan DH. Automated red cell exchange in sickle cell disease. *Br J Haematol* 1997; **97**: 256–8.

45. Lawson SE, Oakley S, Smith NA, Bareford D. Red cell exchange in sickle cell disease. *Clin Lab Haematol* 1999; **21**: 99–102.

46. Vichinsky EP, Earles A, Johnson RA *et al*. Alloimmunization in sickle cell anemia and transfusion of racially unmatched blood. *N Engl J Med* 1990; **322**: 1617–21.

47. Stuart M, Setty BNY. Acute chest syndrome of sickle cell disease. New light on an old problem. *Curr Opin Haematol* 2001; **8**: 111–22.

48. Palmer RMJ, Ashton DS, Moncada S. Vascular endothelial cells synthesize nitric oxide from 1-arginine. *Nature* 1988; **333**: 664–6.

49. Jia L, Bonaventura C, Bonaventura J, Stamler JS. 5-Nitroso-haemoglobin: a dynamic activity of blood involved in vascular control. *Nature* 1996; **380**: 221–6.

50. Gow AJ, Stamler JS. Reactions between nitric oxide and haemoglobin under physiological conditions. *Nature* 1998; **391**: 169–73.

51. Steinberg MH. Management of sickle cell disease. *N Engl J Med* 1999; **340**: 1021–30.

52. Rossaint R, Falke KJ, Lopez F *et al*. Inhaled nitric oxide for the adult respiratory distress syndrome. *N Engl J Med* 1993; **328**: 399–405.

53. Pacilli R, Tarra J, Cook JA, Wink DA, Krishna MC. Hydroxyurea reacts with heme proteins to generate nitric oxide. *Lancet* 1996; **347**: 900.

54. Hart CM. Nitric oxide in adult lung disease. *Chest* 1999; **150**: 1407–17.

55. Head CA, Brugnara C, Martinez Rius R *et al*. Low concentrations of nitric oxide increase oxygen affinity of sickle erythrocytes in vitro and vivo. *J Clin Invest* 1997; **100**: 1193–8.

56. Kinsella JP, Abman SH. Clinical approach to inhaled nitric oxide therapy in the newborn with hypoxemia. *J Pediatr* 2000; **150**: 717–26.

57. Atz AM, Wessel DL. Inhaled nitric oxide in sickle cell disease with acute chest syndrome. *Anesthesiology* 1997; **87**: 988–90.

58. Lian LR, Ollinger FK. Flocor can prevent the development of hypoxia induced ACS in transgenic sickle cell mice. 24th Annual Meeting of the National Sickle Cell Disease Programme, 2000.

Chapter 11
Blood transfusion therapy for haemoglobinopathies

Nay Win

Transfusion support for sickle cell disease

Sickle cell disease (SCD) is characterized by chronic haemolysis and intermittent vaso-occlusion, leading to tissue hypoxia and organ dysfunction.

The mean haemoglobin (Hb) level for SCD (HbSS) is 8 g/dL (range 4.1–13.5) and for sickle beta thalassaemia is 8.9 g/dL (range 6.6–12). HbSS releases oxygen readily to tissue, because of its low affinity to oxygen. Therefore a steady-state Hb level of 5 g/dL is often well tolerated by these patients. However, sustained Hb levels below 5 g/dL should be avoided, as increased cerebral flow and flow velocity associated with severe chronic anaemia may result in watershed infarction [1, 2].

Although red cell transfusions are not usually required in steady-state patients, they remain a mainstay therapy for many complications. There are definite indications for certain clinical situations and some recommendations are based on the findings of design studies and also randomized control trials. However, controversy remains in some areas. Allo-immunization, haemolytic transfusion reactions and iron overload are the distinct adverse effects of red cell transfusions in patients with SCD. Therefore, it is important to understand the aim of transfusion therapy and to be aware of the potential side-effects.

There are several forms of transfusion therapy: simple transfusion, exchange transfusion and chronic transfusion (hypertransfusion regime).

Simple transfusion

This is indicated in episodes of acutely worsening symptomatic anaemia.

Indications for simple transfusion

Aplastic crisis
This is generally caused by the B19 strain of the parvovirus. Aplastic crises are usually transient in nature and do not require transfusion. However, transfusion should be reserved for those who have either evidence of cardiorespiratory compromise or have an Hb level below 5 g/dL with reticulocytopenia [3].

Splenic sequestration
This crisis commonly occurs in infants and young children and is characterized by sudden massive pooling of red cells in the spleen. A major splenic sequestration crisis is defined as an acute fall in Hb level to < 6 g/dL or a fall of Hb > 3 g/dL compared with the baseline value [4].

Hepatic sequestration
This usually occurs in adults and is characterized by a rapid enlargement of the liver [5].

Exchange transfusion

In SCD the blood viscosity is affected by both the haematocrit and the %HbS red cells. At a fixed %HbS, the viscosity increases with the haematocrit and at a fixed haematocrit, the viscosity increases with increasing percentage of HbS [6, 7]. Therefore, if a simple top-up transfusion is given and if the haematocrit rises above 35%, without a significant reduction in the percentage of sickle cells, this could result in a significant increase in blood viscosity [8], and negate improvements in oxygen delivery. Exchange transfusion is implemented to remove sickle cells and to replace them with normal erythrocytes. The aim of exchange transfusion is to reduce the percentage of HbS (usually to < 30%) and to achieve a post exchange Hb of about 12–14 g/dL [9, 10]. This minimizes viscosity changes, enhances blood flow through the microcirculation and improves tissue perfusion.

Exchange transfusions can be performed either manually or by automated cell separator. The manual procedure is a gradual process that requires several exchanges. It is time-consuming and may cause fluctuations in blood volume. The automated method has several advantages over the manual procedure. The patient remains isovolumic with little loss of plasma and platelets. Also the procedure is safe, effective and the mean duration for the procedure is about 2 hours [11].

Indications for exchange transfusion

Acute chest syndrome
In this condition exchange transfusions can be life-saving [12].

Acute multi-organ failure syndrome
There is rapid clinical deterioration and failure of multiple organs (liver, kidney and lung). If untreated the mortality is up to 25% [13].

Priapism
Prolonged priapism may result in erectile impotence. Exchange transfusion has long been advocated for the acute management of priapism. However, exchange transfusion has been associated with neurological events. Oral and intracavernous injections of an alpha adrenergic stimulator have had some reported success in treatment and also prevention of priapism. Therefore, exchange transfusion should be reserved for those who do not respond to medical therapy and other measures [14, 15].

Stroke (cerebrovascular accidents)
These occur commonly in children and recurrence is a prominent feature of this complication. Patients with an acute onset of neurological deficit should be immediately rehydrated, exchange transfused and thereafter investigated [16].

Chronic transfusion therapy (hypertransfusion regime)

This involves an initial exchange transfusion, followed by regular repeated top-up transfusions. The aim is to maintain the HbS level below 30% and the patient's Hb level between 10 and 14 g/dL. This reduces erythropoietic drive and suppresses endogenous erythropoiesis. Thus the majority of circulating cells are transfused normal red cells which will not sickle and this will prevent vaso-occlusion and organ damage. Partial exchange transfusion is necessary when the HbS rises above 30%. Chronic transfusion therapy has now been advocated for the prevention of recurrence of stroke and also primary stroke prevention. The major drawbacks of long-term transfusion therapy are allo-immunization, transfusion reactions and iron overload.

Indications for chronic transfusion therapy

Prevention of recurrence of stroke
Stroke occurs in around 5% of children with SCD, with a high recurrence rate; this can be prevented by a chronic transfusion programme. Without transfusions the risk of recurrence is about 66–90% [17, 18]. Studies have shown that a chronic transfusion regime can reduce the rate of recurrence by 90% [19, 20]. Wilimas *et al.* [21] have reported 70% stroke recurrence after discontinuation of a 1–2-year transfusion programme. The risk of recurrence remains high after cessation of a 5–12-year transfusion regime [22]. So, it is not known how long to keep the patient on a transfusion regime. Presently the recommendations are to either continue indefinitely or to stop the transfusion regime when the patient reaches 18 years of age, provided that at least 3 years of transfusions have been given since the last stroke. It is important to note that a chronic transfusion programme reduces the risk of the

recurrence of stroke but does not eradicate it totally [19, 20].

A retrospective study by Scothorn *et al.* [23] on the risk of recurrent stroke in children with SCD receiving blood transfusions included 137 paediatric patients from 14 centres. The mean age at the time of the first stroke was 6.3 years (1.4–14 years) with a mean follow-up period of 10.1 years (5–24 years). Thirty-one children (22%) had a second stroke (2.2 per 100 patient-years) and the absence of concurrent sickle complications (such as painful crises, chest syndrome, aplastic crisis) with the initial stroke was a major risk factor for a second stroke while receiving chronic transfusions. This was an unexpected finding and demonstrates that additional intervention is required to prevent this devastating complication and further research is required in this area.

Primary prevention of stroke in children (chronic transfusion vs control) [24]
The incidence rates of a first stroke in SCD are 1.02, 0.79 and 0.41 per 100 patient-years for the age groups 2–5 years, 6–9 years and 10–19 years, respectively [25]. The stroke prevention trial (STOP) [24] was a randomized trial that studied 130 children with SCD with ages ranging from 2 to 16 years. Children at risk of stroke were identified by trans-cranial Doppler ultrasonography. It compared the incidence of stroke between two groups: (a) those on chronic transfusion (63 patients), and (b) a control group who had standard medical care (67 patients). During a 20-month median follow-up period, only one stroke was reported in the chronic transfusion group, whereas 11 strokes were reported in the control group. There was a 92% relative risk reduction, therefore the trial was terminated early. Transfusion-related adverse events such as iron overload, red cell allo-immunization and transfusion reactions were recorded in the transfusion group. It is unclear how long transfusion should be continued to prevent stroke and at what stage the transfusion can safely be stopped. The impact of a chronic transfusion programme in the incidence of pain and acute chest syndrome was also evaluated [26]. The result showed that chronic transfusions reduce the frequency of an acute chest syndrome (2.2 vs 15.7 events per 100 patient-years)

and painful crises (9.7 vs 27.1 events per 100 patient-years).

Transfusion therapy in pregnant patients [27]
This study involved 72 patients, 36 in the non-transfused group and 36 who received prophylactic red cell transfusions from 28 weeks gestation. There were no significant differences in perinatal and obstetric outcomes between the two groups. However, there was a significant reduction in painful episodes (14% in the prophylactic group vs 50% in the control group). This demonstrated that in general pregnant patients with SCD do not require routine prophylactic transfusions. This was supported by a recent review [28].

Other indications
Chronic transfusions have been used in some clinical situations, e.g. chronic osteomyelitis, leg ulcers, chronic renal failure and severe recurrent painful episodes. However, far more clinical studies are required to prove that transfusions are effective in these settings.

Peri-operative transfusion management

A comparison of exchange transfusion and simple top-up transfusion was studied in 551 SCD patients [29]. They were randomly assigned to receive either exchange transfusions or simple top-up transfusions. The most common operative procedures were cholecystectomy, ENT and orthopaedic surgery. The aim of exchange transfusion was to achieve a pre-operative Hb level of 10 g/dL with %HbS < 30. The average Hb level and %HbS in this group was 11 g/dL and 31%, respectively. The simple transfusion regime attempted to reach an Hb level of 10 g/dL regardless of the %HbS. The average Hb and %HbS in this group was 10.6 g/dL and 59%, respectively. There were no significant differences in sickle cell-related complications in the two groups. However, haemolytic transfusion reactions and RBC allo-antibody formation were more common in the exchange group than the simple transfusion group (6% vs 1% and 10% vs 5%, respectively). It appears that simple transfusion to a target Hb of 10 g/dL is sufficient in most operative procedures. However, exchange transfusion might still be indicated in high risk operations and for those patients with HbSC [30].

Complications of red cell transfusion in SCD

Red cell allo-immunization

Red cell allo-immunization is common in SCD, with an overall incidence of 18–36% [31–33]. This is due to a lack of phenotypic compatibility between the recipient who is of African and Caribbean descent and the donor who is predominantly Caucasian, with significant differences of antigen frequency in E, C, Kell Fy^a, Fy^b and Jk^b. The risk of allo-immunization is also related to the number of transfusions received [34]. Rh, C, E and Kell are the most commonly formed red cell alloantibodies (66%), as 49% of SCD patients have Rh phenotype Ro (cDe). Davies *et al.* [32] have recommended that newly diagnosed SCD patients or patients with no red cell antibodies should have blood matched for Kell and Rh antigens (other than RhD).

Recent studies have confirmed that matching for major Rh and Kell antigens would have prevented all alloantibody formation in 53.3% of the patients who formed alloantibodies [35]. Further extended typing to include S, Fy^a and Jk^b will prevent allo-immunization in 70.8% of patients who would have formed alloantibodies. However, only 0.6% of random Caucasian donors would match this phenotype. In the STOP trial, 61 patients in the chronic transfusion arm received blood group matched for Rh and Kell antigens. A total of 1830 RBC units were transfused; only five patients developed a clinically significant alloantibody [36]. This rate of allo-immunization (8%) was lower than in another paediatric patient SCD study (29%) in which Rh and Kell matched blood was not provided [37].

All SCD patients should undergo red cell extended phenotyping at diagnosis or before the first transfusion and should receive blood matched for ABO, Rh and Kell type. This will prevent and minimize the risk of red cell allo-immunization. Patients with alloantibodies should receive matched antigen negative units.

In the UK all red cell units are labelled not only for ABO blood groups but also for Rh and Kell, therefore blood banks can easily select the appropriate red cell units for SCD patients.

Delayed haemolytic transfusion reaction (DHTR)

DHTR is a well-known risk in allo-immunized SCD patients who require multiple transfusions. The incidence rates of DHTR in SCD have been reported as 11%, 17% and 22% by various authors [33, 38, 39]. Most reported cases fulfil the criteria for a typical DHTR. It usually occurs 7–10 days after transfusion, with laboratory and clinical evidence of haemolysis: a positive direct antiglobulin test, identification of new red cell antibodies and decreased survival of transfused red cells. DHTR is difficult to prevent, as a third of the antibodies formed are transitory in nature [34]. Therefore the antibody may not be detected in pre-transfusion samples. However, the antibody titre rises rapidly due to anamnestic response after transfusion of incompatible blood. The commonest alloantibodies which cause DHTRs belong to the Rh system (39% anti-C and E) [40].

Hyperhaemolysis syndrome

The hyperhaemolysis syndrome is now well recognized in both paediatric and adult SCD patients [37, 41–43]. It is characterized by severe haemolysis after blood transfusion, significant decrease in reticulocyte count from the patient's steady-state value, hyperbilirubinaemia and haemoglobinuria. The post-transfusion Hb level is always lower than the pre-transfusion level [41, 43]. It differs from a DHTR, as both the patient's and the transfused red cells are destroyed. The direct antiglobulin test may be negative. Some patients have multiple red cell alloantibodies and may also have autoantibodies. In others, no alloantibodies are demonstrable [37, 41–44]. Recovery is associated with reticulocytosis and gradual improvement in Hb level [41, 43]. Further blood transfusion may exacerbate haemolysis, or even cause death [45, 46]. Therefore awareness of this syndrome is important and further transfusions should be withheld if possible. After recovery, haemolysis can recur in some patients following subsequent transfusions [38].

The exact aetiology of hyperhaemolysis is not known. A genetic predisposition theory [47], bystander haemolysis [42], and suppression of erythropoiesis [41], have been proposed. Hyperhaemolysis may be delayed or acute. The delayed form occurs 7–10 days after transfusion and is usually associated with formation of new red cell alloantibodies [37, 41, 42]. Acute hyperhaemolysis occurs < 7 days (usually 48–72 hours) after receiving blood transfusion, and no red cell alloantibodies are demonstrable [37, 43, 44]. The author has reported three cases of acute hyperhaemolysis syndrome in which further transfusions were successfully given under intravenous immunoglobulin (IVIg) and steroid cover [43, 44]. In two cases, HLA antibodies were present. The DAT was negative in two, but was positive in one patient with underlying renal failure. No new red cell alloantibodies were identified in the three cases. All the transfused units were compatible and there was no evidence of red cell antibody-mediated haemolysis. In two cases reticulocytopenia was noted, with a rise in reticulocyte count after treatment with IVIg. In one patient, the bone marrow aspirate showed erythroid hyperplasia. As HbSS red cells and sickle reticulocytes adhere readily to macrophages, the author has suggested that reticulocytopenia in hyperhaemolysis syndrome is not due to suppression of erythropoiesis, but results from destruction by macrophages. This hypothesis is supported by the bone marrow findings, the reticulocyte response to IVIg/steroids, and the lack of evidence of red cell antibody-mediated haemolysis [43]. The association of reticulocytopenia, absence of red cell antibodies and haemolysis has been reported, with radio-isotope studies confirming that the reticulocytes were destroyed by the reticulo-endothelial system [48].

It appears that the pathogenesis of hyperhaemolysis is complex, as it involves not only the destruction of the patient's own cells, but also transfused red cells. In reported cases all red cell units transfused were serologically compatible. This suggests that non-red cell antibodies (e.g. anti-HLA) or bystander haemolysis may contribute to the destruction of the red cells. Sickle cells are highly susceptible to reactive lysis and HLA antibody formation is common among SCD patients. About 73% of red blood cells express the HLA (Bg) antigen, and HLA antibodies can occasionally cause haemolysis. It is possible that transfused erythrocytes expressing HLA antigens are destroyed by HLA antibodies; whereas transfused cells not expressing HLA antigens and the patient's red cells are destroyed by bystander haemolysis [43].

Accelerated destruction of transfused compatible red cells by a hyperactive reticulo-endothelial system has been reported in non-SCD patients [49, 50]. Cessation of haemolysis following treatment with IVIg and steroids may be due to immunomodulation: IVIg blocking the adhesion of sickle red cells and reticulocytes to macrophages, or steroid suppression of macrophage activity [51, 52].

Febrile non-haemolytic transfusion reaction (FNHTR)

The incidence of FNHTR after red cell transfusion is 6.8%. This can be prevented by providing leucocyte-depleted red cell concentrates and has been recommended for use in SCD patients [53]. There are additional benefits of leucocyte-depleted products. In the UK, filtration of white cells is carried out in the blood component processing laboratory under controlled conditions to achieve residual leucocytes of $< 5 \times 10^6$ per unit. All blood components have been leucocyte-depleted since November 1999. This has beneficial effects in prevention of HLA allo-immunization and cytomegalovirus (CMV) infection.

Prevention of HLA allo-immunization

Bone marrow transplantation (BMT) remains the only curative treatment for SCD. HLA antibody formation is not uncommon in SCD, and is directly related to the number of units received. Of those who have received more than 50 RBC units and fewer than 50 RBC units, 85% and 48%, respectively, formed HLA antibodies. HLA antibodies were not demonstrated in those who had not received blood transfusion [54]. An allograft rejection in 4 of 22 SCD patients undergoing BMT was thought to be due to transfusion-induced alloimmunization [55]. The presence of HLA antibodies can also lead to clinical platelet refractoriness, which can complicate the supportive care of BMT patients. The Trial to Reduce Alloimmunization to Platelets (TRAP) [56] showed significant reduction in HLA allo-immunization and platelet refractoriness among leukaemia patients who received transfused leucocyte-depleted blood products. It has been recommended that leucocyte-depleted blood components are provided for those children with SCD who are potential candidates for BMT.

Prevention of CMV infection

SCD children who are seronegative and are potential candidates for BMT should receive CMV seronegative blood components for the prevention of transfusion-transmitted CMV infection. If CMV seronegative blood products are not available, leucocyte-depleted blood components can be used as an alternative [53].

Transfusion support for beta thalassaemia major

Patients with homozygous beta thalassaemia require chronic transfusion support from early childhood. Regular transfusions suppress ineffective erythropoiesis, prevent bone deformity, limit the disfiguring organomegaly, and also promote growth and development. Regular transfusion should be initiated when Hb concentration drops consistently below 7 g/dL [57]. The aim is to maintain pre-transfusion haemoglobin levels of 9.5–10.5 g/dL. The rate of transfusion is 10–15 mL/kg body weight in about 2 hours. These patients usually require transfusion every 4–5 weeks. All patients with thalassaemia should undergo red cell extended phenotyping before transfusions are begun, and should receive blood matched for ABO, Rh and Kell antigens [58]. This recommendation is supported by the finding of Singer et al. [59] that transfusion of leucocyte-depleted blood with limited phenotypic matching (Rh, Kell) is effective in preventing red cell allo-immunization in thalassaemia patients of predominantly Asian descent; (2.8% in patients vs 33.1% in controls` The high incidence of allo-immunization in the control population is mainly due to red cell

phenotype mismatch between the predominantly white donors and Asian recipients. Leucocyte-depleted RBC units are also recommended in thalassaemia patients to prevent FNHTR [53]. Periodic monitoring of the effectiveness of transfusion therapy is necessary. Total volume transfused to maintain pre-transfusions Hb not less than 9.5 g/dL has to be calculated yearly. Blood transfusion requirement > 200 mL/kg/year in the absence of antibody-mediated red cell destruction is suggestive of hypersplenism. All newly diagnosed, seronegative patients should be vaccinated with hepatitis B vaccine [60].

References

1. Prohovnik I, Pavlakis SG, Piomelli S et al. Cerebral hyperemia, stroke and transfusion in sickle cell disease. Neurology 1989; 39: 344.
2. Adams RJ. Neurologic complications. In: Embury SH, Hebbel RP, Mohandas N, Steinberg MH, eds. Sickle Cell Disease: Basic Principles and Clinical Practice. New York: Raven, 1994: 599–621.
3. Rao SP, Miller ST, Cohen BJ. Transient aplastic crisis in patients with sickle cell disease. B19 parvovirus studies during a 7-year period. Am J Dis Child 1992; 146: 1328–30.
4. Vichinsky E, Lubin BH. Suggested guidelines for the treatment of children with sickle cell anaemia. Hematol Oncol Clin North Am 1987; 1: 483.
5. Weatherall DJ. The red cell disorders of the synthesis or function of haemoglobin. In: Weatherall DJ, Ledingham GG, Warrell DA, eds. Oxford Textbook of Medicine. Oxford: Oxford University Press, 1996.
6. Charache S, Conley CL. Rate of sickling of red cells during deoxygenation of blood from persons with various sickling disorders. Blood 1964; 24: 25–48.
7. Schmalzer EA, Lee JO, Brown AK et al. Viscosity of mixtures of sickle and normal red cells at varying hematocrit levels: implications for transfusion. Transfusion 1987; 27: 228–33.
8. Jan K, Usami S, Smith JA. Effects of transfusion on rheological properties of blood in sickle cell anaemia. Transfusion 1982; 22: 17–20.
9. Davies SC, Olatunji PO. Blood transfusion in sickle cell disease. Vox Sang 1995; 68: 145–51.
10. Janes SL, Pocock M, Bishop E, Bevan DH. Automated red cell exchange in sickle cell disease. Br J Haematol 1997; 97: 256–8.
11. Lawson SE, Oakley S, Smith NA, Bareford D. Red cell exchange in sickle cell disease. Clin Lab Haematol 1999; 21: 99–102.

12. Emre U, Miller ST, Gutieriez M *et al.* Effect of transfusion in acute chest syndrome of sickle cell disease. *J Pediatr* 1995; **127**: 901–4.

13. Hassell KL, Eckman JR, Lane PA. Acute multiorgan failure syndrome: a potentially catastrophic complication of severe sickle cell pain episodes. *Am J Med* 1994; **96**: 155–62.

14. Davies SC, Roberts-Harewood M. Blood transfusion in sickle cell disease *Blood Rev* 1997; **11**: 57–71.

15. Telen MJ. Principles and problems of transfusion in sickle cell disease. *Semin Haematol* 2001; **38**: 315–23.

16. Charache S, Lubin B, Reid CD. Stroke. In: Charache S, Lubin B, Reid CD, eds. *Management and Therapy of Sickle Cell Disease*, 3rd edn. Washington: US Department of Health, 1995: 53–8.

17. Powars D, Wilson B, Imbus C, Pegelow C, Allen J. The natural history of stroke in sickle cell disease. *Am J Med* 1978; **65**: 461.

18. Ohene-Frempong K. Stroke in sickle cell disease: demographic, clinical, and therapeutic considerations. *Semin Haematol* 1991; **238**: 213.

19. Russell MO, Goldberg HI, Reis L *et al.* Effect of transfusion therapy on arteriographic abnormalities and on recurrence of stroke in sickle cell disease. *Blood* 1984; **63**: 162–9.

20. Pegelow CH, Adams RJ, McKie V *et al.* Risk of recurrent stroke in patients with sickle cell disease treated with erythrocyte transfusions. *J Pediatr* 1995; **126**: 896–9.

21. Wilimas J, Goff JR, Anderson HR, Langston JW, Thompson E. Efficacy of transfusion therapy for one to two years in patients with sickle cell disease and cerebrovascular accidents. *J Pediatr* 1980; **96**: 205.

22. Wang WC, Kovnar EH, Tonkin IL *et al.* High risk of recurrent stroke after discontinuance of five to twelve years of transfusion therapy in patients with sickle cell disease. *J Pediatr* 1991; **118**: 377–82.

23. Scothorn DJ, Price C, Schwartz D *et al.* Risk of recurrent stroke in children with sickle cell disease receiving blood transfusion therapy for at least five years after initial stoke. *J Pediatr* 2002; **140**: 348–54.

24. Adams RJ, McKie VC, Hsu L *et al.* Prevention of a first stroke by transfusions in children with sickle cell anemia and abnormal results on transcranial Doppler ultrasonography. *N Engl J Med* 1998; **339**: 5–11.

25. Ohene-Frempong K, Weiner SJ, Sleeper LA *et al.* Cerebrovascular accidents in sickle cell disease: rates and risk factors. *Blood* 1998; **91**: 288–94.

26. Miller ST, Wright E, Abboud M *et al.* Impact of chronic transfusion on incidence of pain and acute chest syndrome during the Stroke Prevention Trial (STOP) in sickle-cell anaemia. *J Pediatr* 2001; **139**: 785–9.

27. Koshy M, Burd L, Wallace D, Moawad A *et al.* Prophylactic red-cell transfusions in pregnant patients with sickle cell disease: a randomized cooperative study. *N Engl J Med* 1988; **319**: 1447–52.

28. Mahomed K. Prophylactic versus selective blood transfusion for sickle cell anaemia during pregnancy. *Cochrane Database of Systematic Reviews* 2000; **2**: CD000040.

29. Vichinsky EP, Haberkern CM, Newmayr L *et al.* A comparison of conservative and aggressive transfusion regimens in the perioperative management of sickle cell disease. *N Engl J Med* 1995; **333**: 206–13.

30. Neumayr L, Koshy M, Haberkern C *et al.* Surgery in patients with hemoglobin SC disease. The Preoperative Transfusion to Sickle Cell Disease Study Group. *Am J Hematol* 1998; **57**: 101–8.

31. Orlina AR, Unger PJ, Koshy M. Post-transfusion alloimmunization in patients with sickle cell disease. *Am J Hematol* 1978; **5**: 101–6.

32. Davies SC, McWilliam AC, Hewitt PE *et al.* Red cell alloimmunization in sickle cell disease. *Br J Haematol* 1986; **63**: 241–5.

33. Cox JV, Steane E, Cunningham G, Frenkel EP. Risk of alloimmunization and delayed hemolytic transfusion reactions in patients with sickle cell disease. *Arch Intern Med* 1988; **148**: 2485–9.

34. Rosse WF, Gallagher D, Kinney TR *et al.* The Cooperative Study of Sickle Cell Disease: transfusion and alloimmunization in sickle cell disease. *Blood* 1990; **76**: 1431–7.

35. Castro O, Sandler SG, Houston-Yu P, Rana S. Predicting the effect of transfusion only phenotype-matched RBCs to patients with sickle cell disease: theoretical and practical implications. *Transfusion* 2002; **42**: 684–90.

36. Vichinsky EP, Luban NLC, Wright E *et al.* Prospective RBC phenotype matching in a stroke-prevention trial in sickle cell anemia: a multicenter transfusion trial. *Transfusion* 2001; **41**: 1086–92.

37. Aygun B, Padmanabhan S, Paley C, Chandrasekaran V. Clinical significance of RBC alloantibodies and autoantibodies in sickle cell patients who received transfusions. *Transfusion* 2002; **42**: 37–43.

38. Diamond WJ, Brown FL Jr, Bitterman P *et al.* Delayed haemolytic transfusion reaction presenting as sickle cell crisis. *Ann Intern Med* 1980; **93**: 231–4.

39. Vichinsky EP, Earles A, Johnson RA *et al.* Alloimmunization in sickle cell anaemia and transfusion of racially unmatched blood. *N Engl J Med* 1990; **322**: 1617–21.

40. Garratty G. Severe reactions associated with transfusion of patients with sickle cell disease. *Transfusion* 1997; **37**: 357–61.

41. Petz LD, Calhoun L, Shulman IA *et al.* The sickle cell haemolytic transfusion reaction syndrome. *Transfusion* 1997; **37**: 382–92.

42. King KE, Shirey RS, Lankiewicz MW *et al.* Delayed haemolytic transfusion reactions in sickle cell disease: simultaneous destruction of recipients' red cells. *Transfusion* 1997; **37**: 376–81.

43. Win N, Doughty H, Telfer P *et al.* Hyperhemolytic trans-

fusion reaction in sickle cell disease. *Transfusion* 2001; **41**: 323–8.

44. Cullis JO, Win N, Dudley JM, Kaye T. Post-transfusion hyperhaemolysis in a patient with sickle cell disease: use of steroids and intravenous immunoglobulin to prevent further red cell destruction. *Vox Sang* 1995; **4**: 355–7.

45. Milner PF, Squires JE, Larison PJ *et al*. Post-transfusion crises in sickle cell anaemia: role of delayed hemolytic reactions to transfusion. *South Med J* 1985; **78**: 1462–9.

46. Friedman DF, Kim HC, Manno CS. Hyperhemolysis associated with red cell transfusion in sickle cell disease (abstract). *Transfusion* 1993; **33** (Suppl): 14S.

47. Alarif L, Castro O, Ofosu M *et al*. HLA-B35 is associated with red cell alloimmunisation in sickle cell disease. *Clin Immunol Immunopathol* 1986; **38**: 178–83.

48. Hedge UM, Gordon-Smith EC, Worlledge SM. Reticulocytopenia and absence of red cell auto-antibodies in immune haemolytic anaemia. *BMJ* 1977; **2**: 1444–7.

49. Van der Hart M, Engelfriet CP, Prins HK, Van Loghem JJ. Haemolytic transfusion reaction without demonstrable antibodies *in vitro*. *Vox Sang* 1963; **8**: 363–70.

50. Davey RJ, Gustafson M, Holland PV. Accelerated immune red cell destruction in the absence of serologically detectable alloantibodies. *Transfusion* 1980; **20**: 348–53.

51. Packer JT, Greendyke RM, Swisher SN. The inhibition of erythrophagocytosis *in vitro* by corticosteroids. *Transfusion Association of American Physicians* 1960; **73**: 93–102.

52. Rhoades CJ, Williams MA, Kelsey SM, Newland AC. Monocyte-macrophage system as targets for immunomodulation by intravenous immunoglobulin. *Blood Rev* 2000; **14**: 14–30.

53. British Committee for Standards in Haematology (BCSH), Blood Transfusion Task Force. Guidelines on the clinical use of leucocyte-depleted blood components. *Transfus Med* 1998; **8**: 59–71.

54. Friedman DF, Lukas MB, Jawad A *et al*. Alloimmunization to platelets in heavily transfused patients with sickle cell disease. *Blood* 1996; **88**: 3216–22.

55. Walters MC, Patience M, Leisenring W *et al*. Bone marrow transplantation for sickle cell disease. *N Engl J Med* 1996; **335**: 369–76.

56. Leukocyte reduction and ultraviolet B irradiation of platelets to prevent alloimmunization and refractoriness to platelet transfusions. Trial to Reduce Alloimmunization to Platelets Study Group (TRAP). *N Engl J Med* 1997; **337**: 1861–9.

57. Rebulla P. Blood transfusion in beta thalassemia major. *Transfus Med* 1995; **5**: 247–58.

58. Michail Merianou V, Pamphilip-Panousopoulou L, Piperi-Lowes L *et al*. Alloimmunization to red cell antigens in thalassemia: comparative study of usual versus better-match transfusion programmes. *Vox Sang* 1987; **52**: 95–8.

59. Singer ST, Wu V, Mignacca R *et al*. Alloimmunization and erythrocyte autoimmunization in transfusion-dependent thalassemia patients of predominantly Asian descent. *Blood* 2000; **96**: 3369–73.

60. Pearson HA. Current trends in the management of homozygous β-thalassemia. *Annals of Saudi Medicine* 1996; **16**: 554–8.

Chapter 12

Management of pregnancy in sickle cell disease

Manjiri Khare and Susan Bewley

Introduction

As the life expectancy of children with sickle cell disease (SCD) improves, more reach adulthood, and become parents themselves. Desires for sexual relations, to bear children or to avoid pregnancy are universal and women with SCD require specific advice. This chapter covers aspects of reproductive health relevant to physicians, obstetricians or midwives caring for women with SCD. There is no information about the numbers of sexually active fertile adults with SCD, worldwide or in the UK. It is unknown how many women with SCD become pregnant, or have children. Thus it is difficult to assess the scope of the problem.

Fertility and contraception

The fertility of women with haemoglobinopathies is generally unaffected, except for the usual reasons (e.g. deferred childbearing, poor semen, ovulation disorders, sexually transmitted infection, etc.). Although none of the available methods for contraception are contraindicated, effective contraception is required, especially in view of the additional maternal risks of unwanted pregnancy. The risks of pregnancy are far greater than those of contraceptive methods.

Barrier methods are easily available and widely used. They have minimal side-effects, but carry a higher risk of unwanted pregnancies. Low dose combined contraceptive pills are not contra-indicated in homozygous sickle disease. Indeed, the highly effective protection against unwanted preg-nancy conferred by combined contraceptive pills is a positive advantage. There are no data to suggest that SCD patients have a greater risk than any other patients using low oestrogen preparations [1, 2].

For those who experience difficulty in taking oral contraceptives, for whatever reason, depot progestogens are a good alternative, as there is no medical contraindication to their use. There is some evidence that depot medroxyprogesterone acetate (Depo-Provera®) has a stabilizing action on the red cell membrane [3]. The risk of uterine and tubal infections with intrauterine contraceptive devices (IUCD), particularly in nulliparous women, makes their use relatively contraindicated in SCD, but they may be required in special circumstances for women where other methods are considered unsuitable.

Antenatal screening for haemoglobinopathy

The majority of pregnant women with SCD will al-ready be aware of their haemoglobinopathy status, as they would have suffered from the clinical mani-festations of the disease. Antenatal screening does pick up a small number of new women with milder forms of the disease who can be advised and cared for appropriately. It can be difficult to adjust and cope with a new diagnosis of a chronic disorder during pregnancy.

The main purposes of an antenatal screening pro-gramme are (a) to identify women with SCD who were previously unaware of their status, (b) to identify women with trait or carrier status, (c) to

107

offer testing of the partners of such women, (d) to inform women or couples at high genetic risk about having an affected child and (e) to offer appropriate counselling and, if desired, prenatal diagnosis. Women and men should be advised about their status and the implications if they change partner.

At present antenatal haemoglobinopathy screening programmes vary depending on the local policy. They can be universal (offered to all pregnant women routinely) or selective (offered to all women from at-risk ethnic minorities, or women whose partners are from such groups). Universal antenatal screening is not widely available in the UK, as it is not thought to be entirely cost-effective in populations that are predominantly of Caucasian background with a low prevalence of SCD. However, in certain areas the proportion of ethnic minorities is not low, populations are mixed and prevalence would justify universal as opposed to selective screening. A retrospective review of the organization and cost-effectiveness of universal screening for haemoglobinopathy at a centre in London [4] reported that antenatal screening is likely to be cost-effective at least in areas with haemoglobinopathy traits at or above 2.5%, especially if a high proportion of these were for thalassaemia. At Guy's and St Thomas' Hospitals Trust, London, UK (with a 50% non-Caucasian antenatal population), screening for haemoglobinopathies is offered to all women as recommended by the Department of Health [5].

The laboratory methods of detecting abnormal haemoglobin variants are discussed in Chapter 2.

Prenatal diagnosis

SCD is an autosomal recessive disorder. For women with trait whose partners are unaffected, there is no chance of having an affected offspring, although there is a 50% chance that a child of the couple will have sickle cell trait. For women with trait whose partners are also trait, there is a 25% chance that each offspring will have SCD, 50% of being a carrier and 25% chance of having a genotype HbAA. Women with SCD will either have partners who are AA, and thus all children will have sickle cell trait, or if the partners are carriers, there is a 50% chance that each offspring will have SCD. In the rare

situation of women with SCD whose partners are the same, all children will be affected.

It is important for parents to be aware of the implications of SCD and be prepared before the birth of an affected infant. This preparation can occur if they are counselled and offered the opportunity of antenatal diagnosis (with the possibility of termination of pregnancy if they feel unable to cope with the implications). Ideally, discussions about haemoglobinopathy or carrier status should take place prenatally, so that women can understand and digest information in an unhurried way and consider their options before embarking upon a pregnancy. It is preferable for a partner to be tested to find his haemoglobinopathy status so that counselling of the couple can be more informative.

Some women may not wish to consider or discuss the implications, others will be prepared to have genetic counselling, or consider invasive testing. Cells or tissue for antenatal diagnosis can be obtained by chorion villous sampling (CVS) between 10 and 12 weeks gestation, or by amniocentesis or fetal blood sampling in the late second trimester. With all invasive procedures there is a 1–2% risk of procedure-related loss of the pregnancy. Prenatal diagnosis can be performed by DNA analysis with the polymerase chain reaction (PCR) and Southern blotting [6, 7].

Half the couples at risk of having a child with severe haemoglobinopathy accepted prenatal diagnosis in a prospective regional study by Rowley and colleagues [8]. The rate of uptake of prenatal diagnostic procedures has been found to be higher when performed earlier in pregnancy, and the percentage of terminations of affected pregnancies falls with advancing gestation. Wang *et al.* [9] reported on 500 consecutive prenatal diagnoses of SCD. The first 196 were obtained by Southern blotting and the remaining 304 by PCR. The use of PCR shortened the sampling-to-diagnosis interval to around 6 days in comparison with those from the Southern blotting group that took on average 16 days. This resulted in a fourfold increase in diagnosis, as they also accepted samples in which paternal phenotype was not known. Interestingly, they also showed that an earlier diagnosis (i.e. before 20 weeks of pregnancy) had an odds ratio of termination of pregnancy of 4.7 compared with later diagnosis (after 20 weeks) suggesting that the pregnancy becomes less tentative or more bonded with increasing gestation and fetal maturation. The overall rate of termination of affected pregnancies is around 50% [9–11].

Preimplantation genetic diagnosis (PGD) is an alternative and powerful diagnostic tool for identifying sickle cell status in embryos that uses assisted reproductive techniques in conjunction with modern molecular methods. With PGD, the genetic status of an embryo can be determined before transfer into the uterus after *in vitro* fertilization. This virtually eliminates the risk of bearing a child with the disease. There is a case report of a successful unaffected pregnancy following PGD for sickle cell anaemia [12]. Although prenatal testing is currently available, some couples have strong personal objections to aborting affected fetuses. For these couples, PGD provides a realistic alternative to prenatal testing.

There are concerns about the ethics of termination of pregnancy for what is a chronic medical condition with good treatments, quality of life and life expectancy (at least in the developed world). On the one hand it may be considered 'eugenic' to eliminate genetic diseases. On the other, if abortion is tolerated or legal for all 'unwanted' pregnancies, including social reasons, it can be argued that there are no new ethical issues. Early knowledge enables couples to exercise more reproductive choices. Prenatal diagnosis may enable parents to be more prepared for the birth of an affected and wanted child, or to have children where they may have previously remained voluntarily infertile. If couples are to make informed reproductive choices, they must be well informed before conception, or as early as possible prenatally.

Effect of pregnancy on SCD

Sickle cell crises are unpredictable in or out of pregnancy, although there are well known precipitating factors such as hypoxia, trauma, acidosis, cold, dehydration, alcohol, infection and blood stasis.

Physiological changes of pregnancy that are relevant to SCD include: increased plasma volume, increased red cell mass, decreased peripheral resistance, a sizeable low resistance uteroplacental circulation, less physical movement and an increasing abdominal mass. In addition, there is an increased risk of venous thrombo-embolism, especially in the puerperium. Pregnant women become acidotic more easily and have a tendency to urinary tract infections. Labour, delivery, haemorrhage, and interventions such as vaginal examinations or surgery can cause dehydration and infection. Thus pregnancy and childbirth are potent risk factors for precipitating crises made worse by any obstetric complications.

Crises complicate about 30–88% of HbSS pregnancies and about 30% of HbSC pregnancies in women with SCD [13–25] (see Table 12.1). Crisis may present with general fatigue, illness, joint pains, chest pain, breathlessness or abdominal pain. A problem with the clinical features is that there is overlap of pathological and physiological symptoms of pregnancy. There should be a low threshold for investigation if there is a clinical suspicion.

Sickle cell crises and sequelae of chronic disease may present in a variety of ways in pregnancy. Women may experience their usual painful crises, for example in the extremities and joints, or may have crises in the abdomen or lung. Osteomyelitis may complicate bone pain crisis. Pyelonephritis is common in pregnancy. If women have sickle cell-induced papillary necrosis they may have haematuria on routine dipstick and an increased tendency to dehydration. Haemolysis may lead to jaundice, an increased tendency to gallstones and cholestasis (which has to be distinguished from obstetric causes such as pre-eclampsia, HELLP syndrome, acute fatty liver and obstetric cholestasis). Chronic anaemia can lead to left ventricular hypertrophy or cardiomegaly. Women may develop pulmonary embolus.

A particularly difficult differential diagnosis is that of chest pain or breathlessness, especially in an ill woman. The patient may merely have rib crises (elicited by tenderness over the ribs) or a simple chest infection, but may have acute chest syndrome, pneumonia or pulmonary embolus. Although investigations such as ECG, chest X-ray, blood gases and ventilation–perfusion scans may be diagnostic, on some occasions pathologies may co-exist or patients may be so sick that 'blunderbuss' treatment for all three may be warranted.

Table 12.1 Complications of pregnancy in women with sickle cell disease (1983–2002)

Authors (publication year and country)	Period of study	Total number of pregnancies	Infection n (%)	Painful crisis n (%)	Pre-eclampsia/ PIH n (%)	Anaemia n (%)	Other n (%)
Tuck (1983, UK) [13]	1975–1981	125 SS 54 SC 59 Sβthal 12	UTI N (18) once N (10) recurrent Chest infection and puerperal sepsis N (39) once N (22) recurrent	Antenatal N (38) Postnatal N (22)	Severe pre-eclampsia N (5)	Severe anaemia Hb < 7.5g/dL N (6)	No information given
Powars (1986, USA) [14]	1962–1982	227 SS & Sβ⁰thal 156 SC 44 Sβthal 27	UTI N (22) Pneumonia N (16)	N (44.5)	N (11)	No information given	Thrombophlebitis N (3)
El Shafei (1992, Bahrain) [15]	1986–1988	147 SS 127 Sβthal 11 SD 1 SO 1	3 (2) Type not specified		10 (7)	130 (88)	No information given
Dare (1992, Nigeria) [16]	1980–1988	76 SS 26 SC 19 CC 1	UTI SS 12 (32) SC 13 (38) Puerperal sepsis SS 3 (8) SC 4 (12)	Bone pain crisis SS 18 (49) SC 13 (38) Acute sequestration crisis SS 3 (8) SC 2 (6)	SS 6 (16) SC 5 (15)	Severe anaemia SS 11 (30) SC 5 (15)	Malaria SS 10 (27) SC 8 (23)
Idrisa (1992, Nigeria) [17]	1984–1988	49 type not specified	Bacterial infection Antenatal 9 (22) Postnatal 2 (5)	Bone pain crisis Antenatal 3 (7) Postnatal 5 (12)	1 (2)	Antenatal 21 (51) Postnatal 12 (29)	No information given
Ogedengbe (1993, Lagos, Nigeria) [18]	1985–1989	41 SS 31 SC 10	UTI SS 5 (16) Pyelonephritis SS 1 (3) SC 1(10) Chest SS 2 (7) Wound SS 3(10)	SS 25 (81) SC 3 (30)	SS 5 (16)	No information given	No information given
Seoud (1994, Kansas City, USA) [19]	1981–1991	61 SS 36 SC 22 Sβthal 2 CC 1	UTI SS 6 (30) SC 14 (40) Pneumonia SS 4 (20) SC 5 (14) Postpartum endometritis SS 2 (10) SC 4 (11)	Bone pain crisis SS 10 (50) SC 12 (34) Haemolytic crisis SS 6 (30) SC 3 (9)	SS 4 (20) SC 3 (9)		Deep pelvic thrombosis SS 2 (10)

Study	Period	Number/types					
Howard (1995, UK) [20]	1991–1993	78 singleton (3 twin) SS 39 SC 33 Sβthal 5 Other 1 Type for twins not given	UTI SS 9 (23) SC 1 (3)	Antenatal SS 18 (46) SC 9 (27) Postnatal SS 1 (3) SC 1 (3) Pulmonary complications Antenatal SS 6 (15) SC 2 (6) Postnatal SS 1 (3) SC 1 (3)	SS 3 (8) SC 4 (12)	No information given	No information given
Smith (1996, USA) [21]	1979–1986	286/445 proceeded to delivery SS 320 SC 77 Sβthal 48	Pyelonephritis N (<1)	SS & S β0 thal N (50) SC N (26) Sβ+thal N (46)	N (14)	No information given	No information given
Rahimy (2000, Benin, West Africa) [22]	1994–1997	111 actively managed group (3 twin pregnancies) SS 42 SC 66	UTI SS 7 (17) SC 17 (26) Pulmonary complications SS 2 (5)	Painful SCD crises SS 24 (57) SC 34 (53)	No information given	No information given	*P. falciparum* malaria SS 16 (38) SC 5 (8)
Leborgne-Samuel (2000 Guadeloupe, West Indies) [23]	1993–1997	68 SS 33 SC 30 Sβ+thal 3 Sβ0thal 2	SS 12 (36) SC 7 (23) Sβ+thal 2 (67) Sβ0thal 1 (50)	SS 29 (88) SC 8 (27) Sβ+thal 3 (100)	SS 5 (15) SC 2 (7)	SS 14 (42) SC 1 (3) Sβ+thal 2 (67) Sβ0thal 1 (50)	No information given
Sun (2001, Atlanta, USA) [24]	1980–1999	127 SS 69 SC 58	Pyelonephritis SS n (7) SC n (5) Postpartum infections SS N (22) SC N (10)	Painful crises SS 34 (48) SC 11(19)	SS N (10) SC N (3)	No information given	No information given
*Odum (2002, Nigeria) [25]	1995–1997	SS 66	No information given	No information given	No information given	No information given	Crises, bone pain, haemolytic anaemia or systemic infections N (96)
Total	...	1624	...	...	...	...	...

N, number not given; βthal, beta thalassaemia; UTI, urinary tract infection.
*Results from abstract, actual figures not available.

111

It is important to emphasize to women and their health professionals that the symptoms of pregnancy may overlap with symptoms of crisis, and that the threshold for concern or admission should be lower in pregnancy than outside. In addition, crises may be more severe or may have consequences for the fetus. We recommend that women always seek medical advice in pregnancy for suspicious symptoms and do not stay at home, or 'self-treat', as they might otherwise normally do.

Effect of SCD on pregnancy

General

The documented complications of pregnancy with SCD include miscarriage, urinary tract and pulmonary infections, intrauterine growth restriction, pre-eclampsia, premature labour and delivery, fetal distress, multiple antenatal admissions, raised caesarean section rates, puerperal sepsis and thrombosis. Thus it is not surprising that there are high perinatal and maternal mortality rates. Statistics for maternal mortality and perinatal mortality in women with major SCD before 1970 revealed a maternal mortality of 30–40% and a perinatal mortality of 50–80% [26, 27].

Although the severity of SCD in the non-pregnant state is related to the manifestation during pregnancy, it is unpredictable. HbSS state is generally considered to cause the most severe SCD. The other common variant, HbSC disease, has similar although less severe manifestation in the non-pregnant state. However, the outcome of pregnancy in HbSC women is not necessarily more favourable. Poor obstetric history is important, as is the presence of antibodies (although this may only be a proxy measure of disease severity and requirement for prior treatment). The demands of twin pregnancy make this particularly dangerous [28].

Reports in the literature regarding pregnancy outcome from different centres and over different time periods reflect the dramatic improvement in management of women with SCD and its variants over the last three decades. Whether the improvements are due to specific changes in the care of SCD, better overall health or changes in antenatal man-

agement is not clear. The concept of comprehensive care and multidisciplinary teamworking is gaining acceptance and action in many centres around the world [29].

Table 12.1 summarizes major complications in pregnancy in the published literature (1983–2002). Table 12.2 summarizes the outcome of pregnancies from work published in the last 20 years [13–25].

Miscarriage (spontaneous abortion)

The spontaneous miscarriage rate has been described as about 25% [26, 30]. In the study by Tuck *et al.* [13] in the UK, there was a significantly greater proportion of women (18.4%) who had suffered one previous spontaneous miscarriage as compared with the control group (12.4%). Also there was a significant difference in those with two or more previous spontaneous first trimester miscarriages: 2.4% compared with 1.1% in controls. Powars *et al.* [14] reported a significant decrease in spontaneous miscarriage rates after 1972. Smith *et al.* [21] reported miscarriage rates of 6.5% in 445 pregnancies that included women with sickle cell anaemia, HbSC disease and sickle beta thalassaemia. It is difficult to compare reports of early fetal loss or miscarriage in populations with and without haemoglobinopathy, as diagnostic accuracy of failed pregnancy has improved so much in recent years that earlier detection shows high rates of miscarriage (up to 25%) in normal populations.

Perinatal morbidity

Infants born to mothers with sickle cell anaemia are at increased risk of prematurity, birth weight below the 10th percentile (or small-for-gestational age, SGA), fetal distress in labour and neonatal jaundice [31, 32]. In terms of outcome it is not solely a matter of size, but of underlying disease. Intrauterine growth restriction (IUGR) secondary to placental insufficiency is found more commonly, but not exclusively, in small babies. There is some confusion in the obstetric literature and terminology between absolute small size (SGA) and growth restriction

Table 12.2 Pregnancy outcome and medical interventions in sickle cell disease in pregnancy (1983–2002)

Authors (publication year and country)	Period of study	Total number of pregnancies	Maternal mortality n (%)	Perinatal mortality n (%)	Transfusion n (%)	Caesarean section n (%)
Tuck (1983, UK) [13]	1975–1981	125 SS 54 SC 59 Sßthal 12	Nil	N (5)	N (71)	N (15)
Powars (1986, USA) [14]	1962–1982	227 SS & Sß⁰thal 156 SC 44 Sß⁺thal 27	5 (2.2)	13 (6)	No information given	19 (26)
El Shafei (1992, Bahrain) [15]	1986–1988	147 SS 127 Sßthal 11 SD 1 SO 1	2 (1)	11 (7)	109 (47)	17 (12)
Dare (1992, Nigeria) [16]	1980–1988	76 SS 26 SC 19 CC 1 49	7 (9.2)	11 (13)	No information given	20 (26)
Idrisa (1992, Nigeria) [17]	1984–1988		2 (4)	8 (16) 5 stillbirths 3 NND	No information given	6 (15)
Ogedengbe (1993, Lagos, Nigeria) [18]	1985–1989	41 SS 31 SC 10	5 (14) 3 died undelivered	8 (20) 7 stillbirths 1 NND‡	11 (28) 1 prophylactic partial exchange transfusion in UK	8 (22)
Seoud (1994, Kansas city, USA) [19]	1981–1991	61 SS 36 SC 22 Sßthal 2 CC 1	2 (3) SS 2 1 died undelivered	4 (6) 2 stillbirth 2 NND	25 (43)	23 (42.5)
Howard (1995, UK) [20]	1991–1993	78 singleton (3 twin) SS 39 SC 33 Sßthal 5 Other 1	2 (2.5) SS 1 SC 1	5 (6)	31 (38) singleton 29/78 twins 2/3	38 (49)
Smith (1996, USA) [21]	1979–1986	286/445 proceeded to delivery SS 320 SC 77 Sßthal 48	2 (2.4) SS 2	3/286 (1.0) 3 stillbirths	No information given	No information given
Rahimy (2000, Benin, West Africa) [22]	1994–1997	111 actively managed group (3 twin) SS 42 SC 66	2 (1.8) SC 2	13 (12) SS 9 SC 4	45 (42) SS 23 (54.8) SC 22 (33.3)	38 (35)
Leborgne-Samuel (2000 Guadeloupe, West Indies) [23]	1993–1997	68 SS 33 SC 30 Sßthal 5	1 (1.4) Sßthal	3 (4) All NND	25 (37)	30 (48)
Sun (2001, Atlanta, USA) [24]	1980–1999	127 SS 69 SC 58	Nil	10 (8) SS 8 (11) SC 5 (4)	54 (42) SS 42 (59) SC 12 (21)	N not given SS (36) SC (28)
*Odum (2002, Nigeria) [25]	1995–1997	SS 66	†2 (6.7)	N (12)	N (45) antenatal N (82) postnatal	N (43)
Total	...	1624	32 (0–9.2%)	95§ (1–16%)	28–82%	12–49%

NND, neonatal death, βthal, beta thalassaemia.
*Results from abstract, actual figures not available.
†Number not given in abstract but calculated.
‡3/7 antepartum maternal death.
§Calculation excluding Odum paper [25].

below genetic potential (IUGR). Growth-restricted babies are vulnerable to stillbirth, asphyxia in labour, hypoglycaemia, hypothermia and neonatal death and complications.

In the study by Smith *et al.* [21], 21% of infants born to mothers with HbSS were SGA, although this was not seen commonly in mothers with HbSC [21]. They identified two variables that were risk factors for SGA infants: pre-eclampsia and acute anaemic episodes. As acute anaemic episodes and placental infarcts may occur in early pregnancy, efforts in prevention should be initiated very early in pregnancy.

The increased risk of IUGR might partly be explained by chronic anaemia in the mother or placental damage due to vascular occlusion and sickling in the high capacitance but sluggish utero-placental circulation. The placentas of patients with HbSS disease have been reported as showing infarcts, increased fibrin, abruptions and villous oedema [28, 33–35]. These placentas are small and the associated fetuses have growth restriction. However, Fox [36] did not find these lesions in his study and reported that most of the changes are a result of histological alterations of the intervillous red blood cells. See Chapter 6 for further detailed discussion of pathological changes in SCD.

Perinatal mortality (PNM)

PNM rates are higher in women with haemoglobinopathy, largely due to prematurity and IUGR. Perinatal mortality rates between 50% and 80% were reported before the 1970s [26, 27]. In the study by Powars *et al.* [14], the findings suggested that probability of survival for the fetus of a mother with SCD was significantly higher after 1972 ($P < 0.001$). Table 12.2 shows perinatal mortality statistics published in the literature during the period 1983–2002. There are differences in reported figures of perinatal mortality from different centres across the world, especially between the developed and developing countries. PNM rates reported from the USA and Europe are between 1 and 8%, whereas those from African centres are 12–19%.

In the UK, perinatal mortality rates are at least 4–5 times higher than in women without haemoglo-binopathy. It is difficult to estimate accurately the increased risk related to haemoglobinopathy alone as opposed to adversity related to social factors. However, it must be a cause for concern that Howard *et al.* [20] report an increase in the perinatal mortality rates from 48/1000 to 60/1000 in the last decade in women with SCD, compared with a decrease from 15.5/1000 to 8/1000 in the general obstetric population [37].

Maternal morbidity

The common infections encountered during pregnancy are those involving the urinary tract, pulmonary tree and skeletal tissues. The commonest pathogens are pneumococcus, salmonella and mycoplasma. Urinary tract infections (UTI) are increased in normal pregnancy and may start by being asymptomatic but spread to become pyelonephritis or septicaemia, which are associated with premature labour. Thus it is important to check urine monthly, for culture, and to treat UTIs aggressively. All infections should be promptly treated as the associated fever, dehydration and acidosis predispose women to sickling and painful crises. Due to the physiological changes of pregnancy and labour, women can become dehydrated and acidotic relatively easily. Although many people with SCD manage their crises, fluid intake and analgesia themselves, it is prudent to encourage early admission to hospital with crises in pregnancy, as the ability to monitor fetal well-being is compromised at home and events can deteriorate quickly.

Pregnancy-induced hypertension and pre-eclampsia complicate one-third of pregnancies and so increased surveillance throughout pregnancy is required [20, 38]. Although not highly sensitive or specific, uterine artery Doppler ultrasonography is currently the best screening test for pre-eclampsia [39]. The underlying pathophysiology of placental complications or 'insufficiency' (related to pre-eclampsia, abruption and growth restriction) is failed trophoblast invasion of the spiral arteries in the second trimester. Failed trophoblast invasion may be unrelated to more acute sickle-caused uteroplacental complications. Nevertheless, abnormal uterine Doppler scans (the presence of notching or high resistance indices) are a good reason to be further concerned about an already high risk pregnancy.

Renal manifestations of SCD are common during pregnancy. These include haematuria, progressive inability to concentrate urine, and subtle proton- and potassium-secreting defects. The urinary concentration defect makes pregnant women with the sickling disorder more prone to dehydration.

Labour (particularly if prolonged or induced) is related to stasis, dehydration and infection. Rates of medical interventions are high. There is a trade-off between induction of labour at term (with a higher chance of caesarean section and thus trial of scar and complications in future pregnancies) and awaiting spontaneous labour (with risks of late pre-eclampsia and fetal loss and also high risk of emergency caesarean section for fetal distress). We offer induction routinely at 38 weeks (and certainly by 40 weeks), but tailor individual close monitoring with scans and cardiotocography if women have had few or no crises and are particularly averse to induction. Elective caesarean section is not offered as a routine, partly as it is associated with at least 30% higher severe maternal morbidity even when compared with labour with high emergency caesarean section rates [40] and partly because it should not be performed before 39 weeks as there is a higher risk of neonatal respiratory distress without labour [41]. Increased caesarean section rates of 35–48% have been reported in recent literature [22–25].

The physiological changes in pregnancy produce a hypercoagulable state. There is an increase in fibrinogen levels and clotting factors, particularly factors VIII, IX and X. There is a decrease in fibrinolytic activity, and levels of endogenous anticoagulants, such as antithrombin and protein S, are decreased. All these changes increase the risk of thrombosis in pregnancy and postpartum up to 6 weeks. In women with SCD the risk is further increased owing to anaemia and hyperviscosity of blood and so thromboprophylaxis should be considered when other factors that predispose to thrombosis are present, during any illness or hospitalization, after caesarean sections, and during the puerperium.

Maternal mortality

Increased maternal mortality rates in women with SCD have been reported by various groups (Table 12.2). The mean maternal mortality is 2% (0–9.6%) of pregnancies in women with SCD. The reports before 1970 were based on small numbers of patients from retrospective data. Powars *et al.* [14] summarized the mortality statistics in the literature from 1949 to 1972 and for a decade after 1972. The maternal mortality for 1949–1972 was 43/1000 live births and for 1972–1982 was 60/1000 live births. The overall maternal mortality per pregnancy was 2.2% and the maternal mortality per woman was 4.5%.

In the UK, all maternal deaths are reported to the Confidential Enquiry into Maternal Deaths (CEMD). In the 18 years between 1982 and 1999 inclusively, five maternal deaths in women with SCD were reported [42–44]. As there are no denominator data of numbers of women with SCD of reproductive age or SCD pregnancies over the same time period, a maternal mortality rate cannot be accurately calculated. The five cases reported in recent CEMDs are worth summarizing for lessons they illustrate about care.

1 A multiparous African woman was known to have homozygous SCD. Her antenatal care was uneventful. She was admitted in spontaneous labour and had an emergency caesarean section for fetal distress. On the first postoperative day she developed a chest infection leading to sickle cell crisis. She was transferred for exchange transfusion to a teaching hospital. She died in the third postpartum week following adult respiratory distress syndrome (ARDS). The case highlights the risks of SCD postpartum and especially the need for vigorous treatment of infections. Women should be delivered in centres where the expertise is available.

2 A patient with known SCD presented with breathlessness at 36 weeks of pregnancy. She was seen by the midwife and sent home. Three days later she had worsening breathlessness and abdominal pain. She was diagnosed to have abruption clinically on admission but had a caesarean section 12 hours later and delivered a stillborn baby. She died from renal, hepatic and cardiac failure 8 days later. Post mortem confirmed sickle cell crisis. There should be a low threshold for suspicion of crisis in women with breathlessness and abdominal pain.

3 A patient with HbSS disease had a haemoglobin concentration of 6.8 g/dL in early pregnancy. She was not transfused antenatally. After delivery she developed cough and severe breathlessness and was treated in the intensive care unit for pneumonia. No pathogens were ever grown. She was transfused postnatally and required ventilation. She died from brainstem haemorrhage. She possibly had an acute chest syndrome. She may have benefited from an earlier exchange transfusion but care was not thought to be substandard.

4 A patient had sickle cell/beta thalassaemia and recurrent crises. She had been advised against pregnancy and was offered the option of termination of pregnancy at an early stage of gestation, but declined the offer. She had pseudomonas septicaemia after surgery for common bile duct obstruction with gallstones and preterm delivery at 29 weeks of gestation. She died of liver failure and post-mortem liver biopsy confirmed acute hepatic sequestration crisis. Care was thought to be substandard in terms of the patient's own responsibility.

5 A multigravid Afro-Caribbean woman with known HbSC disease was informed after booking that she was a mild case of sickle cell trait. It is not clear if the medical carers were aware of her HbSC status or did not appreciate the significance of HbSC disease. She was induced for postdates with prostin. Following delay in transfer to the labour ward she was breathless and tachycardic. She was treated for presumed pulmonary embolus, although sickling had been considered and ruled out by the local haematologist. She deteriorated and was transferred to a tertiary unit. Spiral CT scan was negative. She died in spite of haemofiltration. Post mortem confirmed multiorgan failure consequent to sickle cell crisis. There was inappropriate diagnosis following her symptoms.

Role of prophylactic transfusion

The rationale for blood transfusion (exchange or top-up) is to decrease the absolute or relative amount of circulating HbS so that tissue oxygenation is improved and tissue injury due to sickling in the microvasculature is reduced. The major drawbacks of transfusion are the associated risks of transfusion reactions, allo-immunization and risk of exposure to pathogens such as hepatitis and human immunodeficiency viruses, and other uncharacterized new infections. Red cell antibodies were found in 10–22% of transfused women with SCD [20, 28, 45].

Prophylactic transfusion might be considered in an effort to avoid the risks of crises in pregnancy. Although universal prophylactic transfusion is a controversial issue, the evidence from randomized studies shows that there is reduction in the episodes of third trimester crises but no improvement in neonatal outcome [28]. Also, a retrospective multicentre survey in the UK showed that prophylactic transfusion did not improve obstetric outcome compared to those that were not transfused [20]. We reserve transfusion during pregnancy for women with twins, previous poor obstetric history, chest crisis, recurrent crises and severe anaemia.

Practical management of pregnancy

Preconceptual counselling

It is ideal to see women with SCD preconceptually in order to discuss the risks involved and plan the management of pregnancy. If the partner's status is not known it can be checked and prenatal diagnosis can be discussed. The importance of folate supplementation, prophylactic penicillin and analgesia requirements can be discussed. It is important to advise women and health professionals to use folic acid 5 mg per day throughout the pregnancy, as there can be confusion with the general advice to women to take folic acid 400 µg for the first trimester only to prevent neural tube defects. The need for early booking can be encouraged. In some cases, it would be prudent to advise against pregnancy if the risks for the woman are significant even before she embarks upon a pregnancy. Although it is very painful to consider voluntary infertility, having to consider a termination during a planned or wanted pregnancy is also dreadful.

At booking

Women with SCD (and their families) should be advised regarding the increased risk of crisis, intrauterine growth restriction, pre-eclampsia, fetal loss and sickling in uteroplacental circulation. Women should be advised that coping with crises at home is not appropriate during pregnancy, particularly because of the need to monitor the fetus. They should be encouraged to have a low threshold for admission if they think they are starting a crisis. We advise the use of prophylactic penicillin to prevent infection, or erythromycin if allergic to penicillin. An early dating scan is arranged so that accuracy of dates is confirmed and monitoring of growth and timing of delivery can be planned. Hyperemesis in early pregnancy can be a problem, so early prevention of dehydration and control of nausea may reduce the risk of painful episodes in early pregnancy.

Antenatal care

As this is a high risk pregnancy a more frequent schedule of care should be planned between the obstetrician, haematologist and specialist midwives. In the UK, the midwife is the usual lead clinician in pregnancy, and we believe that she should still perform the majority of care even in these high risk pregnancies. Most women do have successful pregnancies and need the usual support in pregnancy, in labour and with their newborn that can be missed if management is 'over-medicalized'. Iron supplementation may be required, but only if the serum ferritin levels are low. A monthly haemoglobin check should be made, and midstream urine should be sent monthly for culture and sensitivity. The fetus should be monitored closely, as there is a higher rate of IUGR and higher perinatal mortality. After the early dating scan (or nuchal translucency scan if this is used for Down's syndrome screening) an anomaly scan is offered at 20 weeks with uterine artery Doppler. This is followed by growth scans at 26, 30, 34 and 38 weeks. Scans may be performed more frequently if there are concerns about growth or liquor volume and umbilical artery Doppler scans may be added. It is vital that the mother understands the risk factors and that there is an open door policy 24 hours, 7 days a week for admission if in pain, sickle cell crises, dyspnoea, pre-eclampsia or if there is any need for blood transfusion.

Intrapartum

The aim is to achieve a safe vaginal delivery when possible. As there is increased perinatal mortality we aim for delivery in our unit between 38 and 40 weeks by induction of labour (IOL). However, the risk–benefit should be individualized, as failed IOL can lead to emergency caesarean section and problems in subsequent pregnancies where IOL is relatively contraindicated in previous scar. The mother should be well hydrated and oxygenated throughout labour. The fetus should be monitored by continuous cardiotocograph, as there is increased risk of fetal distress in labour. Epidural is preferable to general anaesthesia if operative intervention is needed. It is important to avoid hypotensive episodes as these may precipitate a vaso-occlusive crisis. There is an increased risk if postpartum haemorrhage occurs with a background of chronic anaemia and thus the third stage should be actively managed with an oxytocic. Attention to blood loss is especially important if women have become difficult to cross-match or transfuse through the development of antibodies. Throughout labour and delivery a senior midwife and doctor with knowledge of the condition should be responsible for her care so that appropriate timely intervention and management is possible.

Postpartum

Thromboprophylaxis with TED (thromboembolism) stockings and low molecular weight heparin should be considered postnatally, especially with any other risk factor (such as high BMI, operative delivery, high platelet count, HbSC). Early ambulation should be encouraged. Postpartum antibiotics should be given for operative deliveries and there should be a low threshold for treating a suspected infection. The mother should be encouraged to keep well hydrated. The baby should be screened for haemoglobinopathy if prenatal diagnosis was not possible. Cord blood can be collected for screening of the neonate. Contraception should be discussed, and can be prescribed, before discharge.

Multidisciplinary team approach

As these are high risk pregnancies, the importance of a multidisciplinary approach cannot be over-emphasized. The composition of the team involves many professionals such as the haematology doctors and nurses, the obstetrician and midwives, genetic counsellors, laboratory sickle cell specialists, psychologists, anaesthetists, high dependency and intensive care treatment teams. We have no doubt that pregnant women with SCD should be cared for in centres where all the relevant expertise is available. Aside from the membership of the team, frequent non-hurried communication about individual patients, protocols, clinical errors and learning, audit and research must be fostered. There should be updated evidence-based protocols and joint multidisciplinary meetings to maintain high standards of care and effective communication between the team members. An atmosphere of mutual respect must be developed for the different expertise brought to the management of these patients with a complex chronic medical disorder and yet simple and understandable desires for parenting.

References

1. Charache S, Niebyl JR. Pregnancy in sickle cell disease. *Clin Haematol* 1985; **14**: 729–46.
2. Yoong WC, Tuck SM, Yardumian A. Red cell deformability in oral contraceptive pill users with sickle cell anaemia. *Br J Haematol* 1999; **104**: 868–70.
3. De Ceulaer K, Gruber C, Hayes R, Serjeant GR. Medroxyprogesterone acetate and homozygous sickle-cell disease. *Lancet* 1982; **2**: 229–31.
4. Cronin EK, Normand C, Henthorn JS, Graham V, Davies SC. Organisation and cost-effectiveness of antenatal haemoglobinopathy screening and follow up in a community-based programme. *Br J Obstet Gynaecol* 2000; **107**: 486–91.
5. Department of Health. *Working Party of the Standing Medical Advisory Committee on Sickle Cell, Thalassaemia and other Haemoglobinopathies*. London: HMSO, 1993.
6. Lynch JR, Brown JM. The polymerase chain reaction: current and future clinical applications. *J Med Genet* 1990; **27**: 2–7.
7. Husain SM, Kalavathi P, Anandaraj MP. Analysis of sickle cell gene using polymerase chain reaction & restriction enzyme Bsu 361. *Indian J Med Res* 1995; **101**: 273–6.
8. Rowley PT, Loader S, Sutera CJ, Walden M, Kozyra A. Prenatal screening for hemoglobinopathies. I. A prospective regional trial. *Am J Hum Genet* 1991; **48**: 439–46.
9. Wang X, Seaman C, Paik M *et al.* Experience with 500 prenatal diagnoses of sickle cell diseases: the effect of gestational age on affected pregnancy outcome. *Prenat Diagn* 1994; **14**: 851–7.
10. Driscoll MC, Lerner N, Anyane-Yeboa K *et al.* Prenatal diagnosis of sickle hemoglobinopathies: the experience of the Columbia University Comprehensive Center for Sickle Cell Disease. *Am J Hum Genet* 1987; **40**: 548–58.
11. Alter BP. Antenatal diagnosis. Summary of results. *Ann N Y Acad Sci* 1990; **612**: 237–50.
12. Xu K, Shi ZM, Veeck LL, Hughes MR, Rosenwaks Z. First unaffected pregnancy using preimplantation genetic diagnosis for sickle cell anemia. *JAMA* 1999; **281**: 1701–6.
13. Tuck SM, Studd JW, White JM. Pregnancy in sickle cell disease in the UK. *Br J Obstet Gynaecol* 1983; **90**: 112–17.
14. Powars DR, Sandhu M, Niland-Weiss J *et al.* Pregnancy in sickle cell disease. *Obstet Gynecol* 1986; **67**: 217–28.
15. El Shafei AM, Dhaliwal J K, Sandhu AK. Pregnancy in sickle cell disease in Bahrain. *Br J Obstet Gynaecol* 1992; **99**: 101–4.
16. Dare FO, Makinde OO, Faasuba OB. The obstetric performance of sickle cell disease patients and homozygous hemoglobin C disease patients in Ile-Ife, Nigeria. *Int J Gynaecol Obstet* 1992; **37**: 163–8.
17. Idrisa A, Omigbodun AO, Adeleye JA. Pregnancy in hemoglobin sickle cell patients at the University College Hospital, Ibadan. *Int J Gynaecol Obstet* 1992; **38**: 83–6.
18. Ogedengbe OK, Akinyanju O. The pattern of sickle cell disease in pregnancy in Lagos, Nigeria. *West Afr J Med* 1993; **12**: 96–100.
19. Seoud MA, Cantwel, C, Nobles G, Levy DL. Outcome of pregnancies complicated by sickle cell and sickle-C hemoglobinopathies. *Am J Perinatol* 1994; **11**: 187–91.
20. Howard RJ, Tuck SM, Pearson TC. Pregnancy in sickle cell disease in the UK: results of a multicentre survey of the effect of prophylactic blood transfusion on maternal and fetal outcome. *Br J Obstet Gynaecol* 1995; **102**: 947–51.
21. Smith JA, Espeland M, Bellevue R *et al.* Pregnancy in sickle cell disease: experience of the Cooperative Study of Sickle Cell Disease. *Obstet Gynecol* 1996; **87**: 199–204.
22. Rahimy MC, Gangbo A, Adjou R *et al.* Effect of active prenatal management on pregnancy outcome in sickle

cell disease in an African setting. *Blood* 2000; **96**: 1685–9.

23. Leborgne-Samuel Y, Janky E, Venditelli F *et al*. Sickle cell anemia and pregnancy: review of 68 cases in Guadeloupe. *J Gynecol Obstet Biol Reprod [Paris]* 2000; **29**: 86–93.

24. Sun PM, Wilburn W, Raynor BD, Jamieson D. Sickle cell disease in pregnancy: twenty years of experience at Grady Memorial Hospital, Atlanta, Georgia. *Am J Obstet Gynecol* 2001; **184**: 1127–30.

25. Odum CU, Anorlu RI, Dim SI, Oyekan TO. Pregnancy outcome in HbSS-sickle cell disease in Lagos, Nigeria. *West Afr J Med* 2002; **21**: 19–23.

26. Fort AT, Morrison JC, Diggs LW, Fish SA, Berreras L. Counseling the patient with sickle cell disease about reproduction: pregnancy outcome does not justify the maternal risk. *Am J Obstet Gynecol* 1971; **111**: 324–7.

27. Blake PG, Martin JNJ, Perry KG Jr. Disseminated intravascular coagulation, autoimmune thrombocytopenic purpura, and hemoglobinopathies. In: Knuppel RA, Drukker JE, eds. *High-risk Pregnancy. A Team Approach*, 2nd edn. Philadelphia: WB.Saunders, 1993.

28. Koshy M, Burd L, Wallace D, Moawad A, Baron J. Prophylactic red-cell transfusions in pregnant patients with sickle cell disease. A randomized cooperative study. *N Engl J Med* 1988; **319**: 1447–52.

29. Okpala I, Thomas V, Westerdale N *et al*. The comprehensiveness care of sickle cell disease. *Eur J Haematol* 2002; **68**: 157–62.

30. Charache S, Scott J, Niebyl J, Bonds D. Management of sickle cell disease in pregnant patients. *Obstet Gynecol* 1980; **55**: 407–10.

31. Poddar D, Maude GH, Plant MJ, Scorer H, Serjeant GR. Pregnancy in Jamaican women with homozygous sickle cell disease. Fetal and maternal outcome. *Br J Obstet Gynaecol* 1986; **93**: 727–32.

32. Brown AK, Sleeper LA, Miller ST *et al*. Reference values and hematologic changes from birth to 5 years in patients with sickle cell disease. Cooperative Study of Sickle Cell Disease. *Arch Pediatr Adolesc Med* 1994; **148**: 796–804.

33. Anderson M, Went LN, MacIver JE, Dixon HG. Sickle cell disease in pregnancy. *Lancet* 1960; **2**: 516–21.

34. Dunn DT, Poddar D, Serjeant BE, Serjeant GR. Fetal haemoglobin and pregnancy in homozygous sickle cell disease. *Br J Haematol* 1989; **72**: 434–8.

35. Shanklin DR. Clinicopathologic correlates in placentas from woman with sickle cell disease. *Am J Pathol* 1976; **82** (5a).

36. Fox H. *Pathology of the Placenta*. London: Saunders, 1978.

37. Department of Health. *Mortality Statistics: Perinatal and Infant: Social and Biological Factors*, 1991 series DH3 no. 25. London: HMSO, 1993.

38. Horger O III. Sickle cell and sickle cell-hemoglobin C disease during pregnancy. *Obstet Gynecol* 1972; **39**: 873–9.

39. Chapell L, Bewley S. Pre-eclamptic toxaemia: the role of uterine artery Doppler. *Br J Obstet Gynaecol* 1999; **106**: 1328–9.

40. Hofmeyr GJ, Hannah ME. Planned caesarean section for term breech delivery. [Systematic Review] Cochrane Pregnancy and Childbirth Group. *Cochrane Database of Systematic Reviews* 2002; Issue 4.

41. Morrison JJ, Rennie JM, Milton PJ. Neonatal respiratory morbidity and mode of delivery at term: influence of timing of elective caesarean section. *Br J Obstet Gynaecol* 1995; **102**: 101–6.

42. Department of Health. *Report on Confidential Enquiries into Maternal Deaths in the United Kingdom, 1985–87*. London: HMSO, 1991.

43. Department of Health. *Report on Confidential Enquiries into Maternal Deaths in the United Kingdom 1991–93*. London: HMSO, 1996.

44. *Why mothers die. The Fifth Report on Confidential Enquiries into Maternal Deaths in the United Kingdom 1997–99*. London: RCOG Press, 2001.

45. Tuck SM, James CE, Brewster EM, Pearson TC, Studd JW. Prophylactic blood transfusion in maternal sickle cell syndromes. *Br J Obstet Gynaecol* 1987; **94**: 121–5.

Chapter 13
The liver in sickle cell disease

Cage S Johnson

Introduction

The hepatobiliary complications of sickle cell disease (SCD) can be classified as disorders related to chronic haemolysis and its accelerated bilirubin metabolism, to the consequences of transfusion management, to the consequences of vaso-occlusion or to diseases unrelated to haemoglobin S (HbS). Hepatobiliary complications are most common in sickle cell anaemia, but also occur in the doubly heterozygous sickle diseases, HbSC and the HbS thalassaemia syndromes (HbS β^0 thalassaemia and HbS β^+ thalassaemia). Early reports emphasized the classic histological features of Kupffer cell erythrophagocytosis and engorgement of sinusoids as indicative of ischaemic anoxia as the pathophysiology of hepatic dysfunction, but suffer from ascertainment bias due to use of autopsy material or biopsy in advanced disease and to the absence of modern serological testing. More recent reports have emphasized the importance of hepatic disease consequent to disorders unrelated to HbS per se and promote consideration of a wider diagnostic spectrum.

Despite nearly 200 reports in the past 20 years on the hepatobiliary aspects of the sickling disorders, the frequency and pathophysiology of hepatic lesions remains unclear. Consequently, management suffers from the lack of systematic studies that clearly define the pathophysiological processes involved and clarify the therapeutic approach. Data from other patient populations extrapolated to SCD provide support for therapy in certain situations, while treatment approaches for those complications attributed to vaso-occlusion represent the opinions of experts in the field taken from case reports.

Steady-state

In the steady-state, hepatomegaly is present in the majority of patients [1, 2]. Hepatic blood volume and blood flow are increased and contribute to hepatomegaly. Hepatic histology shows varying degrees of Kupffer cell erythrophagocytosis, sinusoidal distension, perisinusoidal fibrosis, extramedullary haematopoiesis and haemosiderosis [3–8]. Chronic congestion due to sinusoidal obstruction and erythrophagocytosis is also thought to contribute to the observed hepatomegaly but has not shown any correlation with clinical state nor with liver tests [3–5]. Shrunken hepatocytes and perivenular necrosis indicative of anoxia and ischaemia are only seen in shock or at post-mortem examinations [4], casting doubt on the concept of anoxia and its pathogenetic significance. The significance of sickled cells in biopsy or autopsy materials is often exaggerated, as post-mortem anoxia and formalin fixation both induce sickling [4]. Hepatic sickling was also found in race–matched controls [3], presumably in individuals with sickle trait, which further decreases its histological significance. The observations that irreversibly sickled cell counts are low in the hepatic vein [9] and that red cell survival studies show rapid hepatic accumulation of the erythrocyte label [10–12] suggest that Kupffer cell erythrophagocytosis may reflect a shift of erythrocyte destruction from the hypo-functioning spleen to the liver, rather than indicate a specific pathogenic mechanism.

Tests of liver function are generally normal other than elevation of unconjugated bilirubin and lactate dehydrogenase (LDH) indicative of haemolysis. The total bilirubin level rarely exceeds 70 µmol/L from haemolysis alone [13, 14]. It is proposed that substrate induction of the conjugating enzyme maintains unconjugated bilirubin at this modest elevation. A study of hepatic UDP-glucuronyl transferase levels confirmed that the enzyme levels are increased in these patients and that low levels during acute hepatitis were associated with very high bilirubin concentrations [15]. Marked increases in the unconjugated fraction have been reported in association with the genetic defect of Gilbert's syndrome [16, 17]. Elevation of aspartate aminotransferase (AST) indicates a contribution from the erythrocyte enzyme due to haemolysis [13]. The correlation of haemoglobin concentration with serum albumin suggests that a slight decrease in albumin concentration may reflect plasma volume expansion [18]. Isolated elevation of alkaline phosphatase is probably of bony origin rather than indicative of liver dysfunction [19, 20].

Vascular occlusion

The 'hepatic crisis', consisting of right upper quadrant pain, fever, jaundice, elevated AST/alanine aminotransferase (ALT) and hepatic enlargement is said to occur in as many as 10% of patients with acute vaso-occlusive crisis (VOC). Right upper quadrant pain and jaundice present a problem in differential diagnosis because of the variety of conditions with prominent abdominal pain reported in sickle cell disease (Table 13.1) [21–27]. Careful evaluation is needed to differentiate this from acute cholecystitis. In 'hepatic crisis', the AST/ALT fall rapidly, as opposed to the slower decline characteristic of acute viral hepatitis, and the γ-glutamyltransferase reportedly decreases [14]. In one study of 30 patients, liver tests taken at the time of uncomplicated VOC and repeated 4 weeks later in the steady-state showed that the alkaline phosphatase was 30% higher

Table 13.1 Unusual causes of right upper quadrant pain or cholestasis reported in the sickling disorders

Cause	Reference*
Biloma	Middleton & Wolper [21]
Focal nodular hyperplasia	Heaton et al. [22]
Fungal ball	Ho et al. [23]
Hepatic infarct/abscess	Chong et al. [24]
Hepatic vein thrombosis	Sty [25]
Mesenteric/colonic ischaemia	Gage & Gagnier [26]
Pancreatitis	
Peri-colonic abscess	
Pulmonary infarct/abscess	
Renal vein thrombosis	
Retained intrahepatic stones	

*A representative reference is provided; the remainder have been reviewed in Magid et al. [27].

during VOC. In addition, the ALT was threefold higher, and the bilirubin was elevated by twofold, primarily due to elevation of the conjugated fraction [20].

Hepatic sequestration

Hepatic sequestration is a rare complication of VOC; in one study, there was one case in 161 consecutive hospital admissions [28]. Undoubtedly mild episodes are not recognized. This syndrome is characterized by a rapidly enlarging liver accompanied by a fall in haemoglobin and a rise in reticulocyte count [1, 29–34]. The liver is smooth and variably tender. The bilirubin may be as high as 450 µmol/L with a predominance of the conjugated fraction. The alkaline phosphatase can be as high as 650 IU/L but may be normal; the transaminases are only minimally elevated (< 110 IU) and often normal. Recurrence is common. Ultrasonography and computed tomography (CT) scanning show only diffuse hepatomegaly. Liver biopsy shows massively dilated sinusoids with sickled erythrocytes and Kupffer cell erythrophagocytosis. Intrahepatic cholestasis with bile plugs in canaliculi may be seen. Hepatocyte necrosis is unusual. The pathophysiology is believed to be obstruction of sinusoidal flow by the masses of sickled erythrocytes, causing trapping of red blood cells (RBCs) within the liver and compression of the biliary tree.

Successful resolution of hepatic sequestration has been seen with either simple or exchange transfusion, as well as with supportive care alone. In one case, treated with simple transfusion, resolution of sequestration was accompanied by a rapid increase in the haemoglobin concentration, representing return of sequestered RBCs to the circulation, resulting in a fatal acute hyperviscosity syndrome [33]. Because of this risk, exchange transfusion is preferred.

Cholestasis

Cholestasis may occur when the hepatic vein pressure abruptly increases, exceeding the maximal bile secretory pressure of 20 mmHg, as in passive congestion or biliary obstruction [35]. It is seen with drugs that affect the $Na^+ K^+$ ATPase activity, such as phenothiazines, androgens or oestrogens, or with drugs (like indomethacin), which affect the bile acid-binding cytosolic proteins. In sepsis, endotoxin decreases bile flow. Thus, acute and chronic cholestatic syndromes can be caused by a wide variety of clinical entities in sickle cell patients. The term sickle cell intrahepatic cholestasis (SCIC) has recently been applied to the cholestatic syndromes; however, the use of one term for this complex problem obscures the differences in presentation and clinical course between clinically 'benign' types of cholestasis and more serious forms.

A benign cholestatic picture has been described in which there are striking elevations of bilirubin (up to 1000 µmol/L) with only modest elevations of alkaline phosphatase (< 2× normal) and transaminases (< 500 IU/L). Importantly, the hepatic synthetic function is not impaired, as reflected by serum albumin or coagulation times, and platelet counts are normal to increased. The patients are asymptomatic other than profound jaundice. Fever, abdominal pain, altered mental status and bleeding are conspicuously absent. Drug-induced cholestasis can be implicated in some cases. In the 14 cases with these characteristics, only 3 were older than 15 years. Resolution of cholestasis occurred within weeks to months in all cases in the absence of specific therapy. The longest course was seen in the patient for whom androgen therapy was implicated as the cause of cholestasis [13, 36–38].

In contrast, a progressive cholestasis in the absence of cirrhosis has been reported in 29 instances. These cases are characterized by right upper quadrant pain, progressively increasing elevations of bilirubin (up to 2500 µmol/L), striking elevation of alkaline phosphatase (> 3× normal) and variable elevation of transaminases (90–6700 IU/L). This syndrome occurs primarily in adults but has been reported in children as young as 6 years. Importantly, fever, hepatic encephalopathy, elevated ammonia, renal failure and thrombocytopenia (< 150 × 10^5/µl) are often present. Declining hepatic protein synthesis is universal, with falling albumin and severe prolongation of coagulation times unresponsive to vitamin K administration.

Liver histology in both benign and progressive forms of cholestasis shows intrasinusoidal sickling and Kupffer cell hyperplasia with phagocytosis of sickled erythrocytes but fails to explain the difference in clinical course. Percutaneous liver biopsy carries a high risk of bleeding, possibly related to hepatic venous congestion, and the trans-jugular approach should be considered [39]. Mortality due to uncontrollable bleeding or to hepatic failure occurred in 17 of the 29 cases [13, 38, 40–48]. These case reports often lack sufficient information to exclude hepatic sequestration and benign, immune or drug-induced cholestasis from consideration, making full interpretation difficult [13, 41, 49, 50]. These syndromes attributable to intrahepatic vaso-occlusion are best treated with exchange RBC transfusion because of the potential risk of acute hyperviscosity [33]. Plasmapheresis and platelet transfusion are useful in controlling haemostatic failure. Several patients responded to liver transplantation but often required continuing hypertransfusion [45, 48]. The prolonged course in some cases suggests that future studies are indicated to test the hypothesis that hepatic damage might release immunogenic material into the circulation [50].

Viral hepatitis

The hepatic complications due to the anaemia are essentially those consequent to transfusion therapy: transmission of viral infection and iron overload.

As transfusion therapy is applied for an increasing number of indications, the risk for transmission of current and emerging infectious agents needs continuing surveillance. Acute viral hepatitis has the same clinical course in the sickling disorders as in the general population, other than a higher peak bilirubin level because of haemolysis.

Surveys for serological evidence of hepatitis B infection show a range of prevalence from 3% to 46% [13, 14, 51, 52, 53, 54] related to local endemicity as well as to past transfusion practice. Because chronicity is inversely related to age, vaccination is indicated early in life [55, 56]. Similar surveys for hepatitis C infection indicate prevalence rates from 2% to 26% [14, 53, 54, 57, 58] with a clear relationship to transfusion practice. In studies of patients with persistent elevations of AST/ALT, biopsy frequently shows evidence of chronic hepatitis [4, 5, 52], indicating the overall importance of hepatitis C infection. End-stage liver disease requiring liver transplant has been reported in these patients [59]. Treatment of chronic viral hepatitis is based upon data that sustained suppression of viral replication reduces the inflammatory process and decreases the subsequent development of cirrhosis and hepatocellular carcinoma. The management of chronic hepatitis requires close co-ordination with gastroenterology to guide diagnostic and therapeutic decision making.

Indications for treatment of hepatitis B include HBsAg positivity for more than 6 months, evidence for active virus replication by HbeAg and HBV DNA positivity and evidence of active liver disease by persistent elevation of ALT and/or biopsy evidence of chronic hepatitis. Therapy with 5 million units of alpha-interferon daily or 10 million units three times weekly for 16 weeks is effective; treatment data in SCD are lacking but should be similar to that for the general population [35].

In hepatitis C, persistent elevation of AST/ALT, positive PCR for viral RNA and/or biopsy evidence of chronic hepatitis are indications for treatment. The treatment schedule is alpha-interferon, 3 million units three times weekly, plus ribavarin 1 g orally per day for 48 weeks in those infected with genotype 1 and for 24 weeks for those with genotypes 2 or 3 [35]. Reports of successful therapy in SCD are just appearing [60]. Careful monitoring of haemoglobin is necessary, as ribavarin causes a haemolytic anaemia attributed to oxidative damage to the RBC membrane [61].

Other hepatitides

Autoimmune hepatitis has been reported in five patients [49, 62, 63]. This diagnosis is suggested in the setting of painless jaundice and a marked polyclonal gammopathy. Serological tests for ANA (antinuclear antibody) and SMA (serum mitochondrial antibody) are variably positive. This disorder is characterized by dense T-cell infiltrates in the peri-portal areas with bridging fibrosis and piecemeal necrosis. Extrahepatic manifestations of arthropathy, rash and leg ulcers may occur. Treatment with prednisone (10–60 mg per day) and azathioprine (50 mg per day) for 24 months induces a clinical remission, followed by biochemical then histological remission.

Granulomatous hepatitis due to tuberculosis, sarcoidosis, or viral infection has been reported in a number of cases [4, 39], for which specific anti-tuberculous or immunosuppressive therapy would be used. These cases, as well as others showing the changes of alcoholism [4, 13, 39], indicate the necessity of a broad diagnostic consideration in sickle cell patients. Persistent elevation of serum ferritin above 500 mg/L that is unexplained by transfusion history is a useful indication of significant liver disease and can guide the clinician in the judicious use of liver biopsy [13, 14].

Haemosiderosis/haemochromatosis

Iron overload and cirrhosis develop as a consequence of frequent transfusion [64], although there is one case report of genetic haemochromatosis [65]. Iron overload is suggested by a transfusion history of 50 units or more, serum ferritin values of > 1500 mg/L and a transferrin saturation in excess of 50% [64]. A single serum ferritin value may be elevated out of proportion to the degree of iron stores because of its acute phase reactant property as well as other factors, such as ascorbate status or liver disease [13, 14, 66]. Acute vaso-occlusive crisis transiently raises the ferritin value sixfold so that multiple measurements during the steady-state are needed for full interpretation [64]. Definitive assessment requires liver biopsy for quantification of tissue iron burden. Magnetic resonance imaging, comparing the signal intensity of liver, pancreas and spleen to that of muscle, is able to detect iron overload but is not very sensitive to gradations of iron load [67].

The relationship of transfusion to tissue iron burden is illustrated by studies during transfusion therapy. In women receiving supportive transfusion during pregnancy, incidental liver biopsy performed at abdominal surgery showed that two-thirds had significant hepatocyte iron accumulation after an average transfusion burden of 13.6 units [68]. In patients receiving transfusion for the prevention of stroke, the serum ferritin rose 10-fold at an average follow-up of 42 months and was associated with an eightfold rise in AST/ALT [69]. A similar stroke study demonstrated that, after a mean of 15.4 transfusions over 21 months, the hepatic iron level was 9.4 mg/g, dry weight, and that one-third of patients had portal fibrosis. After 4 years of transfusion and chelation therapy, the mean hepatic iron rose to 14.1 mg/g, dry weight [70]. The author concluded that portal fibrosis occurs in these patients at tissue iron burden levels of 7 mg/g liver, similar to those reported in thalassaemia and haemochromatosis.

The standard subcutaneous regimens for desferrioxamine therapy are as effective in these patients as in thalassaemia [71]. Complications of therapy include ophthalmic toxicity or ototoxicity, allergic reactions, growth failure and unusual infections (*Yersinia*, fungi). Because of poor patient compliance, periodic intensive intravenous therapy can be given. Aggressive chelation with intravenous doses of 6–12 g daily have shown rapid declines in serum ferritin and ALT and are associated with clinical improvement in cardiac function and other indices [72, 73]. Adverse effects have not been noted in short-term therapy, although zinc excretion is increased. This intensive intravenous approach is attractive because of the claims of improved compliance and efficacy [73].

Gall bladder

Chronic haemolysis with its accelerated bilirubin turnover leads to a high incidence of biliary sludge and pigment gallstones. The gall bladder concentration of both conjugated and unconjugated bilirubin metabolites is increased in patients with SCD but are not different between those with or without cholelithiasis [74, 75]. Thus, stone formation appears to require additional pathogenic factors over and above the poor solubility of bilirubin. A careful study of biliary function in sickle cell patients indicates that there is an enlarged fasting, as well as post-prandial, gall bladder volume consistent with stasis of bile [76]. This incomplete emptying may allow the precipitation of bilirubin and initiate the process of sludge and/or stone formation. Patients with a more severe clinical course had the largest gall bladder volumes, suggesting that sickling and ischaemia might be responsible for the altered gall bladder function.

Biliary sludge is a complex mixture of mucus, calcium bilirubinate and cholesterol, forming a viscous material detectable by non-acoustic shadowing on ultrasonography [77] and may be a precursor of gallstone development. Certain antibiotics seem to promote sludge formation [78]; such compounds are theorized to crystallize in the gall bladder, forming a nidus for stone formation. Differences in the use of such antibiotics could account for some of the geographic variation in choleli-thiasis frequency. Studies in patients with SCD indicate that sludge is often found with or without concomitant stones. The finding of sludge alone is believed to predict a high likelihood of subsequent stone formation, but serial ultrasound studies have found that sludge may or may not progress to stone formation and may clear [79, 80–82].

Ultrasound surveys of patient populations indicate that the onset of cholelithiasis is as early as 2 years of age and that cholelithiasis progressively increases in prevalence with age [79, 83–85], reaching nearly 30% frequency by age 18 and a higher prevalence in adults [86, 87]. Cholelithiasis is associated with a higher sickle disease morbidity [88, 89], but there is considerable controversy as to whether the cholelithiasis is responsible for the increased disease severity or is a reflection of overall disease severity. African populations appear to have a substantially lower prevalence than that in Jamaican or North American patients [84, 90]; this difference has been attributed to differences in dietary cholesterol and/or fibre but other factors (genetic or environmental) may have an influence on stone formation.

The co-inheritance of alpha thalassaemia appears to reduce the frequency of stones as the result of a lesser degree of haemolysis [91]. Common duct obstruction can be partial, as pigment stones are small, and may allow bile flow [92]. Gallstones have been known to pass without inducing pancreatitis or other acute symptomatology [93, 94].

Cholecystitis

Fever, nausea, vomiting and abdominal pain are common events in SCD. Establishing the aetiology of these symptoms can be difficult and requires consideration of acute vaso-occlusion as well as a wide variety of other disorders that have been reported in these patients with symptoms mimicking cholecystitis (Table 13.1). A careful clinical evaluation is necessary to establish a clear diagnosis. Ultrasound examination is often definitive in diagnosis. In confounding situations, biliary scintigraphy might be helpful; however, its use is controversial because of a high false positive rate and low positive predictive value. A normal study indicating that the cystic duct is patent is useful because of its negative predictive value [95]. False positives can result from prolonged fasting, severe hepatocellular disease, extrahepatic obstruction, chronic cholecystitis or narcotic-induced spasm of the sphincter of Oddi [96]. The Tc-99 RBC scan may prove more useful in detecting the hyperaemia of acute cholecystitis, but its use has not been reported in these patients [97]. CT scans can be helpful in clarifying confounding clinical situations (Table 13.1) [27]. Treatment of acute cholecystitis with antibiotics and supportive care does not differ from that in the general population, and elective cholecystectomy after the acute episode subsides is appropriate.

Cholecystectomy

As biliary sludge may clear in as many as 20% of patients [81, 82], it is best observed. Serial ultrasound examinations at 12–24-month intervals can assess for clearance of sludge or for progression to stone formation. Should cholestasis due to thickened sludge occur [98], cholecystectomy is indicated. The Jamaican data [85] provide the strongest argument for a conservative approach, but Jamaican patients seem to be substantially less symptomatic than North American ones. An aggressive approach provides the benefit of reducing the risk of the morbid complications of cholelithiasis, as well as eliminating gall bladder disease as a confounding item in the differential diagnosis of right upper quadrant pain [94, 99–101]. It should be noted that some patients remain symptomatic after cholecystectomy, further indicating a cautious approach to surgery in these patients [87, 102]. For asymptomatic patients, there is considerable support for a conservative approach [93, 103], as it is estimated that symptoms occur at a rate of only 1% per year [104]. Bacteraemia, ascending cholangitis, empyema and other hyper-acute biliary complications require surgery on a more urgent basis consistent with good surgical practice [101].

Laparoscopic cholecystectomy on an elective basis in a well prepared patient has become the standard approach to symptomatic patients [101, 105] because of the shortened hospital stay, lower cost and fewer immediate surgical complications. Identification of common duct stones at the time of surgery is often done with intra-operative cholangiography (IOC). However, IOC has a false positive rate estimated at 25%, so that endoscopic retrograde cholangiopancreatography at the time of laparoscopic cholecystectomy is preferred, but IOC is still useful in delineating the anatomy of the cystic duct and its artery [94, 106, 107].

The hepatobiliary dysfunction in SCD has long been attributed to anoxia secondary to sinusoidal obstruction and Kupffer cell erythrophagocytosis. The absence of shrunken hepatocytes and the lack of correlation between the transaminase levels and the liver histology are evidence against that concept. Thus, the pathogenesis of the cholestatic syndromes remains unexplained, nor is there a unifying hypothesis for the differences in clinical course. Further studies are needed to understand why some patients progresss to hepatic insufficiency or necrosis while others improve. Importantly, liver disease in SCD is often explained by disorders other than intrahepatic sickling, so that careful evaluation of these patients and judicious use of liver biopsy is necessary to establish a correct diagnosis and determine the appropriate course of treatment.

References

1. Hernandez P, Dorticos E, Espinosa E, Gonzalez X, Svarch E. Clinical features of hepatic sequestration in sickle cell anaemia. *Haematologia* 1989; **22**: 169–74.
2. Serjeant GR. *Sickle Cell Disease*, 3rd edn. Oxford: Oxford University Press, 2001.
3. Bauer TW, Moore GW, Hutchins GM. The liver in sickle cell disease: a clinicopathologic study of 70 patients. *Am J Med* 1980; **69**: 833–7.
4. Omata M, Johnson CS, Tong MJ, Tatter D. The pathological spectrum of liver diseases in sickle cell disease. *Dig Dis Sci* 1986; **31**: 247–56.
5. Mills LR, Mwakyusa D, Milner PF. Histopathologic features of liver biopsy specimens in sickle cell disease. *Arch Pathol Lab Med* 1988; **112**: 290–4.
6. Aken'ova YA, Olasode BJ, Ogunbiyi JO, Thomas JO. Hepatobiliary changes in Nigerians with sickle cell anaemia. *Ann Trop Med Parasitol* 1993; **87**: 603–6.
7. Charlotte F, Bachir D, Nenert M *et al.* Vascular lesions of the liver in sickle cell disease. A clinicopathological study in 26 living patients. *Arch Pathol Lab Med* 1995; **119**: 46–52.
8. Teixeira AL, Viana MB, Roquette MLV, Toppa NH. Sickle cell disease: a clinical and histopathologic study of the liver in living children. *J Pediatr Hematol Oncol* 2002; **24**: 125–9.
9. Serjeant GR, Petch MC, Serjeant BE. The *in-vivo* sickle phenomenon: a reappraisal. *J Clin Lab Med* 1973; **81**: 850–6.
10. McCurdy PR. Erythrokinetics in abnormal hemoglobin syndromes. *Blood* 1962; **20**: 686–99.
11. Malamos B, Belcher EH, Gyftaki E, Binopoulos D. Simultaneous radioactive tracer studies of erythropoiesis and red-cell destruction in sickle-cell disease and sickle-cell haemoglobin/thalassaemia. *Br J Haematol* 1963; **9**: 487–98.
12. Hathorn M. Patterns of red cell destruction in sickle-cell anaemia. *Br J Haematol* 1967; **13**: 746–51.
13. Johnson CS, Omata M, Tong MJ *et al.* Liver involve-

14. Richard S, Billett HH. Liver function tests in sickle cell disease. *Clin Lab Haematol* 2002; **24**: 21–7.
15. Maddrey WC, Cukier JO, Maglalang AC, Boitnott JK, Odell GB. Hepatic bilirubin UDP-glucuronyltransferase in patients with sickle cell anemia. *Gastroenterology* 1978; **74**: 193–5.
16. Lin J, Johnson CS, Liebman HA. *Gilbert's syndrome in sickle cell anemia*. Annual Meeting of the National Sickle Cell Disease Program, Washington, DC, 15–20 September, 1997.
17. Passon RG, Howard TA, Zimmerman SA, Schultz WH, Ware RE. Influence of bilirubin uridine diphosphate-glucuronosyltransferase 1A promoter polymorphisms on serum bilirubin levels and cholelithiasis in children with sickle cell anemia. *J Pediatr Hematol Oncol* 2001; **23**: 448–51.
18. El-Hazmi MAF, Al-Swailem AR, Warsy AS. Liver function tests in sickle cell anemia patients: a case control study in Saudi Arabia. *Am J Med Sci* 1987; **30**: 371–6.
19. Brody JI, Ryan WN, Haldar MA. Serum alkaline phosphatase isoenzymes in sickle cell anemia. *JAMA* 1975; **232**: 738–41.
20. Ojuawo A, Adeoyin MA, Fagbule D. Hepatic function tests in children with sickle cell anaemia during vaso occlusive crisis. *Cent Afr J Med* 1994; **40**: 342–3.
21. Middleton JP, Wolper JC. Hepatic biloma complicating sickle cell disease. *Gastroenterology* 1984; **86**: 743–4.
22. Heaton ND, Pain J, Cowan NC, Salisbury J, Howard ER. Focal nodular hyperplasia of the liver: a link with sickle cell disease? *Arch Dis Child* 1991; **66**: 1073–4.
23. Ho F, Snape WJ Jr, Venegas R, Lechago J, Klein S. Choledochal fungal ball. An unusual cause of biliary obstruction. *Dig Dis Sci* 1988; **33**: 1030–4.
24. Chong SKF, Dick MC, Howard ER, Mowat AP. Liver abscess as an unusual complication in sickle cell anemia. *J Pediatr Gastroenterol Nutr* 1993; **16**: 221–2.
25. Sty JR. Ultrasonography: hepatic vein thrombosis in sickle cell anemia. *Am J Pediatr Hematol Oncol* 1982; **4**: 213–15.
26. Gage TP, Gagnier JM. Ischemic colitis complicating sickle cell crisis. *Gastroenterology* 1983; **84**: 171–4.
27. Magid D, Fishman EK, Charache S, Siegelman SS. Abdominal pain in sickle cell disease: the role of CT[1]. *Radiology* 1987; **163**: 325–8.
28. Davies SC, Brozovic M. Acute admissions of patients with sickle cell disease who live in Britain. *BMJ* 1987; **294**: 1206–8.
29. Hatton CSR, Bunch C, Weatherall DJ. Hepatic sequestration in sickle cell anaemia. *BMJ* 1985; **290**: 744–5.
30. Gutteridge C, Newland AC, Sequeira J. Hepatic sequestration in sickle cell anaemia. *BMJ* 1985; **290**: 1214–15.
31. Sarma PSA. Hepatic sequestration of red cells in

sickle cell anaemia. *J Assoc Physicians India* 1987; **35**: 384–6.

32. Koduri PR, Patel AR, Pinar H. Acute hepatic sequestration caused by parvovirus B19 infection in a patient with sickle cell anemia. *Am J Hematol* 1994; **47**: 250–1.

33. Lee ESH, Chu PCM. Reverse sequestration in a case of sickle cell crisis. *Postgrad Med J* 1996; **72**: 487–8.

34. Singh NK, El-Mangoush M. Hepatic sequestration crisis presenting with severe intrahepatic cholestatic jaundice. *J Assoc Physicians India* 1996; **44**: 283–4.

35. Schiff ER, Sorrell MF, Maddrey WC. *Schiff's Diseases of the Liver*. Philadelphia: Lippincott, Williams & Wilkins, 2003.

36. Buchanan GR, Glader BE. Benign course of extreme hyperbilirubinemia in sickle cell anemia: analysis of six cases. *J Pediatr* 1977; **91**: 21–4.

37. Mallouh AA, Asha ML. Acute cholestatic jaundice in children with sickle cell disease: hepatic crisis or hepatitis. *Pediatr Infect Dis J* 1988; **7**: 689–92.

38. Kaine WN, Udeozo OK. Sickle cell hepatic crisis in Nigerian children. *J Trop Pediatr* 1988; **34**: 59–64.

39. Zakaria N, Knisely A, Portmann B *et al*. Acute sickle cell hepatopathy represents a potential contraindication for percutaneous liver biopsy. *Blood* 2003; **101**: 101–3.

40. Rigano P, Renda D, Calabrese A, Spinello M, Pinzello G, Maggio A. Acute liver failure in sickle cell/β-thal disease solved by intensive transfusional regimen. *Am J Hematol* 1994; **46**: 372–3.

41. Shao SH, Orringer EP. Sickle cell intrahepatic cholestasis: approach to a difficult problem. *Am J Gastroenterol* 1995; **90**: 2048–50.

42. Stephan JL, Merpit-Gonon E, Richard O, Raynaud-Ravni C, Freycon F. Fulminant liver failure in a 12-year old girl with sickle cell anaemia: favourable outcome after exchange transfusions. *Eur J Pediatr* 1995; **154**: 469–71.

43. O'Callaghan AO, O'Brien SGO, Ninkovic M *et al*. Chronic intrahepatic cholestasis in sickle cell disease requiring exchange transfusion. *Gut* 1995; **37**: 144–7.

44. Betrosian A, Balla M, Kafiri G, Palamarou C, Sevastos N. Case report: reversal of liver failure in sickle cell vaso-occlusive crisis. *Am J Med Sci* 1996; **311**: 292–5.

45. Emre S, Kitibayashi K, Schwartz M *et al*. Liver transplantation in a patient with acute liver failure due to sickle cell intrahepatic cholestasis. *Transplantation* 2000; **69**: 675–6.

46. Ross AS, Graeme-Cook F, Cosimi AB, Chung RT. Combined liver and kidney transplantation in patient with sickle cell disease. *Transplantation* 2002; **73**: 605–8.

47. Khurshid I, Anderson L, Downie GH, Pape GS. Sickle cell disease, extreme hyperbilirubinemia, and pericardial tamponade: case report and review of the literature. *Crit Care Med* 2002; **30**: 2363–7.

48. Gilli SCO, Boin IFS, Leonardi LS *et al*. Liver transplantation in a patient with Sβ⁰-thalassemia. *Transplantation* 2002; **74**: 896–8.

49. Svarch E, Gonzalez A, Villaescusa R, Basanta P. Plasma exchange for acute cholestasis in homozygous sickle cell disease. *Haematologia* 1986; **19**: 49–51.

50. Villaescusa R, Santos MN, Espinosa E, Hernandez P. Circulating immune complexes in sickle cell anaemia. *Haematologia* 1986; **19**: 185–91.

51. Abiodun PO, Fatunde OJ, Flach KH, Buck T. Increased incidence of hepatitis B markers in children with sickle-cell anemia. *Blut* 1989; **58**: 147–50.

52. Gomer GM, Ozick LA, Sachdev RK *et al*. Transfusion-related chronic liver disease in sickle cell anemia. *Am J Gastroenterol* 1991; **86**: 1232–4.

53. DeVault KR, Friedman LS, Westerburg S *et al*. Hepatitis C in sickle cell anemia. *J Clin Gastroenterol* 1994; **18**: 206–9.

54. Samperi P, Consalvo C, Romano V *et al*. Liver involvement in white patients with sickle-cell disease. *Arch Pediatr Adolesc Med* 1996; **150**: 1177–80.

55. Sarnaik SA, Merline JR, Bond S. Immunogenicity of hepatitis B vaccine in children with sickle cell anemia. *J Pediatr* 1988; **112**: 429–30.

56. Mok Q, Underhill G, Wonke B *et al*. Intradermal hepatitis B vaccine in thalassaemia and sickle cell disease. *Arch Dis Child* 1989; **64**: 535–40.

57. King SD, Dodd RY, Haynes G *et al*. Prevalence of antibodies to hepatitis C virus and other markers in Jamaica. *West Indian Med J* 1995; **44**: 55–7.

58. Hasan MF, Marsh F, Posner G *et al*. Chronic hepatitis C in patients with sickle cell disease. *Am J Gastroenterol* 1996; **91**: 1204–6.

59. Kindscher JD, Laurin J, Delcore R, Forster J. Liver transplantation in a patient with sickle cell anemia. *Transplantation* 1995; **60**: 762–4.

60. Swaim MW, Agarwal S, Rosse WF. Successful treatment of hepatitis C in sickle-cell disease. *Ann Intern Med* 2000; **133**: 750–1.

61. De Franceschi L, Fattovich G, Turrini F *et al*. Hemolytic anemia induced by ribavirin therapy in patients with chronic hepatitis C virus infection: role of membrane oxidative damage. *Hepatology* 2000; **31**: 997–1004.

62. El Younis CM, Min AD, Fiel MI *et al*. Autoimmune hepatitis in a patient with sickle cell disease. *Am J Gastroenterol* 1996; **91**: 1016–18.

63. Chuang E, Ruchelli E, Mulberg AE. Autoimmune liver disease and sickle cell anemia in children: a report of three cases. *J Pediatr Hematol Oncol* 1997; **19**: 159–62.

64. Ballas SK. Iron overload is a determinant of morbidity and mortality in adult patients with sickle cell disease. *Semin Hematol* 2001; **38** (Suppl 1): 30–6.

65. Conrad ME. Sickle cell disease and hemochromatosis. *Am J Hematol* 1991; **38**: 150–2.

66. Brittenham GM, Cohen AR, McLaren CE *et al.* Hepatic iron stores and plasma ferritin concentration in patients with sickle cell anemia and thalassemia major. *Am J Hematol* 1993; **42**: 81–5.

67. Siegelman ES, Outwater E, Hanau CA *et al.* Abdominal iron distribution in sickle cell disease: MR findings in transfusion and nontransfusion dependent patients. *J Comput Assist Tomogr* 1994; **18**: 63–7.

68. Yeomans E, Lowe T, Eigenbrodt EH, Cunningham FG. Liver histopathologic findings in women with sickle cell disease given prophylactic transfusion during pregnancy. *Am J Obstet Gynecol* 1990; **163**: 958–64.

69. Harmatz P, Butensky E, Quirolo K *et al.* Severity of iron overload in patients with sickle cell disease receiving chronic red blood cell transfusion therapy. *Blood* 2000; **96**: 76–9.

70. Olivieri NF. Progression of iron overload in sickle cell disease. *Semin Hematol* 2001; **38** (Suppl 1): 57–62.

71. Cohen AR, Martin MB. Iron chelation therapy in sickle cell disease. *Semin Hematol* 2001; **38** (Suppl 1): 69–72.

72. Cohen AR, Mizanin J, Schwartz E. Rapid removal of excessive iron with daily, high-dose intravenous chelation therapy. *J Pediatr* 1989; **115**: 151–5.

73. Silliman CC, Peterson VM, Mellman DL *et al.* Iron chelation by desferoxamine in sickle cell patients with severe transfusion-induced hemosiderosis: a randomized double-blind study of the dose-response relationship. *J Clin Lab Med* 1993; **122**: 48–54.

74. Soloway RD, Trotman BW, Ostrow JD. Progress in gastroenterology. Pigment gallstones. *Gastroenterology* 1977; **72**: 167–82.

75. Trotman BW, Soloway RD. Pigment gallstone disease: summary of the National Institutes of Health – international workshop. *Hepatology* 1982; **2**: 879–84.

76. Everson GT, Nemeth A, Kourourian S *et al.* Gallbladder function is altered in sickle hemoglobinopathy. *Gastroenterology* 1989; **96**: 1307–16.

77. Lee SP, Maher K, Nicholls JF. Origin and fate of biliary sludge. *Gastroenterology* 1988; **94**: 170–6.

78. Schaad UB, Wedgewood-Krucko J, Tschaeppeler H. Reversible ceftriaxone-associated biliary pseudolithiasis in children. *Lancet* 1988; **2**: 1411–13.

79. Sarnaik S, Slovis TL, Corbett DP, Enami E, Whitten CF. Incidence of cholelithiasis in sickle cell anemia using the ultrasonic gray-scale technique. *J Pediatr* 1980; **96**: 1005–8.

80. Winter SS, Kinney TR, Ware RE. Gallbladder sludge in children with sickle cell disease. *J Pediatr* 1994; **125**: 747–9.

81. Walker TM, Serjeant GR. Biliary sludge in sickle cell disease. *J Pediatr* 1996; **129**: 443–5.

82. Al-Salem AH, Qaisruddin S. The significance of biliary sludge in children with sickle cell disease. *Pediatr Surg Int* 1998; **13**: 14–16.

83. Rennels MB, Dunne MG, Grossman NJ, Schwartz AD. Cholelithiasis in patients with major sickle hemoglobinopathies. *Am J Dis Child* 1984; **138**: 66–7.

84. Billa RF, Biwole MS, Juimo AG, Bejanga BI, Blackett K. Gall stone disease in African patients with sickle cell anaemia: a preliminary report from Yaounde, Cameroon. *Gut* 1991; **32**: 539–41.

85. Walker TM, Hambleton IR, Serjeant GR. Gallstones in sickle cell disease: observations from the Jamaican cohort study. *J Pediatr* 2000; **136**: 80–5.

86. McCall IW, Desai P, Serjeant BE, Serjeant GR. Cholelithiasis in Jamaican patients with homozygous sickle-cell disease. *Am J Hematol* 1978; **3**: 15–21.

87. Bond LR, Hatty SR, Horn MEC *et al.* Gall stones in sickle cell disease in the United Kingdom. *BMJ* 1987; **295**: 234–6.

88. Karayalcin G, Hassani N, Abrams M, Lanzkowsky P. Cholelithiasis in children with sickle cell disease. *Am J Dis Child* 1979; **133**: 306–7.

89. Webb DKH, Darby JS, Dunn DT, Terry SI, Serjeant GR. Gall stones in Jamaican children with homozygous sickle cell disease. *Arch Dis Child* 1989; **64**: 693–6.

90. Nzeh DA, Adedoyin MA. Sonographic pattern of gallbladder disease in children with sickle cell anaemia. *Pediatr Radiol* 1989; **19**: 290–2.

91. Haider MZ, Ashebu S, Aduh P, Adekile AD. Influence of α-thalassemia on cholelithiasis in SS patients with elevated Hb F. *Acta Haematol* 1998; **100**: 147–50.

92. Gholson SF, Grier JF, Ibach MB *et al.* Sequential endoscopic/laparoscopic management of sickle hemoglobinopathy-associated cholelithiasis and suspected choledocholithiasis. *South Med J* 1995; **88**: 1131–5.

93. Ariyan S, Shessel FS, Pickett LK. Cholecystitis and cholelithiasis masking as abdominal crises in sickle cell disease. *Pediatrics* 1976; **58**: 252–8.

94. Ware RE, Schultz WH, Filston HC, Kinney TR. Diagnosis and management of common bile duct stones in patients with sickle hemoglobinopathies. *J Pediatr Surg* 1992; **27**: 572–5.

95. D'Alonzo WA Jr, Heyman S. Biliary scintigraphy in children with sickle cell anemia and acute abdominal pain. *Pediatr Radiol* 1985; **15**: 395–8.

96. Serafini AN, Spoliansky G, Sfakianakis N, Montalvo B, Jensen WN. Diagnostic studies in patients with sickle cell anemia and acute abdominal pain. *Arch Intern Med* 1987; **147**: 1061–2.

97. Rachlin S, Sarkar SD, McCarthy CS *et al.* Detection of acute cholecystitis on Tc-99m RBC scintiscans for hemangioma. *Clin Nuclear Med* 1994; **19**: 163–4.

98. Muirhead EE, Halden ER, Wilson BJ. Recurrent crises in sickle cell anemia responding to cholecystectomy: a syndrome apparently based on cholecysto- and choledochostasis. *Am J Med* 1956; **20**: 953–4.

99. Rambo WM, Reines HD. Elective cholecystectomy for the patient with sickle cell disease and asymptomatic cholelithiasis. *Am Surg* 1986; **52**: 205–7.

100. Malon BS, Werlin SL. Cholecystectomy and cholelithiasis in sickle cell anemia. *Am J Dis Child* 1988; **142**: 799–800.

101. Ware RE, Kinney TR, Casey JR, Pappas TN, Meyers WC. Laparoscopic cholecystectomy in young patients with sickle hemoglobinopathies. *J Pediatr* 1992; **120**: 58–61.

102. Johna S, Shaul D, Taylor EW, Brown CA, Bloch JH. Laparoscopic management of gallbladder disease in children and adolescents. *Journal of the Society for Laparoendoscopic Surgery* 1997; **1**: 241–5.

103. Manno CS, Cohen AR, Schwartz E. Sickle cell anemia and cholelithiasis. *Pediatr Radiol* 1988; **18**: 178.

104. Singhal A, Raju N, Serjeant GR. Empyema of the gallbladder in a child with homozygous sickle-cell disease. *West Indian Med J* 1990; **39**: 243–4.

105. Jawad AJ, Kurban K, El-Bakry A *et al*. Laparoscopic cholecystectomy for cholelithiasis during infancy and childhood: cost analysis and review of current indications. *World J Surg* 1998; **22**: 69–74.

106. Tagge EP, Othersen HB, Jackson SM *et al*. Impact of laparascopic cholecystectomy on the management of cholelithiasis in children with sickle cell disease. *J Pediatr Surg* 1994; **29**: 209–13.

107. Al-Salem AH, Nourallah H. Sequential endoscopic /laparoscopic management of cholelithiasis and choledocholithiasis in children who have sickle cell disease. *J Pediatr Surg* 1997; **32**: 1432–5.

Chapter 14

Pulmonary hypertension: a complication of haemolytic states

Iheanyi E Okpala

Introduction

High blood pressure in the vessels of the lungs is an increasingly recognized feature of conditions in which there is premature destruction of erythrocytes [1]. So, it is not only a complication of the haemoglobinopathies sickle cell disease (SCD) and thalassaemia, but also paroxysmal nocturnal haemoglobinuria (PNH). It is important to identify people with SCD and thalassaemia complicated by pulmonary hypertension (PHT) because it has a poor prognosis and may be life-threatening [2]. The normal pulmonary artery blood pressure is about 25/15 mmHg, with a mean of 18 mmHg. PHT may be defined as pulmonary artery systolic pressure (PASP) > 30 mmHg, or mean pressure > 25 mmHg. Alternatively, a tricuspid valve regurgitant jet velocity up to 2.5 m/s could be taken as diagnostic of PHT, if tricuspid valve regurgitation is present. However, the absence of a tricuspid regurgitant jet does not rule out pulmonary high blood pressure.

Pathogenesis

The pathogenesis of PHT in SCD and other haemolytic states is probably multifactorial and mediated via different mechanisms. Intravascular haemolysis is considered to have an important role in the development of raised blood pressure [1]. Destruction of erythrocytes within the blood vessels releases haemoglobin into the plasma. Free plasma haemoglobin consumes nitric oxide (NO) about a thousand times faster than Hb inside red blood cells. In addition, the enzyme arginase released from lysed red blood cells converts arginine to urea and ornithine. Arginine is the natural precursor that is normally converted to NO by the enzyme NO synthase. The two pathological processes of consumption of NO by free plasma haemoglobin and diversion of arginine to urea and ornithine reduce the amount of NO in the blood vessels. The potent vasodilator effect of NO is lost, leading to vasoconstriction and a rise in blood pressure. There is evidence in support of the importance of intravascular haemolysis in the pathogenesis of PHT in SCD [1]. The severity of PHT in SCD correlates with indices of haemolysis: directly with levels of plasma Hb, bilirubin, ferritin and iron; inversely with the amount of haemoglobin inside the red blood cells. Also, SCD patients with PHT have significantly raised serum arginase levels (from lysed red blood cells) compared with healthy HbAA control individuals.

Apart from intravascular haemolysis, other pathogenetic mechanisms may contribute to high blood pressure in haemolytic disorders. Hypoxia and high blood flow through the lungs (which receive the entire cardiac output) lead to a rise in pressure within the pulmonary vascular bed. In SCD, ischaemic damage to lung tissue leading to healing by fibrosis in and around blood vessels might increase vascular resistance to blood flow and raise pulmonary blood pressure. Such lung parenchymal tissue damage and vasculopathy could result from recurrent embolism of marrow fat or thrombi, acute chest syndrome, chronically low oxygen saturation and sleep-induced hypoxia [2–4]. While the histological changes found in affected patients may be the results of PHT or other pathological processes, some of them would have the effect of increasing resistance to blood flow and, ultimately, the blood pressure. For example, the peripheral pulmonary arteries are obliterated, there is fibrosis in the tunica intima of the pulmonary veins, and the structure of the pulmonary artery changes to resemble that of the aorta, with smooth muscle hypertrophy.

Prevalence of pulmonary hypertension in SCD

Studies of the magnitude of the problem in SCD have given variable reports, probably as a result of different methods used to examine the issue. However, it is generally evident that the prevalence of PHT in SCD increases with age. In this context, it is pertinent to bear in mind that pulmonary blood pressure normally increases with age. Ataga and colleagues observed a prevalence rate of 40% in adult SCD patients aged 21–64 years [5]. Others found prevalence rates from < 4.3% to 32% [6, 7]. Low prevalence rates were observed from investigations based on autopsy findings consistent with PHT, whereas prospective clinical observations or community-based screening programmes noted higher prevalence.

Features of pulmonary hypertension

The clinical features of PHT include fatigue, chest pain, dyspnoea on exertion, syncopal attacks, a loud pulmonary component of the second heart sound, pansystolic murmur if there is tricuspid regurgitation, and reduced oxygen saturation. The patient is at risk of sudden death from cardiac arrhythmia or pulmonary thrombo-embolism. Evidence of right ventricular hypertrophy is detected on echocardiography or electrocardiography. Right ventricular failure may occur. Diagnosis is usually based on estimation of the pulmonary artery pressure from the echocardiogram. A tricuspid regurgitant velocity ≥ 2.5 m/s is also taken as indicative of PHT.

Prognosis

The outcome for people with SCD complicated by PHT is poor. In one hospital series of 17 patients, 9 (53%) had died 4 years after the diagnosis of PHT; the median survival was 1 year [6]. The poor prognosis associated with PHT makes it necessary to recognize and treat this life-threatening complication of haemolytic states.

Treatment

Until recently, antihypertensive drugs that lower (systemic) blood pressure were the only medications available for the treatment of PHT in SCD. This situation presents the physician with a dilemma. Systemic blood pressure is usually lower in SCD patients compared with HbAA controls [8]. For example, it is not unusual to record a blood pressure of 90/55 mmHg in an adult female who has SCD. Antihypertensive drugs given for PHT lower the systemic blood pressure even further, with a risk of undesired hypotension. Fatal hypotension has been reported in an individual who had SCD complicated by severe PHT that was treated with hydrallazine [9]. Calcium channel blockers like nifedipine were used, although it was uncertain if people with PHT secondary to SCD can tolerate the high doses effective in primary PHT without a dangerous fall in systemic blood pressure. There are a number of promising new treatment modalities for PHT in SCD, although none has attained general use. The rationale for each therapeutic intervention is to disrupt the pathogenesis of PHT as described previously.

Regular exchange blood transfusion

A programme of exchange blood transfusion reduces intravascular haemolysis by replacing erythrocytes containing HbS with normal red cells. This reduces the concentration of free plasma haemoglobin that avidly consumes NO. NO is then available to exert its potent vasodilator effect, and lowers pulmonary blood pressure. In addition to reducing the high pulmonary blood pressure in SCD, regular exchange blood transfusion confers other benefits, such as reduction in the number of sickle cell crises and prevention of stroke.

Inhalation of NO gas

Inhaled NO replaces the endogenous product consumed by haemoglobin free in plasma. This treatment corrects the relative NO deficiency in SCD, stimulates vasodilation and reduces pulmonary blood pressure [10].

Administration of oral arginine

The natural substrate for the formation of NO by NO synthase, arginine given orally at a dose of 0.1 g/kg three times a day reduced the pulmonary blood pressure in nine (100%) SCD patients with PHT [11]. This treatment modality is more convenient and apparently more effective than inhalation of NO gas, which requires special equipment and trained staff.

L-Carnitine therapy

A derivative of the naturally occurring amino acid carnitine, laevo-carnitine is thought to stabilize the cell membrane of erythrocytes, and so reduce haemolysis. Orally administered L-carnitine at a dose of 1 g three times daily reduced the mean pulmonary artery pressure from 40.2 ± 7.2 mmHg to 32 ± 6.5 mmHg in 14/18 (78%) SCD patients aged 4–16 years [12]. In our centre, anecdotal use of L-carnitine with regular exchange blood transfusion reduced the high pulmonary blood pressure in two SCD patients.

Oxygen therapy

Home oxygen therapy decreases the high pulmonary blood pressure in SCD patients who have low oxygen saturation (< 90%) during steady-state, and in those whose pressure was reduced by oxygen administration during cardiac catheterization. Oxygen therapy may be combined with other treatment modalities to achieve greater benefit. There is a risk of explosion if oxygen gas cylinders are used by people who smoke at home.

Conclusion

There is no universal standard treatment for PHT secondary to SCD and thalassaemia. Exchange blood transfusion, arginine, NO and L-carnitine have shown promise.

References

1. Reiter CD, Wang X, Tanus-Santos JE *et al*. Cell-free hemoglobin limits nitric oxide bioavailability in sickle cell disease. *Nature Med* 11 Nov 2002; Online.
2. Powars D, Weidman JA, Odom-Maryon T *et al*. Sickle cell chronic lung disease: prior morbidity and the risk of pulmonary failure. *Medicine (Baltimore)* 1988; **67**: 66–76.
3. Samuels MP, Stebbens VA, Davies SC *et al*. Sleep related upper airway obstruction and hypoxaemia in sickle cell disease. *Arch Dis Child* 1992; **67**: 925–9.
4. Yung GL, Channick RN, Fedullo PF *et al*. Successful pulmonary thromboendarterectomy in two patients with sickle cell disease. *Am J Respir Crit Care Med* 1998; **157**: 1690–3.
5. Ataga KI, Kelly EA, Santucci S *et al*. Prevalence of pulmonary hypertension in sickle cell disease. *Blood* 2002; **100** (Suppl): 451a.
6. Castro O. Systemic fat embolism and pulmonary hypertension in sickle cell disease. *Hematol Oncol Clin North Am* 1996; **10**: 1289–303.
7. Gladwin MT, Castro O, Jison M *et al*. A prospective clinical study of the prevalence and etiology of secondary pulmonary hypertension in sickle cell anemia. *Abstract Book of the National Sickle Cell Conference of USA*, Washington, DC, 17–23 September, 2002, p. 55.
8. Johnson CS, Giorgio AJ. Arterial blood pressure in adults with sickle cell disease. *Arch Intern Med* 1981; **141**: 891–3.
9. Hammond TG, Mosesson MW. Fat small bowel necrosis and pulmonary hypertension in sickle cell disease. *Arch Intern Med* 1989; **149**: 447–8.
10. Coles W, Nicolas JS, Smatlak PK *et al*. A clinical study of the efficacy of nitric oxide delivery via portable versus conventional systems to reduce secondary pulmonary hypertension in sickle cell anemia. *Abstract Book of the National Sickle Cell Conference of USA*, Washington, DC, 17–23 September, 2002, p. 54.
11. Morris CR, Hagar W, vam Warmerdam J *et al*. Arginine therapy improves pulmonary artery

pressures in patients with sickle cell disease and pulmonary hypertension. *Blood* 2002; **100** (Suppl): 452a.

12. El-Beshlawy A, Abdelaouff E, Hassan F, Bebawy I. Pulmonary hypertension in sickle cell disease. *Abstract Book of the 25th Meeting of the International Society of Haematology (African & European Division)*, Durban, South Africa, 18–23 September, 1999, p. 120.

Chapter 15
Stroke in sickle cell disease

Janet Kwiatkowski and Kwaku Ohene-Frempong

Introduction

Stroke (or cerebrovascular accident) is one of the common complications of severe sickle cell disease (SCD). It also serves as a prototypical manifestation of the disease because it demonstrates the combined effects of both small and large vessel damage and chronic anaemia. It is now evident that cerebral pathology in SCD ranges from 'silent' parenchymal infarct with little or no evidence of large vessel disease but demonstrable deterioration in neurocognitive function to overt stroke associated with stenosis and occlusion of multiple large vessels and cerebral cortical infarcts. Management of overt stroke has become somewhat standardized, even in the absence of controlled clinical trials. However, the management of 'silent' infarcts or demonstrable vascular pathology is evolving and currently under study. In this chapter, we present briefly the incidence and prevalence of stroke, its known risk factors, and a review of the current management.

Pathophysiology of stroke

Stroke in SCD is caused primarily by damage to small and large cerebral vessels complicated by severe anaemia. Small vessels in the arterial border zones are presumed to be lost early in the genesis of cerebrovascular pathology in SCD. The loss of these vessels is thought to lead to the deep white matter infarcts ('silent' infarcts) and changes in perfusion seen even in neurologically asymptomatic patients with SCD [1, 2]. However, overt stroke in

SCD is typified by stenosis and occlusion of large cerebral arteries, particularly those of the circle of Willis. Microscopically, these large vessels show various degrees of intimal hyperplasia that may be severe enough to occlude the vessel [2]. Thus infarction of brain tissue results either from ischaemic damage resulting from the *in situ* occlusion of a damaged artery or distal embolization of a thrombus formed in the damaged vessel. These vessels also show increased formation of aneurysms, perhaps as advanced manifestation of the same vasculopathy [3, 4]. In addition, moyamoya disease, the formation of a mass of small friable blood vessels, is a common consequence of stenosis of large cerebral vessels in SCD [5]. Rupture of the aneurysms or the friable vessels in moyamoya is the usual cause of haemorrhagic stroke in SCD. The bleeding is commonly subarachnoid but may be intraventricular or parenchymal.

Incidence and prevalence

Although there are many sophisticated techniques of neuroimaging and assessment of cerebral perfusion, stroke remains a clinical diagnosis. The index of suspicion of stroke is raised more by demonstration of motor deficits and less by changes in personality, intellectual (or academic) performance, and memory. In SCD, where stroke is common in young children, non-motor signs of stroke are likely to be missed as they may not be as easily demonstrable in or expressed by children as they would by adults. The USA Co-operative Study of Sickle Cell Disease (CSSCD) classified SCD-related stroke into three types: infarctive, haemorrhagic and transient ischaemic attack (TIA) (as uncompleted stroke).

The CSSCD reported overall stroke prevalence at enrolment of its large cohort of subjects of all ages and genotypes to be 4%, and 5% in those with homozygous beta-S (SCD-SS). Stroke was seen in all the common genotypes; however, it was more frequent in subjects with SCD-SS. The annual incidence of first stroke was approximately 0.6 per 100 patient-years in SCD-SS. The highest incidence (1.02 per 100 patient-years) was seen in children 2–5 years of age with SCD-SS. However, stroke occurred in all age groups and the cumulative risk of stroke increased with age: 11% by age 20, 15% by 30, and 24% by 45 years of age. The clinical impact of this cumulative risk is devastating considering the tendency of stroke to leave permanent physical and neurocognitive impairment.

The silent infarct

Earlier studies in many SCD patients after stroke using standard angiography and post-mortem examination of cerebral vessels had shown more extensive vascular damage than could explain the clinical presentation [6]. This finding suggested that some of the cerebrovascular damage in SCD can be clinically 'silent'. In 1988, Pavlakis *et al.* reported the presence of cerebral infarcts in SCD patients who had not had a clinical stroke [1]. In the magnetic resonance imaging (MRI) studies of children aged ≥ 6 years in the CSSCD cohort without a history of clinical stroke, as many as 25% (62 of 248) had developed 'silent' infarcts after 5.2 (+ 2.2) years of observation following the initial study [7]. Compared with those with normal MRI, the children with 'silent' infarct had a 14-fold increase in the risk for overt stroke. The actual risk may be higher if children 2–5 years of age, the period of highest incidence of stroke, had been included in the study. Longitudinal observational studies of children with silent infarcts who do not receive treatment suggest that there is an increased risk of developing new or larger silent infarcts [8]. The silence of these infarcts is placed in serious doubt by the demonstration of greater degrees of neurocognitive abnormalities in children with infarcts than in those without [9, 10].

The pathophysiology of silent cerebral infarction may differ from that of overt stroke. This is supported by a lack of concordance between transcranial Doppler (TCD) and MRI findings in the multicentre primary stroke prevention trial (STOP) [11]. In that report on 78 older children (mean age 11 years) with no history of overt stroke, of 61 subjects with normal MRI, 11 (18%) had conditional or abnormal TCD results, while among 17 subjects with silent infarction, 5 (29%) had conditional or abnormal TCD velocity. Thus, TCD and MRI results were discordant in 23 patients: 12 with normal TCD and abnormal MRI, and 11 with elevated TCD and normal MRI. In children with no history of overt stroke, the deep white matter infarcts on MRI may be demonstrating the results of small vessel occlusive disease, while TCD may be demonstrating large vessel disease.

Risk factors for stroke

In examining its large body of clinical data, the CSSCD was able to identify disease-associated risk factors for stroke in its cohort [12]. Factors associated with infarctive stroke included the following: prior TIA, history of meningitis, increased systolic blood pressure, increased steady-state leucocyte count, the 2-week period following acute chest syndrome, increased rate of acute chest syndrome, and low steady-state Hb level. In multivariate analysis, prior TIA, low steady-state Hb level, high systolic blood pressure and the two factors related to acute chest syndrome were found to be significant risks for infarctive stroke. Similarly, low steady-state Hb level and high leucocyte count were found to be significant risk factors for haemorrhagic stroke. Alpha thalassaemia (of any degree) was found to protect SCD patients from infarctive stroke through its positive effect on steady-state haemoglobin levels.

Following the CSSCD report several other risk factors for stroke in SCD have been identified. Among these, elevated cerebral blood flow velocity as measured through TCD [13], and nocturnal hypoxaemia measured by pulse oximetry [14], have had practical application. Genetic predisposition to cerebrovascular disease and stroke in SCD has been suggested by familial clustering of stroke [15],

A. Initial assessment and care
  1. Brief history and physical examination (including careful neurological examination)
    – distinguish between symptoms due to pain and those due to weakness
  2. Stabilization, support and monitoring of vital signs as necessary; maintain euthermia
  3. Good oxygenation
  4. Careful intravenous hydration at maintenance level or less
B. Laboratory evaluation
  1. Complete blood count with differential and reticulocyte count
  2. Coagulation studies – PT, PTT
  3. Blood to blood bank for typing and cross-match
    a. Obtain extended antigen profile for previously untransfused patient
    b. Request phenotypically matched red blood cells, if available
  4. Blood chemistry
  5. Evaluation for meningitis
    – if physical examination raises that suspicion and neurological examination
    (or neuroimaging)
    – assures the safety of a lumbar puncture
C. Neuroimaging
  1. CT scan as soon as possible to rule out haemorrhage
  2. MRI/MRA to define both parenchymal and vascular lesions
    – diffusion-weighted MRI is highly sensitive in detecting early ischaemic changes
D. Red cell transfusion
  1. Initial transfusion
    a. Simple transfusion
      – goal is to raise Hb to about 10 g/dL but NOT higher
      – do not exceed 15 mL/kg in a single transfusion
      – allow equilibration (2–3 hours), check Hb level, and give more red cells, if necessary
    b. Exchange transfusion (manual or automated)
      – goal is to raise Hb to 10–12 g/dL and lower HbS to < 30%
      – do not delay initial transfusion if exchange is not readily available

Table 15.1 Management of the SCD patient with acute stroke symptoms

presence of HLA types associated with increased rates of stroke [16], higher homocysteine levels in SCD patients with stroke compared with those without [17], and sibling concordance in TCD results [18].

Clinical presentation of stroke in SCD

As in others, infarctive stroke in SCD patients presents typically with hemiparesis, aphasia, monoparesis, or seizure. In young children, subtle changes in motor performance, such as painless limp, are likely to be missed as signs of stroke except by the keen observer. Haemorrhagic stroke often presents with severe headache. Rarely, a patient with either type of stroke has presented in coma. The clinical diagnosis of stroke is often substantiated with neuroimaging studies, such as MRI or computerized tomography (CT), that show haemorrhage and infarcts, and magnetic resonance angiography (MRA) that can demonstrate evidence of large vascular disease. The CT may be negative within the first several hours following acute infarctive stroke. Diffusion-weighted MRI is most sensitive in detecting early ischaemic damage. The management of a patient presenting with acute neurological symptoms is outlined in Table 15.1.

Treatment

Management of acute stroke

Red blood cell transfusion

No clinical trials have investigated the optimal acute management of ischaemic stroke in SCD and it is unclear if the initial management affects long-term outcome. Thus, clinical management in the acute period is empiric (Table 15.1). Red cell transfusion to lessen the anaemia, reduce tissue hypoxia and reduce the percentage of HbS is the mainstay of treatment. Manual or automated exchange transfusion, when available, is often employed in the initial management. The goal is to reduce the %HbS to < 30% of the total haemoglobin and to raise the haemoglobin level to about 10–12 g/dL. Oxygen-carrying capacity is increased and potentially harmful sickle cells are removed while minimizing rapid shifts in fluid and blood pressure changes that could be detrimental in the presence of acute ischaemia. This form of transfusion, therefore, may be preferable to simple transfusion. The downside to exchange transfusion involves the need for large intravenous access – often a central line must be placed acutely – and lack of ready access to apheresis teams, which can prolong the time to treatment. A simple transfusion to raise the haemoglobin level to no higher than 10 g/dL should be given if exchange transfusion cannot be performed within a few hours of pre-sentation.

Supportive therapy

Although not formally studied, some of the principles of supportive therapy employed for ischaemic stroke in the non-sickle cell patient are utilized in initial management. Supportive therapy should be aimed at avoiding hypotension and maintaining adequate hydration. Fever is associated with worse outcome in patients without SCD with ischaemic stroke, and therefore euthermia should be maintained [19]. The use of antifibrinolytic agents, such as t-PA, although standard care in adults without SCD with non-haemorrhagic stroke of < 3 hours duration, has not been studied in SCD [20]. Furthermore, because of the occurrence of haemorrhagic stroke in SCD, there is concern about increased risk of haemorrhagic transformation. Therefore, no clear recommendation can be made regarding the use of antifibrinolytics in ischaemic stroke for patients with SCD.

Long-term management

The goals of long-term management of stroke are to prevent stroke recurrence, allo-immunization and iron overload (Table 15.2). Without treatment, there is a high risk of recurrent stroke in SCD. In one cohort study of 35 sickle cell patients with stroke by Powars *et al.*, 67% of long-term survivors who were not treated with chronic transfusions experienced a recurrent stroke [21]. A Jamaican study reported a recurrence rate of 47% in untreated SCD-SS patients with stroke; however, the follow-up time was not specified [22]. Stroke recurrences often happen in the first few years following the initial event. In the Powars study, 80% of the recurrences occurred within 3 years of the initial event, and many occurred within 1–2 years. Multiple recurrent strokes may occur and the rate of permanent neurological deficit appears to increase with subsequent strokes [22].

Chronic transfusion therapy is the most effective known method to reduce recurrences of stroke. The initial goal of transfusion therapy is to maintain %HbS < 30%. Although this number is somewhat arbitrary, *in vitro* viscosity studies have shown favourable flow conditions when %HbS is < 40% [23]. This can often be accomplished by simple red cell transfusion every 3–4 weeks. The target post-transfusion haemoglobin level goal is usually 10–12 g/dL; higher haemoglobin levels should be avoided because the viscosity of blood containing sickled cells increases with increasing haemoglobin levels. Although sickle trait (AS) red cells can be safely transfused, donor red cells that do not contain HbS should be utilized to allow for accurate monitoring of HbS levels.

Although red cell transfusion has not been studied in a randomized controlled clinical trial, data from several case series [6, 24, 25] as well as a multicentre retrospective study [26] support its beneficial effect. In one series, only 2 of 27 (7.4%) patients with a history of stroke experienced recurrences while on transfusion therapy [24], a rate that is substantially lower than historical untreated controls [21]. Furthermore, 12 of the 27 (44%) patients had experienced a recurrent stroke before beginning transfusion therapy, and thus transfusion therapy was associated with a significant reduction in stroke recurrence in this cohort. In a more recent multicentre retrospective study, only 8 of 60 (13.3%) subjects receiving chronic transfusion had stroke recurrences [26]. This included six

Table 15.2 Long-term management of stroke in SCD

A. Chronic red cell transfusion (RCT) therapy
   1. Goal: maintain pre-transfusion Hb level of 8–10 g/dL and %HbS of < 30%
      a. Check Hb level before each transfusion to determine RBC volume to give
      b. Check %HbS before each transfusion to help determine interval and RBC volume for
         future transfusion
      c. Post-transfusion blood tests usually not necessary
      d. Monitor for hepatitis, HIV and other transfusion-transmissible infections
      e. Monitor for iron overload
         – maintain record of cumulative volume of RBC transfused
         – iron studies at least every 6 months
         – consider liver biopsy when ferritin exceeds 2000 ng/mL or cumulative RBC transfused reaches 120 mL/kg body weight to determine
           need for chelation therapy
   2. Management of iron overload
      a. Prevention
         – early institution of exchange transfusion programme can prevent iron overload
         – allowing HbS level to rise to < 50% after initial 3–4 years of transfusion without neurological events will reduce rate of iron
           accumulation
      b. Treatment of iron overload
         – start iron chelation therapy when cumulative iron load exceeds 120 mL/kg body weight
         – use desferrioxamine or other approved iron chelators
   3. Management of allo-immunization
      a. Prevention
         – use RBC matched closely to those of patient (for people of tropical African ancestry, give RBC negative (at least) for C, E and Kell
           antigens)
         – encourage blood donation by members of the patient's genetic community
      b. Treatment of multiply allo-immunized stroke patient
         – monitor carefully (Hb level, %HbS, RBC antibodies, conjugated bilirubin level) the survival of transfused cells
         – weigh the benefit of continued RBC exposure against risk of transfusion failure in a life-threatening situation
         – if compatible RBC units are too difficult to find, consider hydroxyurea therapy as an experimental alternative to chronic RBC therapy
B. Neuropsychological evaluation
   1. Obtain initial evaluation within weeks of acute event
   2. Institute interventions to improve neurocognitive losses
   3. Monitor every 6–12 months if abnormal
C. Physical, occupational, speech and other therapies
   1. Obtain initial evaluation within days of acute event
   2. Institute interventions to improve outcomes as necessary
D. Neuroimaging
   MRI/MRA annually
   – assess progression of vascular disease: aneurysms, moyamoya disease, and other lesions that may be amenable to surgical intervention

infarctions and two intracranial haemorrhages. An additional multicentre retrospective study by Scothorn and others found a recurrence rate of 22% in 137 paediatric patients who had been on chronic red cell transfusions for a minimum of 5 years after the initial stroke [27]. In that report, recurrence rate for children who had an antecedent medical event including fever, hypertension, acute chest syndrome, severe anaemia or exchange transfusion, was significantly lower after the initial 2 years of transfusion than in those whose infarcts were not temporally associated with such a medical event.

Recurrence risk may be increased with higher levels of HbS. In the Sarnaik study, the 2 of 27 children who had stroke recurrences had HbS levels of 48% and 80%, respectively, at the time of recurrence [24]. In the multicentre retrospective study, in five of the six patients with recurrent infarctions, HbS levels were ≥ 30% at the time of occurrence [26]. None the less, despite adequate chronic transfusion therapy, some patients will experience recurrent cerebral infarctions even with very low HbS levels. One case series described three children with stroke recurrences when HbS levels were between 17% and 33.5% [28]. Furthermore, five of six children in the Scothorn report had HbS percentages < 30% at the time of recurrence [27]. It is unclear if this subset of patients would benefit from alternative therapies such as antiplatelet agents or stem cell transplant. There are no reports of the efficacy of transfusions in preventing haemorrhagic stroke. Haemorrhages occurred even with lower %HbS, suggesting that transfusion may not be as effective for this type of stroke. An earlier report suggesting that transfusion therapy may be associated with amelioration of cerebral vascular damage, or at least with a halt in progression of disease, has not been substantiated [29].

The optimal duration of transfusion therapy is currently undetermined. Although most stroke recurrences happen within a few years of the initial event, an attempt to discontinue transfusions after a period of 1–2 years resulted in a 70% recurrence rate within a year of discontinuing transfusions [25]. An additional report showed a 50% rate of recurrence within 12 months when transfusions were discontinued after a substantially longer period of 5–12 years [30]. However, in another series of nine patients in whom transfusion therapy was discontinued after 1.5–16.5 years, no patient experienced recurrent ischaemia, although one patient died from a cerebral haemorrhage [31]. However, six of the nine patients began hydroxyurea therapy, which may have affected stroke risk, at a median of 4 years after discontinuing red cell transfusion.

Significant complications of chronic transfusion therapy include infection, red blood cell allo-immunization and transfusional iron overload. Unfortunately, the most commonly used drug for iron chelation, desferrioxamine, is given as a subcutaneous or intravenous infusion. It is administered over several hours, usually 10–12 hours per day, because of its short half-life. Non-compliance is high, leading to toxicity from iron overload and/or eventual discontinuation of transfusion therapy. In an attempt to reduce iron loading, modified methods of red cell transfusion have been employed. One method is to allow HbS levels to rise to < 50% pre-transfusion [32, 33]. Because stroke recurrences often occur within the first 3 years of the initial event, this method is usually only employed after 3–4 years of transfusion therapy with an 'aggressive' HbS target of < 30%. In a study of 15 patients with SCD-SS and history of cerebrovascular accident, patients without history of neurological progression on chronic transfusion therapy for a minimum of 4 years with a target %HbS of 30%, had the target pre-transfusion HbS level raised to < 50% [32]. During a median follow-up period of 84 months (range 14–130 months), there were no recurrent infarctive strokes. However, two patients had fatal intracranial bleeds. One patient had an intraventricular haemorrhage 1 day after a transfusion (pre-transfusion HbS = 30%) and an additional pregnant patient had a subarachnoid haemorrhage with a %HbS of 29%. Another patient had a recurrent infarction 3 months after discontinuing transfusion therapy, which she had received for 9 years (4 years with an HbS target of < 50%). Transfusion requirements were significantly reduced with a mean reduction of 30% after increasing the target HbS level to 50%. A second study reported no stroke recurrence after 12–27 months of observation following relaxation of the pre-transfusion HbS level to the 40–60% range in patients transfused aggressively for 4.5–13.7 years [33].

An additional method of reducing net transfusional requirements involves either manual or automated partial red cell exchange (erythrocytapheresis). When used in combination with a higher target %HbS, this technique can greatly reduce iron accumulation. In a study of 14 subjects with SCD who were receiving chronic red cell transfusion therapy including 11 subjects with a history of stroke, erythrocytapheresis was used to maintain a target %HbS of < 50%. Annual net red cell transfusion requirements were reduced by 87% in seven patients previously receiving conventional simple transfusions (HbS < 30%) and by 81% in seven patients previously receiving modified simple transfusions (HbS < 50%) [34]. The mean annual iron load was 19 mg iron/kg/year with this approach, compared with 144 mg iron/kg/year and 107 mg iron/kg/year for those previously receiving simple or modified transfusion regimens, respectively. Of note, four subjects were able to discontinue desferrioxamine chelation therapy and an additional two subjects were able to avoid starting chelation therapy with this treatment approach. If exchange transfusion is not available, chelation therapy should be strongly considered when the cumulative volume of red cells transfused reaches or exceeds 120 ml/kg of body weight or when the liver iron exceeds 7 mg/g dry weight [35].

Allo-immunization is a common complication of chronic red cell transfusion in SCD. This risk may be minimized through careful matching of donor and recipient antigens. In the USA it is recommended that SCD patients, mostly of African ancestry, receive blood that is phenotypically matched for C, E and Kell antigens [36].

Hydroxyurea therapy

The use of hydroxyurea therapy as an alternative to red cell transfusion for secondary stroke prevention has been studied in one clinical centre. In a series of 16 patients with SCD and a history of stroke, red cell transfusions were discontinued after a mean duration of 56 ± 36 months [37]. Reasons for discontinuation of transfusions included red cell alloantibody or autoantibody formation, stroke recurrence on transfusion therapy, iron overload, and non-compliance with transfusions or chelation therapy. Three patients (19%) had recurrent ischaemic stroke at 3–4 months after discontinuation of transfusions. No haemorrhagic neurological complications occurred. Additionally, 14 patients tolerated phlebotomy while on hydroxyurea therapy and had a significant reduction in iron overload. The authors postulate that the early stroke recurrences may have been due to an incomplete effect of hydroxyurea in the first few months of treatment. Hydroxyurea use was associated with an amelioration of vasculopathy as documented by serial MRA in one patient who was treated with hydroxyurea for secondary stroke prevention due to religious considerations [38]. However, this patient had progression of diffuse cerebral atrophy, suggesting that hydroxyurea therapy may not treat brain parenchymal disease. Furthermore, concern about the use of hydroxyurea therapy for stroke prevention has been brought on by a report of two patients who developed intracranial haemorrhage (fatal in one) while being treated with this medication [39]. Thus, the use of hydroxyurea for secondary stroke prevention in patients with SCD is an enticing alternative therapy that requires further study.

Stem cell transplantation

Stem cell transplantation has also been utilized for patients with SCD who have experienced stroke. In the USA, cerebrovascular disease is the most common clinical eligibility factor for bone marrow transplantation (BMT) in SCD [40, 41]. However, it is estimated that only 18% of children with SCD in the USA have an HLA-matched sibling, limiting the broad application of this therapy [42].

The rate of neurological complications after transplantation appears to be higher in children with SCD than in those who receive BMT for other indications. In an early report of the Multicenter Investigation of Bone Marrow Transplantation for Sickle Cell Disease, 3 of 21 patients experienced intracranial haemorrhage [40]. All these patients had a history of clinical stroke prior to transplant, although intracranial haemorrhage in the peritransplant period has been reported in a patient without prior history of stroke [43]. In the former report, intracranial haemorrhages occurred between 8 and 243 days after transplant and the event was fatal in two patients [40]. Additionally, seizures occurred in 6 of the 21 patients, 3 of whom had a prior history of stroke. Hypertension, thrombocytopenia and/or relative polycythaemia were present in many of the subjects who experienced neurological events. Subsequently, additional supportive measures in the peri-transplant period were instituted. These included improved blood pressure control, anticonvulsant prophylaxis, prompt correction of magnesium deficiency, and maintenance of platelet counts $> 50\,000/mm^3$ and haemoglobin levels between 9 and 11 gm/dL [41]. No further intracranial bleeding was observed on that study following these new interventions; however, seizures occurred in 9 of 43 patients. Furthermore, subarachnoid haemorrhage has been reported in a patient undergoing BMT despite similar interventions [43]. Thus, these modifications may reduce but have not eliminated neurological complications in this patient population.

The results to date suggest that BMT may have promising results in the prevention of stroke recurrence. In a subsequent report of the Multicenter Investigation of Bone Marrow Transplantation for Sickle Cell Disease 13 patients with SCD and a history of stroke had undergone BMT, 3 patients had developed graft rejection, 1 of whom had a stroke recurrence when the HbS level was 60% [41]. The two others resumed red cell transfusion therapy and did not experience recurrent strokes. Ten of the 13 patients had stable engraftment, and none has had clinical stroke after transplantation. Similarly, in another report [44], five of six patients with SCD and a history of stroke who underwent BMT had stable engraftment and none of those five patients had stroke recurrence.

It remains unclear whether BMT can reverse existing cerebrovascular disease in patients with SCD. The 2000 report of the Multicenter Investigation of Bone Marrow Transplantation for Sickle Cell Disease suggests that radiographic abnormalities may stabilize or improve after BMT [41, 43]. In that report, serial MRA were examined in four consecutive patients who underwent allogeneic BMT. Two of these patients had pre-existing vessel stenosis by MRA that improved in most but not all of the vessels involved after BMT. In other reports of two other patients, however, a worsening of cerebral vasculopathy after BMT occurred [45, 46].

Primary stroke prevention

The advent of TCD ultrasonography has allowed for the non-invasive detection of cerebral vasculopathy in children with SCD. Elevated cerebral blood flow velocity in the terminal internal carotid artery (t-ICA) and/or middle cerebral artery (MCA) predicts an increased risk of stroke [13, 47]. The results of TCD studies can be divided into three stroke risk categories: abnormal (≥ 200 cm/s), conditional (170–199 cm/s) and normal (< 170 cm/s) [48]. Abnormal TCD studies are associated with a 40% risk of stroke, while normal studies carry only a 2% risk

of stroke over a 3-year period [47]. Thus, this technique allows the identification of children who are at high risk of developing a first stroke, creating the potential for intervention to decrease the risk of first stroke. The Stroke Prevention Trial in Sickle Cell Anemia was a multicentre randomized controlled trial that studied the use of red cell transfusions to prevent first stroke in children with abnormal TCD studies [48]. Blood transfusion was chosen as a therapy based on the effectiveness of this therapy for secondary stroke prevention in SCD. The study began in 1995 and a total of 130 children were enrolled; 63 children were randomly assigned to receive red cell transfusions and 67 to receive standard care (no stroke prevention treatment). Red cell transfusions were administered at a mean interval of 25 ± 8 days with a goal of maintaining the pre-transfusion %HbS at < 30% of total haemoglobin. There were 11 strokes in the standard care group and only one in the transfused group ($p < 0.001$). The rate of stroke in the untransfused group was 10% per year. The significant reduction in stroke risk with red cell transfusions led to early termination of the trial in September 1997, so that all children with abnormal TCD could be offered red cell transfusion. Various institutions have adopted their own protocols for screening children with SCD with TCD, MR and neurocognitive studies in order to provide them with advice on possible stroke prevention therapy. The screening protocol followed at the Sickle Cell Center, the Children's Hospital of Philadelphia is outlined in Figure 15.1.

Haemorrhagic stroke

There has been no special approach to the management of haemorrhagic stroke in SCD. Chronic red cell transfusion has not been demonstrated to be as effective in prevention of recurrent haemorrhagic stroke as it has in infarctive stroke. In fact, some patients on long-term chronic red cell transfusion following infarctive stroke have developed haemorrhagic stroke [3, 32, 49]. It is important to establish early in the course of evaluating a patient with a new stroke event that there is no haemorrhagic component to the lesion. A bleeding aneurysm may require prompt neurosurgical intervention such as clipping or coil embolization [50]. In rare case

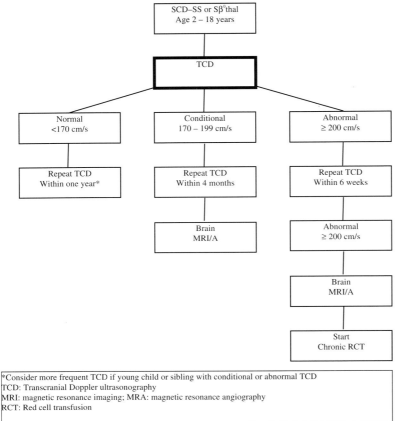

Fig. 15.1 Protocol used for transcranial Doppler (TCD) ultrasonographic screening of children with sickle cell disease in the Children's Hospital of Philadelphia, USA. MRI/A, magnetic resonance imaging/angiography; RCT, red cell transfusion.

reports, patients with SCD who have developed moyamoya disease have undergone bypass procedures to improve perfusion to the brain [51].

Silent cerebral infarction

Limited information is available about the natural course of silent cerebral infarction because of its relatively recent discovery [1]. There have been no randomized controlled studies of the treatment of silent cerebral infarction in SCD. None the less, it is reasonable to expect that treatments that have been effective in the prevention of overt stroke might also be beneficial in the treatment of silent cerebral infarction or abnormal TCD, as both processes may progress to overt stroke.

The effect of red cell transfusion therapy in the prevention of progression of silent infarction or development of new stroke was assessed as a secondary aim in the STOP study [52]. This was limited to the evaluation of children with abnormal TCD results who were treated with chronic transfusion therapy or observation. Among the patients with silent infarction on baseline MRI, none of the 18 treated with transfusions developed new or progressive silent infarcts or developed overt stroke. In contrast, 6 of 29 developed new or progressive silent infarcts and 9 subjects developed overt stroke in the group with baseline silent infarcts who did not receive transfusions (p < 0.001). Further studies are required to determine if this benefit will hold for those with normal TCD velocities and silent cerebral infarction. The use of hydroxyurea for treatment of silent cerebral infarction has not been formally studied.

References

1. Pavlakis SG, Bello J, Prohovnik I *et al*. Brain infarction in sickle cell anemia: magnetic resonance imaging correlates. *Ann Neurol* 1988; **23**: 125–30.

2. Merkel KH, Ginsberg PL, Parker JC Jr *et al*. Cerebrovascular disease in sickle cell anemia: a clinical, pathological and radiological correlation. *Stroke* 1978; **9**: 45–52.

3. Oyesiku NM, Barrow DL, Eckman JR *et al*. Intracranial aneurysms in sickle-cell anemia: clinical features and pathogenesis [see comments]. *J Neurosurg* 1991; **75**: 356–63.

4. Diggs LW, Brookoff D. Multiple cerebral aneurysms in patients with sickle cell disease [see comments]. *South Med J* 1993; **86**: 377–9.

5. Seeler RA, Royal JE, Powe L *et al*. Moyamoya in children with sickle cell anemia and cerebrovascular occlusion. *J Pediatr* 1978; **93**: 808–10.

6. Russell MO, Goldberg HI, Reis L *et al*. Transfusion therapy for cerebrovascular abnormalities in sickle cell disease. *J Pediatr* 1976; **88**: 382–7.

7. Miller ST, Macklin EA, Pegelow CH *et al*. Silent infarction as a risk factor for overt stroke in children with sickle cell anemia: a report from the Cooperative Study of Sickle Cell Disease. *J Pediatr* 2001; **139**: 385–90.

8. Pegelow C, Reed G, Moser F *et al*. Natural history of silent infarct in children with sickle cell anemia. *Blood* 1999; **94** (Suppl 1): 199a.

9. Armstrong FD, Thompson RJ Jr, Wang W *et al*. Cognitive functioning and brain magnetic resonance imaging in children with sickle cell disease. Neuropsychology Committee of the Cooperative Study of Sickle Cell Disease. *Pediatrics* 1996; **97**: 864–70.

10. Brown RT, Davis PC, Lambert R *et al*. Neurocognitive functioning and magnetic resonance imaging in children with sickle cell disease. *J Pediatr Psychol* 2000; **25**: 503–13.

11. Wang WC, Gallagher DM, Pegelow CH *et al*. Multicenter comparison of magnetic resonance imaging and transcranial Doppler ultrasonography in the evaluation of the central nervous system in children with sickle cell disease. *J Pediatr Hematol Oncol* 2000: **22**: 335–9.

12. Ohene-Frempong K, Weiner SJ, Sleeper LA *et al*. Cerebrovascular accidents in sickle cell disease: rates and risk factors. *Blood* 1998; **91**: 288–94.

13. Adams R, McKie V, Nichols F *et al*. The use of transcranial ultrasonography to predict stroke in sickle cell disease. *N Engl J Med* 1992; **326**: 605–10.

14. Kirkham FJ, Hewes DK, Prengler M *et al*. Nocturnal hypoxaemia and central-nervous-system events in sickle-cell disease. *Lancet* 2001; **357**: 1656–9.

15. Driscoll MC, Hurlet A, Styles L *et al*. Stroke risk in siblings with sickle cell anemia. *Blood* 2003; **101**: 2401–4.

16. Hoppe C, Klitz W, Noble J *et al*. Distinct HLA associations by stroke subtype in children with sickle cell anemia. *Blood* 2003; **101**: 2865–9.

17. Houston PE, Rana S, Sekhsaria S *et al*. Homocysteine in sickle cell disease: relationship to stroke. *Am J Med* 1997; **103**: 192–6.

18. Kwiatkowski JL, Hunter JV, Smith-Whitley K *et al*. Transcranial Doppler ultrasonography in siblings with sickle cell disease. *Br J Haematol* 2003; **121**: 932–7.

19. Reith J, Jorgensen S, Pedersen PM *et al*. Body temperature in acute stroke: relation to stroke severity, infarct size, mortality, and outcome. *Lancet* 1996; **347**: 422–5.

20. Tissue plaminogen activator for acute ischemic stroke. The National Institute of Neurological Disorders and Stroke rt-PA Stroke Study Group. *N Engl J Med* 1995; **333**: 1581–7.

21. Powars D, Wilson B, Imbus C *et al*. The natural history of stroke in sickle cell disease. *Am J Med* 1978; **65**: 461–71.

22. Balkaran B, Char G, Morris JS *et al*. Stroke in a cohort of patients with homozygous sickle cell disease. *J Pediatr* 1992; **120**: 360–6.

23. Murphy JR, Wengard M, Brereton W. Rheological studies of HbSS blood: influence of hematocrit, hyperviscosity, separation of cells, deoxygenation, and mixture with normal cells. *J Lab Clin Med* 1976; **87**: 475.

24. Sarnaik S, Soorya D, Kim J *et al*. Periodic transfusions for sickle cell anemia and CNS infarction. *Am J of Dis Child* 1979; **133**: 1254–7.

25. Wilimas J, Goff JR, Anderson HR Jr *et al*. Efficacy of transfusion therapy for one to two years in patients with sickle cell disease and cerebrovascular accidents. *J Pediatr* 1980; **96**: 205–8.

26. Pegelow CH, Adams RJ, McKie V *et al*. Risk of recurrent stroke in patients with sickle cell disease treated with erythrocyte transfusions. *J Pediatr* 1995; **126**: 896–9.

27. Scothorn DJ, Price C, Schwartz D *et al*. Risk of recurrent stroke in children with sickle cell disease receiving blood transfusion therapy for at least five years after initial stroke. *J Pediatr* 2002; **140**: 348–54.

28. Buchanan GR, Bowman WP, Smith SJ. Recurrent cerebral ischemia during hypertransfusion therapy in sickle cell anemia. *J Pediatr* 1983; **103**: 921–3.

29. Russell MO, Goldberg HI, Hodson A *et al*. Effect of transfusion therapy on arteriographic abnormalities and on recurrence of stroke in sickle cell disease. *Blood* 1984; **63**: 162–9.

30. Wang WC, Kovnar EH, Tonkin IL *et al*. High risk of recurrent stroke after discontinuance of five to twelve years of transfusion therapy in patients with sickle cell disease. *J Pediatr* 1991; **118**: 377–82.

31. Rana S, Houston PE, Surana N *et al*. Discontinuation of

long-term transfusion therapy in patients with sickle cell disease and stroke. *J Pediatr* 1997; **131**: 757–60.

32. Cohen AR, Martin MB, Silber JH *et al.* A modified transfusion program for prevention of stroke in sickle cell disease. *Blood* 1992; **79**: 1657–61.

33. Miller ST, Jensen D, Rao SP. Less intensive long-term transfusion therapy for sickle cell anemia and cerebrovascular accident. *J Pediatr* 1992; **120**: 54–7.

34. Kim HC, Dugan NP, Silber JH *et al.* Erythrocytapheresis therapy to reduce iron overload in chronically transfused patients with sickle cell disease. *Blood* 1994; **83**: 1136–42.

35. Vichinsky E. Consensus document for transfusion-related iron overload. *Semin Hematol* 2001; **38**: 2–4.

36. Vichinsky EP. Current issues with blood transfusions in sickle cell disease. *Semin Hematol* 2001; **38**: 14–22.

37. Ware RE, Zimmerman SA, Schultz WH. Hydroxyurea as an alternative to blood transfusions for the prevention of recurrent stroke in children with sickle cell disease. *Blood* 1999; **94**: 3022–6.

38. Helton KJ, Wang WC, Wynn LW *et al.* The effect of hydroxyurea on vasculopathy in a child with sickle cell disease. *Am J Neuroradiol* 2002; **23**: 1692–6.

39. Vichinsky EP, Lubin BH. A cautionary note regarding hydroxyurea in sickle cell disease. *Blood* 1994; **83**: 1124–8.

40. Walters MC, Sullivan KM, Bernaudin F *et al.* Neurologic complications after allogeneic marrow transplantation for sickle cell anemia. *Blood* 1995; **85**: 879–84.

41. Walters MC, Storb R, Patience M *et al.* Impact of bone marrow transplantation for symptomatic sickle cell disease: an interim report. *Blood* 2000; **95**: 1918–24.

42. Mentzer WC, Heller S, Pearle PR *et al.* Availability of related donors for bone marrow transplantation in sickle cell anemia. *Am J Pediatr Hematol Oncol* 1994; **16**: 27–9.

43. Steen RG, Helton KJ, Horwitz EM *et al.* Improved cerebrovascular patency following therapy in patients with sickle cell disease: initial results in 4 patients who received HLA-identical hematopoietic stem cell allografts. *Ann Neurol* 2001; **49**: 222–9.

44. Vermylen C, Cornu G. Bone marrow transplantation for sickle cell disease: the European experience. *Am J Pediatr Hematol Oncol* 1994; **16**: 18–21.

45. Abboud MR, Jackson SM, Barredo J *et al.* Neurologic complications following bone marrow transplantation for sickle cell disease. *Bone Marrow Transplant* 1996; **17**: 405–7.

46. Kalinyak KA, Morris C, Ball WS *et al.* Bone marrow transplantation in a young child with sickle cell anemia. *Am J Hematol* 1995; **48**: 256–61.

47. Adams RJ, McKie VC, Carl EM *et al.* Long-term stroke risk in children with sickle cell disease screened with transcranial Doppler. *Ann Neurol* 1997; **42**: 699–704.

48. Adams RJ, McKie VC, Brambilla D *et al.* Stroke prevention trial in sickle cell anemia. *Control Clin Trials* 1998; **19**: 110–29.

49. Anson JA, Koshy M, Ferguson L *et al.* Subarachnoid hemorrhage in sickle-cell disease [published erratum appears in *J Neurosurg* 1992; **76**: 726]. *J Neurosurg* 1991; **75**: 552–8.

50. McQuaker IG, Jaspan T, McConachie NS *et al.* Coil embolization of cerebral aneurysms in patients with sickling disorders. *Br J Haematol* 1999; **106**: 388–90.

51. Vernet O, Montes JL, O'Gorman AM *et al.* Encephalo-duroarterio-synangiosis in a child with sickle cell anemia and moyamoya disease. *Pediatr Neurol* 1996; **14**: 226–30.

52. Pegelow CH, Wang W, Granger S *et al.* Silent infarcts in children with sickle cell anemia and abnormal cerebral artery velocity. *Arch Neurol*, 2001; **58**: 2017–21.

Chapter 16

Iron chelation therapy in beta thalassaemia major

Beatrix Wonke

Introduction

Iron overload may develop as a consequence of increased absorption of iron over a prolonged period, as in hereditary haemochromatosis, thalassaemia intermedia, sideroblastic anaemia, pyruvate kinase deficiency and others; or from repeated red cell transfusions, as in thalassaemia syndromes and sickle cell disease (SCD). The latter two groups accumulate iron at a rate of approximately 0.5 mg/kg/day. This iron is deposited in almost all tissues, but the bulk is found in the reticulo-endothelial cells, in the spleen, liver, bone marrow and parenchymal tissue, primarily in the hepatocytes and endocrine glands. The iron in the reticulo-endothelial cells is relatively harmless. Parenchymal siderosis, however, results in significant organ damage. In multiple red cell transfusions, the primary site of iron accumulation is in the reticulo-endothelial cells. In gross iron overload, however, redistribution of iron occurs in all tissues, reticulo-endothelial cells and parenchymal cells, with time. This iron is toxic to the endocrine organs, liver and eventually to the heart, causing cardiac failure and death. Patients treated with repeated red cell transfusion will therefore require iron chelation therapy. Most of our knowledge in this field has been obtained from patients with beta thalassaemia major treated with desferrioxamine for the last three decades and deferiprone for the last 15 years. This chapter will discuss the beneficial and toxic effects of these drugs in the context of this disease.

Assessment of iron overload

The human body is designed to conserve as much iron as possible; hence there is no mechanism for iron excretion. In children with beta thalassaemia major (a hyperactive bone marrow disorder), tissue damage from iron may be present from very early in life, and regular iron chelation should begin at the 10th to 12th blood transfusion [1]. Careful planning and assessment of iron burden are important, as if not used judiciously iron chelators can have many side-effects (see toxic effects of desferrioxamine and deferiprone below). Serum ferritin concentration is well correlated with hepatic and macrophage iron stores, less well with pituitary or cardiac iron. It is measured by immunoassay technology as a convenient, non-invasive measure of iron. Normal concentration of serum ferritin has a wide range from 15 to 350 µg/L and in patients on regular blood transfusions the goal of iron chelation therapy is to prevent or reduce and maintain the iron overload to a serum ferritin level of around or below 1000 µg/L. The importance of maintaining consistently low serum ferritin levels in a clinical setting is illustrated in Fig. 16.1. Serial serum ferritin levels, four or more assessments yearly in individual patients, usually give an indication of whether the iron burden in that patient is static, increasing or decreasing. Single or sporadic measurement of serum ferritin alone may be a poor indication of iron burden. This is because ferritin synthesis is influenced by factors other than iron; in particular, it acts as an acute phase reactant in many inflammatory diseases, and because damage to ferritin-rich organs can release large amounts of

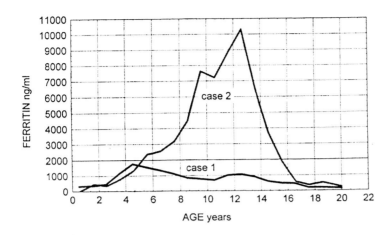

Fig. 16.1 Serial serum ferritin concentrations in two patients with transfusion-dependent thalassaemia. (Data collated by Dr Antonio Piga, Centro Microcitemie, Dipartimento Di Scienze Pediatriche E Dell' Adolescenza, Torino, Italy; reproduced with permission.)

tissue ferritin into the plasma. Increased serum ferritin concentrations have also been reported in malignancy, in which redistribution of iron from haemoglobin to macrophage stores may occur, or some tumours may produce their own ferritin. Ascorbate deficiency on the other hand can lower serum ferritin concentration.

In iron overload, transferrin becomes completely saturated with iron with the formation of non-transferrin-bound iron. Non-transferrin-bound iron assay in the plasma relies on the use of a large excess of a low affinity ligand, which removes and complexes low molecular weight iron and iron non-specifically bound to serum protein. Non-transferrin-bound iron concentrations are between 1 and 10 µM in the plasma. Once transferrin becomes saturated in the blood in iron overload, non-transferrin-bound iron becomes elevated in plasma and because it is not tightly co-ordinated to a ligand or within an iron-containing protein, is potentially available to redox cycle with the generation of free radicals. The loss of an electron by iron results in the gain of an electron by other molecules, resulting in free radical formation and oxidative tissue damage. This oxidative tissue damage accounts for most of the myocardial damage associated with iron overload. For this reason it is important to monitor and accurately quantify this potentially toxic iron fraction [2]. Several centres are currently engaged in measuring low molecular weight iron in tissue fluids and assessing the progress of chelation therapy in iron overloaded disorders. However, this assay is not in routine use but rather a research tool.

Liver biopsy allows direct examination of total body iron stores by histological staining for iron or by chemical quantitative measurement of iron. Liver iron is normally found in the hepatocytes and macrophages, with normal values of 0.5–2.0 mg/g/dry weight. Serial liver biopsies and quantitative liver iron estimation in beta thalassaemia major in the absence of cirrhosis or focal liver lesions can accurately assess total body iron stores, provided that the liver biopsy sample is at least 1.0 mg/g/dry weight [3]. Total body iron stores can then be calculated from the following formulae:

Total body iron stores $= (10.6) \times$ hepatic iron concentration

mg/kg/body weight = mg/kg/dry weight

Liver fibrosis and cirrhosis are well known complications in beta thalassaemia major. The role of iron overload in the natural history of liver fibrosis has only recently been elucidated [4]. One hundred and eleven patients cured by bone marrow transplantation had serial liver biopsies for a median follow-up of 64 months. None of the hepatitis C-negative patients with hepatic iron content < 16 mg/g/dry weight showed progression to fibrosis. However, patients co-infected with hepatitis C virus and those with a liver iron > 22 mg/g/dry weight showed progression to liver fibrosis. Iron overload and hepatitis C infection are independent co-factors for liver fibrosis. Co-infection with hepatitis C and high liver iron levels are the most likely predisposing factors for the development of liver cirrhosis. Therefore all patients with active hepatitis C infection should be de-ironed to a near normal liver iron level. Serial liver biopsies are used not only in predicting the progression to liver cirrhosis but also in monitoring the effect of iron chelation on the liver. Several beta thalassaemia patients cured by bone marrow transplantation and successfully de-ironed by venesections and treated with antiviral treatment for hepatitis C showed marked improvement in their cirrhosis. This suggests that fibrosis in the liver may be reversible, if the underlying profibrotic conditions are eliminated [5].

While serial liver biopsies seem to have a great value in predicting the severity of total body iron burden, progression to liver fibrosis and monitoring the beneficial effect of treatment, quantification of liver iron from a single liver biopsy in the long term has little value in predicting complications of iron overload [6].

Diagnostic accuracy and safety of consecutive percutaneous liver biopsies in adults [7] and children [8] have been assessed and in the latter group it was found to be safe, with a complication rate of 0.5% without ultrasound guidance and < 0.1% with ultrasound guidance. However, the procedure requires general anaesthesia in all patients under the age of 10 years and local anaesthesia for older children. The technique is invasive, painful and unpleasant, necessitating clotting studies before the procedure and administration of vitamin K if the prothrombin activity or activated partial thromboplastin times are prolonged. Low platelet count could exclude patients from liver biopsy, or necessitate platelet transfusion. Reported complications associated with liver biopsies are: haemoperitoneum, pericholecystic haematoma, kidney haematoma, bile peritonitis and others.

Superconducting quantum-interference-device (SQUID) [9] and magnetic resonance imaging (MRI) [10, 11] techniques are non-invasive magnetic measurements of hepatic iron stores. SQUID is routinely used in monitoring iron chelation programmes in Switzerland, Germany, Italy and the USA. It is non-invasive, reproducible, accurate and particularly useful in monitoring iron chelation programmes in children. The MRI technique, measuring signal intensity ratio between liver and skeletal muscle [11], also offers a safe and reproducible non-invasive method for the determination of liver iron concentration, within a wide range of iron overloaded diseases. This method is especially indicated in those patients where a non-invasive determination of liver iron concentration is preferable and histological information is not required.

However, the methods discussed above are unsuitable for the accurate assessment of cardiac iron loading, the commonest cause of morbidity and mortality in beta thalassaemia major. A modification of the MRI technique using gradient echo T_2 star (T_2^*) measurements to quantify cardiac iron loading has recently been reported to be an accurate technique with a high degree of reproducibility in the heart (coefficient of variation 0.5%) [12]. Using MRI T_2^* technology, liver iron, left ventricular ejection fraction, left ventricular end diastolic volume, left ventricular end systolic volume and left ventricular mass can be accurately and reproducibly measured and related to cardiac iron overload. This technique is by far the most advanced in diagnosing tissue iron loading and the response to iron chelation, and assessing the effects of different iron chelators and the rates at which they remove iron from the heart [13].

Iron chelators

Desferrioxamine mesylate is a natural siderophore produced by *Streptomyces pilosus*. It is a water-soluble compound, stable in solution up to 3 weeks at room temperature or at 4 °C. It has a high affinity for ferric (Fe^{3+}) iron, to which it combines at a 1 : 1 molar ratio with a high stability constant. It also has a low affinity to zinc and other metal ions. The half-life of desferrioxamine in plasma when the drug is injected is only 60 minutes. The gastrointestinal absorption of desferrioxamine is poor and therefore it is only given parenterally. The mechanism by which desferrioxamine works once injected is by combining with the labile iron pool (or chelatable iron pool). Storage iron, ferritin and haemosiderin are not static in the liver and other storage organs, but are turned over and degraded every few days with resulting increased fluxes of labile or chelatable iron in iron overload. Once desferrioxamine combines with the chelatable iron it forms ferrioxamine (desferrioxamine iron complex), a stable complex resistant to enzymic degradation. It is distributed in the extracellular space and is unable to penetrate cells; most of the ferrioxamine is excreted in the urine, while hepatocellular iron is confined to the bile and excreted in the faeces.

Desferrioxamine therapy

In view of its short plasma half-life, it is recommended that the drug is infused subcutaneously by slow infusion, either over 8–12 or 24 hours, or intravenously continuously. Several syringe driver pumps are available, all capable of slow delivery of desferrioxamine, usually through a needle inserted in the subcutaneous tissue. The longer the duration of desferrioxamine administration, the greater is the efficacy. The dose of desferrioxamine should be adjusted according to body iron load. When starting after the ferritin level has reached 1000 µg/L, the dose should be 20 mg/kg body weight, up to 50 mg/kg daily in grossly iron overloaded patients. Calculating the therapeutic index helps to prevent under- or over-dosing with desferrioxamine.

$$\text{Therapeutic index} = \frac{\text{mean daily dose mg/kg}}{\text{ferritin } \mu g/L}$$

The aim is to keep the index < 0.025 at all times. Vitamin C increases iron excretion by increasing the availability of chelatable iron. It should be given orally in doses of 2–3 mg/kg at the time of the desferrioxamine infusion. Desferrioxamine has been in clinical use for over 30 years in the developed countries for the treatment of iron overload. Recently published survival data of beta thalassaemia major patients from the UK [14] show that 50% of patients can comply conscientiously with desferrioxamine treatment and they have a long-term survival and good quality of life. Unfortunately the other half of the patients cannot achieve this because iron chelation with subcutaneous desferrioxamine is burdensome, painful, time-consuming and unending. During their lifetime beta thalassaemia patients whose compliance is erratic will develop a number of endocrine complications, liver problems and eventually cardiomyopathy leading to early death (Fig. 16.1).

Figure 16.1 illustrates the problem in two patients. Patient one has a good quality of life as a consequence of persistent iron chelation. Patient two is non-compliant and developed gonadal failure, short stature, hypothyroidism, diabetes and at the age of 14 years heart failure, necessitating continuous intravenous delivery of desferrioxamine at a high cost of morbidity.

There are several new approaches for increasing the tolerability of desferrioxamine treatment, which includes the use of local anaesthetic cream applied to the skin and covered by a see-through plaster 60 minutes before injection. This is particularly helpful in a paediatric setting.

The use of a small subcutaneous needle (Thalaset), replacing the large butterfly needle (Fig 16.2) and the introduction of home delivery disposable Baxter desferrioxamine balloon pumps (Fig 16.3), have helped to improve compliance with desferrioxamine treatment.

Conventional subcutaneous desferrioxamine chelation therapy requires aseptic dilution of the drug by the patient, which is time-consuming. The battery-operated pump is noisy and cumbersome to carry; moreover, infusions are not given continuously, allowing non-transferrin-bound iron to accumulate in the plasma in the absence of the drug. In the UK, with the help of Baxter Healthcare Ltd, we have developed a special desferrioxamine infuser, which is light, silent, pre-filled and disposable [15] (Fig 16.3). The desferrioxamine is in the balloon reservoir, which provides continuous pressure. Preset flow rates are controlled by the flow restrictor. A variety of flow rates are available – 12, 24, 48 hours and even a 7-day infuser. The device allows continuous infusion of desferrioxamine, either by subcutaneous or intravenous route. Compliance with this treatment modality has much improved and plasma non-transferrin-bound iron levels fall significantly with the treatment, compared with the overnight intermittent desferrioxamine. However, there is a substantial cost involved with the use of these disposable infusers and therefore its use is selective to patients with gross iron overload.

Intravenous desferrioxamine treatment is recommended for patients with massive cardiac iron loading, or for those who are allergic to subcutaneous desferrioxamine. The treatment requires the inser-

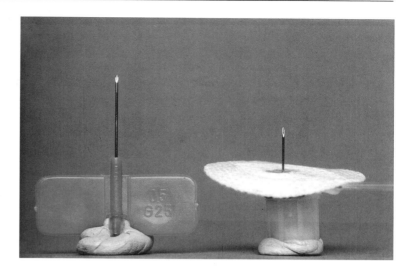

Fig. 16.2 Small subcutaneous needle (Thalaset) replacing large butterfly needle.

tion of an intravenous catheter by a specialist under general anaesthesia and the full anticoagulation of the patient. Insertion of needles or connecting the cannulas requires strict aseptic techniques. The long-term benefit of this treatment is improvement in the actuarial survival of cardiac disease in beta thalassaemia patients to 62% at 13 years, compared with 3.6 years with subcutaneous desferrioxamine treatment [16]. Intravenous desferrioxamine with blood transfusions is a convenient, although not universally practised treatment. When intravenous desferrioxamine is infused at the time of blood transfusions in doses of 500 mg – 2 g/unit of blood, the excretion of urinary iron is substantially increased in iron overloaded patients [17]. There is no need to give this treatment in well chelated patients.

Desferrioxamine is a remarkably safe drug, allowing for the fact that it is given from early childhood throughout life in considerable quantities. However, its long-term and in some cases inappropriate use has led to the following side-effects in some patients: local skin reactions at the site of the infusion, hypersensitivity to desferrioxamine, ophthalmic toxicity and ototoxicity, pseudorickets-type skeletal changes, platyspondylosis of the spine with associated disproportionate growth and tendency to *Yersinia* spp. septicaemia.

The local skin reactions may be solved either by the addition of small doses of hydrocortisone

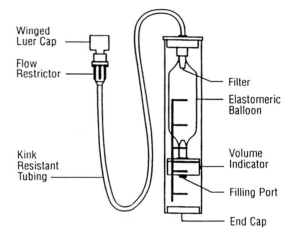

Fig. 16.3 Home delivery disposable Baxter desferrioxamine balloon pump.

(1–2 mg per syringe) to the desferrioxamine, or by increasing the volume of solution to desferrioxamine ration (desferrioxamine infuser where the drug is diluted in 60 ml of water for injection). Hypersensitivity to desferrioxamine is rare, desensitization is possible but recurrences are common. Ophthalmic toxicity and ototoxicity if severe will require the use of a hearing aid and regular yearly testing. Changing iron chelating agent from desferrioxamine to the oral chelator is advisable. Skeletal changes associated with disproportional growth (short spine, long extremities) occur mainly in patients who started iron chelation in their first year of life when the iron burden was minimal or in those who are hypersensitive to the drug. The exact mechanism of the drug's toxicity is poorly understood; it may be related to the chelation of trace elements in critical iron-dependent enzymes such as ribonucleotide reductase or alkaline phosphatase. Changing from desferrioxamine to the oral chelator has been reported to reverse bone deformities without correcting the final standing height [18].

Yersinia infection is not uncommon in iron overloaded and desferrioxamine-treated patients. The *Yersinia* family of bacteria has low pathogenicity but an unusually high requirement for iron as they do not secrete siderophore but have receptors for ferrioxamine. They become pathogenic in iron overload, and thus present an important hazard to any patient receiving desferrioxamine. Clinicians should be alert to the possibility of *Yersinia* infection in iron overloaded patients presenting with abdominal pain, diarrhoea, vomiting, as well as fever and sore throat. Desferrioxamine should be stopped immediately, stool cultures or blood serology undertaken and co-trimoxazole or aminoglycoside treatment given empirically.

Deferiprone, the oral iron-chelating drug, has been in clinical use mainly as a research tool since 1987; however, the drug was licensed for the treatment of iron overload in thalassaemia in India in 1994 and in the European Union in 1999 for patients unable to use desferrioxamine without serious side-effects. Deferiprone is an oral iron chelator, rapidly absorbed, reaching a peak plasma level within 45–60 minutes of ingestion. It has a very high affinity to bind iron in a 3 : 1 complex. It also binds zinc, aluminium and other metals. The deferiprone iron complex is eliminated from plasma within 5–6 hours of ingestion. Deferiprone is inactivated by glucuronidization in the liver, which makes the compound inactive for further iron chelation. The speed of glucoronidization affects the chelation efficiency of the drug and this may explain patients' individual responses to it. Most of the deferiprone iron complex and free drug is excreted in the urine, with a negligible amount in the faeces. Urine iron excretion in response to deferiprone has not been found to be consistently affected by co-administration of vitamin C, or by

giving in 2, 3 or 4 divided daily doses with food or fasting. The recommended dose of deferiprone for patients with minimal iron loading is 75 mg/kg/day – those with gross iron overload may need up to 100 mg/kg/day.

The effectiveness of deferiprone to remove tissue iron has been the subject of many reports and an extensive review on this subject has recently been published in *Blood* [19]. SQUID and MRI T_2* studies suggest that deferiprone is less effective in removing iron from the liver than desferrioxamine but it is clearly more effective than desferrioxamine at removing cardiac iron [13]. MRI T_2* studies [12, 13] undertaken on a large number of iron-chelated beta thalassaemia major patients revealed that the iron pools in the heart and liver are separate and both need careful assessment. One cannot extrapolate from liver iron quantification to cardiac iron loading and vice versa. Assessment of cardiac iron loading is particularly relevant, considering that myocardial iron loading leading to heart failure is a major cause of death in patients with beta thalassaemia.

As deferiprone is less effective in removing iron from the liver and desferrioxamine in removing iron from the heart, the author and others have reassessed the current iron chelation regimens and introduced a combination of the two drugs to achieve optimal effect [20–22]. The beneficial effects of using these drugs is based on the ability of deferiprone to enter cells to remove iron from within the cells, from cell membrane and from transferrin and transfer it to desferrioxamine, a 'shuttle' effect, which is particularly efficient at removing iron from the heart even before overall body iron burden is substantially reduced [23, 24]. Combined therapy is an option for chelation in beta thalassaemia patients suffering from severe cardiac failure. Daily subcutaneous continuous desferrioxamine 50 mg/kg/day and daily deferiprone 75 mg/kg/day can in the author's experience (unpublished data) replace intensive intravenous desferrioxamine chelation. Successful reversal of cardiomyopathy is safer and more rapid with this approach than continuous intravenous desferrioxamine alone.

Patients with moderately severe cardiac iron and minimal liver iron loading may comply better with daily deferiprone and 1 or 2 days a week of desferrioxamine treatment. To date, this combination therapy has shown no unanticipated side-effects.

Iron chelation needs to be reassessed in view of recent findings and in each patient after careful assessment of tissue iron loading, iron chelation treatment has to be individually tailored to achieve the maximum benefit.

Deferiprone toxicity

Agranulocytosis occurs in 0.5% of patients, arthropathy in 25%; however, the most common complication is nausea and gastrointestinal symptoms. Zinc deficiency and fluctuating liver function tests have also been reported. Agranulocytosis is preceded by neutropenia and it is therefore advisable to monitor weekly blood counts at the start of treatment, and when neutrophil counts are below 1.0×10^9/L discontinue the drug. Agranulocytosis and neutropenia are reversible on discontinuation of the drug, although some patients may require granulocyte-colony stimulating factor (G-CSF). Agranulocytosis is an idiosyncratic toxicity of unknown cause. Milder forms of neutropenia may be related to hypersplenism and intercurrent infections rather than drug toxicity. Side-effects other than neutropenia, arthropathy and very severe nausea may require discontinuation of therapy. Liver fibrosis with time does not occur in patients on deferiprone treatment who are hepatitis C virus-negative [25].

Conclusion and future prospects

Much is known about the efficacy and toxicity of desferrioxamine and deferiprone. Deferiprone used at a dose of 75 mg/kg/body weight per day appears, on average, to be about 65% as effective as desferrioxamine, with wide individual patient variation. Compliance with deferiprone is better and for patients already committed to regular transfusions for whom deferiprone is equally as effective as desferrioxamine, it is clearly preferable to take an orally active drug rather than subcutaneous infusion. Furthermore, with the emergence of the advanced cardiac MRI technique, it is now possible to accu-

rately and reproducibly assess tissue iron loading. This will enable physicians to introduce better and more innovative iron chelation programmes, either by giving desferrioxamine alone to its maximum therapeutic dose intravenously or subcutaneously without causing toxic side-effects, or using oral chelation with deferiprone with doses up to 100 mg/kg body weight, or the combination of the two. Improved treatment options and better techniques for the assessment of tissue iron overload will improve the quality of life of beta thalassaemia major patients and prolong their survival worldwide. It is to be hoped that other orally active iron chelators will become available for clinical use and so further improve iron chelation treatment of beta thalassaemia major and other diseases treated with regular transfusions.

References

1. *Guidelines for the Clinical Management of Thalassaemia*. Nicosia, Cyprus: Thalassaemia International Federation, 2000.
2. Singh S, Hider RC, Porter JB. A direct method for quantification of non-transferrin bound iron. *Anal Biochem* 1990; **186**: 320–33.
3. Angelucci E, Brittenham GM, McLaren CE *et al*. Hepatic iron concentration and total body iron stores in thalassaemia major. *N Engl J Med* 2000; **343**: 327–31.
4. Angelucci E, Muretto P, Nicolucci A *et al*. Effects of iron overload and hepatitis C virus positivity in determining progression of liver fibrosis in thalassaemia following bone marrow transplantation. *Blood* 2002; **100**: 17–21.
5. Muretto P, Angelucci E, Lucarelli G. Reversibility of cirrhosis in patients cured of thalassaemia by bone marrow transplantation. *Ann Intern Med* 2002; **136**: 667–72.
6. Telfer PT, Prescott E, Holden S *et al*. Hepatic iron concentration combined with long-term monitoring of serum ferritin to predict complications of iron overload in thalassaemia major. *Br J Haematol* 2000; **110**: 971–7.
7. Piccinino F, Sagnelli E, Pasquale G, Giusti G. Complication following percutaneous liver biopsy: a multicentric retrospective study of 68276 biopsies. *J Hepatol* 1986; **2**: 165–73.
8. Angelucci E, Baronciani D, Lucarelli G *et al*. Needle liver biopsy in thalassaemia: analyses of diagnostic accuracy and safety in 1184 consecutive biopsies. *Br J Haematol* 1995; **89**: 757–61.
9. Brittenham GM, Farrell DE, Harris JW *et al*. Magnetic-susceptibility measurement of human iron stores. *N Engl J Med* 1982; **307**: 1671–5.

10. Kaltwasser JP, Goltchalk R, Schalk KP, Hartl W. Non-invasive quantitation of liver iron-overload by magnetic resonance imaging. *Br J Haematol* 1990; **74**: 360–3.

11. Jensen PD, Jensen FT, Christensen T, Ellegard J. Non-invasive assessment of tissue iron overload in the liver by magnetic resonance imaging. *Br J Haematol* 1994; **87**: 171–84.

12. Anderson LJ, Holden S, Davis B *et al.* Cardiovascular T_2 star (T_2*) magnetic resonance for the early diagnosis of myocardial iron overload. *Eur Heart J* 2001; **22**: 2171–9.

13. Anderson LJ, Wonke B, Prescott E *et al.* Comparison of effects of oral deferiprone and subcutaneous desferrioxamine on myocardial iron concentrations and ventricular function in β thalassaemia. *Lancet* 2002; **360**: 516–20.

14. Modell B, Khan M, Darlison M. Survival in β Thalassaemia Major in the United Kingdom: data from UK Thalassaemia Register. *Lancet* 2000; **355**: 2051–2.

15. Araujo A, Kosaryan M, MacDowell A *et al.* A novel delivery system for continuous desferrioxamine infusion in transfusional iron overload. *Br J Haematol* 1996; **93**: 835–7.

16. Davis BA, Porter JB. Long term outcome of continuous 24-hour desferrioxamine infusion via indwelling intravenous catheters in high-risk β thalassaemia. *Blood* 2000; **95**: 1229–36.

17. Modell CB, Beck J. Long term desferrioxamine therapy in thalassaemia. *Ann N Y Acad Sci* 1974; **232**: 201–10.

18. Mangliagli A, De Sanctis V, Campisi S, Di Silvestro G, Urso L. Treatment with deferiprone (L_1) in a thalas-saemic patient with bone lesions due to desferrioxamine. *J Pediatr Endocrinol Metab* 2000; **13**: 677–80.

19. Hoffbrand AV, Cohen A, Hershko C. The role of deferiprone in chelation therapy for transfusional iron overload. *Blood* 2003; **103**: 17–24.

20. Wonke B, Wright C, Hoffbrand AV. Combined therapy with deferiprone and desferrioxamine. *Br J Haematol* 1998; **103**: 361–4.

21. Aydinok Y, Nisli G, Kavakli K *et al.* Sequential use of deferiprone and desferrioxamine in primary school children with thalassaemia major in Turkey. *Acta Haematol* 1999; **102**: 17–21.

22. Balveer K, Pyar K, Wonke B. Combined oral and parenteral iron chelation in β thalassaemia major. *Med J Malaysia* 2000; **55**: 493–7.

23. Link G, Konijn AM, Breuer W, Cabantchik I, Hershko G. Exploring the 'iron shuttle' hypothesis in chelation therapy: effects of combined desferrioxamine and deferiprone treatment in hypertransfused rats with labelled iron stores and in iron-loaded rat heart cells in culture. *J Lab Clin Med* 2001; **138**: 130–8.

24. Grady RW, Bordoukas V, Rachmilewitz EA *et al.* Iron chelation therapy: metabolic aspects of combining deferiprone and desferrioxamine (abstract). *11th International Conference on oral chelation in the treatment of thalassaemia major and other diseases*, Catania, 2001, pp. 74–8.

25. Wanless IR, Sweeney G, Dhillon AP *et al.* Lack of progressive hepatic fibrosis during long-term therapy with deferiprone in subjects with transfusion dependent beta thalassaemia. *Blood* 2002; **5**: 1566–9.

Chapter 17
Renal manifestations of sickle cell disease

Ian Abbs

Introduction

The recognition that sickle cell disease (SCD) can affect the kidney is not new. In the original report by Herrick of 'Peculiar elongated and sickle-shaped red blood cells in a case of severe anaemia' in the *Archives of Internal Medicine* he noted that the illness was associated with the passage of an increased volume of urine of low specific gravity [1]. It is now recognized that SCD is associated with a spectrum of renal anatomical and functional abnormalities [2–4]. The increased survival of patients with SCD, due to advances in haemoglobinopathy management, has allowed the full expression of the renal manifestations of this illness to be determined. Early features of SCD in the kidney are decreased urinary concentrating ability, initially reversible by exchange transfusion, and defects of urinary acidification. Children and young adults with sickle cell anaemia may have increased total renal blood flow and increased glomerular filtration rates. In some patients sickling of red blood cells in nutrient blood vessels results in ischaemia of the central (medullary) region of the kidney. This causes damage to the juxtamedullary nephrons and decreased urinary concentrating ability that cannot be reversed by exchange transfusion. Continued ischaemic damage to the renal tubules may be associated with progressive renal impairment. Pathologically, a common feature is medullary fibrosis and loss of the network of blood vessels supplying the inner kidney. The renal complications of sickle cell anaemia include the development of end-stage renal disease (ESRD) with the requirement for dialysis and transplantation, treatments that pose particular challenges in this complex patient group.

Pathogenesis

The kidney is a harsh environment for a red blood cell and in a patient with SCD the renal circulation provides conditions ideally suited to promote sickling of erythrocytes. The normal environment of the renal medulla promotes erythrocyte sickling as it is an area of low oxygen tension, of high osmolality (that increases the HbS concentration in the red blood cell by promoting water movement out of the cell), and of relatively low pH. Sickling of erythrocytes in the vasa recta capillaries of the medulla causes congestion and stasis and this further impairs medullary blood flow and leads to an ischaemic cycle that promotes tissue injury. Important mediators of injury in the kidney in sickle cell nephropathy (SCN) include free radicals, generated following ischaemia-reperfusion [5], that increase oxidative stress [6] and up-regulation of nitric oxide (NO) synthase [7]. Inhibition of HbS polymerization and of sickle cell ischaemia–reperfusion injury may prevent the development of SCN. Recent demonstration, in a mouse model of SCN, that inhibition of HbS polymerization by gene therapy prevented development of the urine concentration defect is encouraging [8]. However, factors not directly related to the polymerization of HbS and cell sickling, such as the up-regulation of pro-inflammatory cytokine and adhesion molecules and activation of inflammatory and endothelial cells, are also likely to be of importance in the generation of the renal lesions of SCN [9, 10] and strategies that block these pathways may be of therapeutic importance.

Repeated episodes of ischaemia lead to haemorrhage and ischaemic necrosis and, eventually, to interstitial inflammation and fibrosis. Ischaemic disruption of the counter-current multiplication and exchange system results in early abnormalities of tubular function. Ultimately tubular atrophy, papillary infarcts and irreversible loss of renal function occur. Microradiographic studies in younger patients with SCD of the blood flow to the medulla demonstrate a reduction in the number of vasa recta capillaries and dilatation and partial obliteration of those remaining. In older patients such radiographic studies may show complete obliteration of the vasa recta capillary system. Although the lesions associated with repeated cycles of ischaemia are most marked in the kidneys of patients with homozygous (HbSS) SCD, they are also seen in patients win HbSC disease and other variant sickle haemoglobinopathies and, to a lesser extent, in patients with sickle cell trait. In a small study of patients dying of renal failure in association with sickle cell anaemia, the kidneys were found to be small at autopsy, suggesting that continued ischaemia eventually results in a reduction in renal mass.

Clinical manifestations

Ischaemic injury to the kidney in patients with sickle cell anaemia results in a spectrum of renal disorders that may be subclinical or that may present with overt clinical symptoms and signs.

Disorders of renal tubular function

Ischaemic disruption of the physiology of the renal tubule results in decreased urinary concentrating ability, probably as a result of disruption of the counter-current exchange mechanism. This may present as enuresis in childhood and as nocturia and frequency in adults. In early childhood this defect may be reversed by exchange transfusions but by late childhood the condition is irreversible [11]. By the age of 15 years patients with SCD have a fixed urine output of approximately 4000 ml per day, often associated with complaints of nocturia. They are unable to concentrate their urine under conditions of water deprivation and can achieve a maximum urine osmolality of only 400–450 milliosmoles per kg, about 50% of normal [2]. Patients with SCD are therefore unable to defend body volume homeostasis in conditions of volume loss such as gastrointestinal upset, high environmental temperature or fever or enforced fluid deprivation.

Disruption of the physiology of the distal renal tubule in SCD may result in a defect of the acidification of urine and is manifest as incomplete distal renal tubular acidosis (RTA). Acidosis is not usually apparent unless conditions of stress such as infection occur, or in patients with established renal impairment. Patients have a hyperchloraemic acidosis [12] and are unable to excrete an acid load.

Distal tubular dysfunction is also manifest as impaired potassium excretion. This defect, similar to the defect of acidification, is not usually clinically apparent. However, in situations of stress or in patients with renal impairment, the defect may result in hyperkalaemia. Some buffering of hyperkalaemia occurs because of increased beta-adrenergic drive in patients with SCD causing excess potassium to pass into cells.

Patients with SCD may exhibit supranormal proximal tubular function manifest by increased secretion of creatinine and by reabsorption of phosphorus and beta(2)-microglobulin [4]. Increases in proximal tubular creatinine secretion in SCD reduces the usefulness of creatinine clearance as a measure of renal function in these patients, as this investigation will therefore overestimate renal function measured against true glomerular filtration rate (GFR).

Bleeding

Haematuria is common in patients with SCD and may be present as microscopic or gross macroscopic bleeding. Gross haematuria is a relatively common complaint in patients with SCD, presumably as a result of papillary infarcts and ischaemic necrosis. It is usually mild, does not require transfusion and is self-limiting, although it may continue for some weeks. Occasionally bleeding may be more severe and patients may present with renal colic and with ureteric obstruction. Treatment is supportive, with hydration and transfusion if required, and intervention is rarely needed. Bleeding may also be seen in patients with sickle cell trait and papillary necrosis has been described. Expression in heterozygotes presumably reflects the harsh environment of the renal medulla for red blood cells with even low concentrations of HbS.

Papillary necrosis

Of all areas of the kidneys, the harshest environment for a SCD red blood cell is the ischaemic, hypertonic and acid medullary pyramid. Severe ischaemia of the medullary pyramid results in papillary necrosis and, as above, can be seen in both SCD and sickle cell trait. The incidence of papillary necrosis has been reported as between 23% and 67% in different series. Patients may be asymptomatic or may present with bleeding, renal colic or ureteric obstruction. Infection may complicate papillary necrosis and, in this setting, acute renal failure has been described.

Medullary carcinoma

Renal medullary carcinoma is an aggressive tumour found most commonly in black patients with sickle cell haemoglobinopathy, most commonly as sickle cell trait and HbSC disease [13]. It presents with loin pain, haematuria, a possible history of weight loss and a palpable flank mass may be present. The tumour has often metastasized by the time of presentation and complete surgical removal is seldom successful. Response to chemotherapy or radiotherapy is poor and survival time from diagnosis ranges from 1 to 7 months.

Acute renal failure

Acute renal failure (ARF) has been described in SCD but it is not as common as may be predicted by the patient population. ARF has been described as complicating sickle cell crises, usually in the context of volume depletion, extreme fever and infection.

The importance of non-traumatic rhabdomyolysis in the pathogenesis of ARF in SCD should not be overlooked. Early detection of this in at-risk patients may offer a therapeutic window for treatment that may prevent the development of established, dialysis-dependent ARF that carries a high morbidity and mortality. Rhabdomyolysis as a causative factor in ARF in patients with sickle cell trait undertaking extreme exertion has been described. ARF has also been described following complications of pregnancy in women with SCD. In patients with ARF who fail to recover renal function, subsequent histological examination has revealed cortical necrosis, the extreme result of ischaemic injury.

Hypertension

The blood pressure profiles of patients with sickle cell anaemia are different to those of Afro-Caribbean patients without sickle cell anaemia. The blood pressure of patients attending the comprehensive sickle cell clinic tends to be lower than average and blood pressures of 100/70 mmHg are common, reflecting the lower prevalence of hypertension in these patients. In a study of a Los Angeles sickle cell population involving 180 patients, the prevalence of hypertension was only 3.2% compared with an expected prevalence of 30%. The mean blood pressure for the sickle cell anaemia group was 116/70 mmHg. Adjusting for age and gender there were large differences in blood pressure (10–20 mmHg for both systolic and diastolic blood pressures in all age groups) between sickle cell patients and normal individuals. Age-related blood pressure increases are not observed in the sickle cell group. However, hypertension is a feature of patients with established renal failure. The cause of these differences is unclear but it may reflect generalized up-regulation of vasodilator compounds. The observation that the usual blood pressure for patients with SCD is lower than the population average is of importance. SCD patients may be inappropriately labelled as normotensive when their blood pressures are inappropriately elevated. This is of particular importance in the assessment of women during pregnancy in whom a blood pressure still in the normal range but high for SCD may herald the onset of pre-eclampsia.

Glomerular abnormalities in SCD

A variety of glomerular abnormalities have been described in SCD. These range from glomerular hypertrophy through a number of specific histological entities to glomerular obsolescence in ESRD due to SCN. Specific histological abnormalities described include focal segmental glomerular sclerosis (FSGS), a relatively common biopsy appearance in SCN. Mesangio-capillary glomerulonephritis (MCGN) with or without immune deposits and membranous glomerulonephritis have also been described. The mechanisms that cause glomerular scarring in SCD and that lead to the common finding of FSGS are of potential therapeutic importance [14]. Initial glomerular injury may occur as a result of ischaemia following capillary occlusion by erythrocytes or as a result of a haemodynamic injury as a consequence of glomerular hyperperfusion and hypertension under the control of vasodilator prostaglandins and NO. Nephron loss as a consequence of ischaemic and hyperfiltration injury results in increased workload falling on the remaining, intact, glomeruli. Such increased load is manifest by a further increase in glomerular pressure that accelerates glomerular injury. Such a vicious circle has been proposed as an important mechanism of disease progression in a number of models of chronic renal failure (CRF). That this may be operating in SCD accelerating renal functional loss, may be of importance as it offers a therapeutic opportunity [15], treatment with drugs that block the renin–angiotensin axis, as discussed below.

Not all patients with sickle haemoglobin develop nephropathy. Factors that influence the development of focal segmental lesions include the type of haemoglobinopathy present (the incidence of FSGS is lower in HbSC disease than in HbSS: 2.4% vs 4.2%) and non-haemoglobin genetic markers (the Bantu haplotype is associated with more aggressive renal disease). Inheritance of deletions in the alpha globin genes may offer a reno-protective effect and reduce the likelihood of development of sickle nephropathy [16].

Proteinuria

The finding of proteinuria in patients with SCD is ominous as it implies the onset of sickle nephropathy. It suggests the presence of a significant renal lesion and is usually the manifestation of glomerular pathology. The detection of proteinuria is important as it may offer a treatment opportunity if found at an early stage in the development of renal disease. Microalbuminuria (MA) has been described as an early and sensitive marker for renal involvement in diabetes mellitus before the development of frank proteinuria and it has been used as a prompt for early therapeutic intervention. In diabetic nephropathy (DN), there is strong evidence that early intervention with drugs that block the renin–angiotensin axis is of use. There are similarities in the glomerular pathology in DN and SCN and there is a clinically coherent rationale for the early use of angiotensin-converting enzyme inhibitors and of angiotensin II receptor antagonists in patients with the early manifestations of SCN. The detection of herald proteinuria in SCN, similar to that of the early proteinuria that heralds the onset of DN, may be used to determine those patients who may benefit from drug intervention. Elevated urinary microalbumin/creatinine ratios are reported in 39–43% of adults with HbSS and the overall prevalence of MA in children with HbSS has been reported as 26.5%. There appears to be a strong correlation between patient age and MA, with a prevalence of MA in children between the ages of 10 and 18 years of 46%, similar to the prevalence in adults [17]. Patients may benefit from early intervention with drugs that block the renin–angiotensin axis but more studies are needed to see if this hypothesis is valid.

Proteinuria, detected by stick testing of the urine, usually points to eventual progressive decline in renal function and the development of end-stage renal failure. The prevalence of proteinuria detected by urine dipstick in sickle cell anaemia varies in studies between 15% and 30%. There is an age gradient in the reported prevalence of proteinuria with approximately 22% in the age range 21–30 years, 35% in the age range 31–40 years and 55% in those patients over 40 years testing positive for protein.

The presence of proteinuria is usually associated with a serum creatinine increased above the normal range. Once present, proteinuria usually progresses and patients may develop frank nephrotic syndrome. Fortunately, the time course of the decline in function is measured in years rather than months. Nephrotic syndrome, the co-incidence of heavy proteinuria, oedema and hypo-albuminaemia, has been described in approximately 4–5% of patients with SCD. Proteinuria and the nephrotic syndrome strongly predict the subsequent development of ESRD in patients with SCD.

SCN and the development of ESRD

Early in the clinical course of patients with SCD the GFR is paradoxically raised and may be as high as 150% of normal [14]. The mechanism of GFR elevation is unclear but it may be a reflection of the release of vasodilator prostaglandins via an indomethacin-sensitive pathway and/or as a result of NO-mediated vasodilatation. The potential role of NO has been highlighted by work that demonstrated that the inducible form of NO synthetase is up-regulated in the glomeruli and distal nephrons of HbSS transgenic mice [18]. That this process occurs early in life is highlighted by the finding of glomerular hypertrophy in children as young as 2 years of age. With older age, however, GFR falls in patients with sickle nephropathy. The previously elevated GFR may fall into the normal range by the age of 20. In some patients GFR continues to decline and by the age of 30–40 years a number of patients with SCD will have CRF.

The prevalence and natural history of chronic and end-stage renal failure in patients with sickle cell anaemia are now being described as patients survive into middle age due to improvements in haemoglobinopathy management. The reported prevalence of renal insufficiency to date is low compared with the prevalence of proteinuria. In a study of 368 patients reported in 1990 [19], the prevalence of chronic renal insufficiency was 4.6% overall. In a prospective 25-year longitudinal study of 725 patients with sickle cell anaemia and HbSC disease, approximately 4.2% of patients with SCD progressed to end-stage renal failure [20]. This study suggested that the Bantu beta S haplotype was associated with more aggressive disease. The relative risk for mortality in the group of sickle cell anaemia patients with renal impairment was 1.42. The Co-operative Study of SCD enrolled 3764 patients and found that CRF was implicated in 22 of 38 deaths due to organ failure [21].

Additional factors in renal disease progression in SCN

The role of non-steroidal anti-inflammatory drugs (NSAIDs) in the progression of CRF in SCD is of importance. NSAIDs are nephrotoxic and have been implicated in the progression of CRF, presumably as a consequence of inhibition of vasodilator prostaglandin production and promotion of ischaemia. While they may be useful in patients without evidence of renal disease, they may promote the development of CRF in patients with diminished GFR and they should be avoided if possible. Recurrent urinary tract infections should be investigated and treated and, if possible, prevented by the use of prophylactic antibiotics. Patients with SCD may, of course, have any of the more common causes of renal impairment, such as urinary outflow obstruction in men due to prostatic hypertrophy, and these should be excluded by appropriate investigation. If necessary, renal biopsy should be performed to confirm the presence of SCN and to exclude other parenchymal renal diseases.

The management of patients with ESRD due to SCD

The management of patients with ESRD due to SCD requiring dialysis and transplantation is complex. The available treatment options for patients with ESRD are essentially those of dialysis or renal transplantation. Dialysis is a method of artificially cleaning the blood, but all methods are relatively inefficient and should be regarded as palliation of renal failure rather than cure. Dialysis may be either as haemodialysis or as continuous ambulatory peritoneal dialysis (CAPD). Haemodialysis involves the removal of blood from the circulation and the passage of that blood through an artificial kidney. Semipermeable membranes in the artificial kidney allow the passage of toxic products from the blood into the waste removal section of the dialyser. Clean blood is then returned to the patient. The main difficulty of haemodialysis is creating access to the bloodstream to enable blood to pass to the artificial kidney and subsequently be returned to the circulation. Commonly, access is provided by the creation of an artificial blood vessel, commonly an arteriovenous fistula, large enough to allow needles to be repeatedly placed in the circulation. Creation of an arteriovenous fistula requires the anastomosis of an artery to a vein. This may be difficult if the veins have been damaged and in these circumstances it is possible to create access using artificial vessels anatomized between an artery and vein, but such artificial access has a higher failure and infection rate than native vessels. Haemodialysis usually lasts for 4 hours and is required three times per week. It is usually carried out in hospital. Surprisingly, sickle cell crises are not common during haemodialysis despite the removal of blood into the artificial environment of the dialysis kidney. Peritoneal dialysis requires a flexible tube to be placed in the abdomen. Fluid can be introduced into the abdominal cavity through the tube and the membrane lining the cavity acts as a filter, across which unwanted solutes pass from the bloodstream into the fluid. Removal of the fluid from the abdomen removes unwanted waste products of metabolism. Peritoneal dialysis is an effective method of treatment, but it does have complications, including repeated infections. Dialysis, either as haemodialysis or CAPD, is required to continue for life or until a renal transplant becomes available. Without dialysis patients die in a matter of days.

Preferably patients at risk of the complications of SCD should be managed in a combined clinic with specialist renal input [22]. Early referral to a nephrologist is of great importance to the eventual outcome of ESRD treatment in all patients. This is particularly true for patients with SCD in whom there may be particular challenges to optimum management. For example, the creation of haemodialysis access may be particularly difficult in a patient who has had multiple cannulations of arm veins. Such patients need early onward referral to a surgeon with specialist experience of dialysis access. Both haemodialysis and peritoneal dialysis have been used in patients with ESRD due to SCD, although the total number of patients reported in the literature is small. Analysis of 375 152 patients in the US Renal Data System who started ESRD therapy between 1 January 1992 and 30 June 1997 described 397 (0.11%) with SCN, of whom 93% were African-American. The mean age at presentation to ESRD was 40.68 ± 14.00 years. SCN patients had an independently increased risk of mortality (hazard ratio 1.52, 95% CI: 1.27–1.82) compared with other patients, including those with diabetes [23].

Complications of CRF and ESRD

The kidney has a central role in the production of red blood cells by the bone marrow as it is the site of production of erythropoietin. This hormone is responsible for driving the precursors of red blood cells in the bone marrow to multiply and to pass into the bloodstream. Lack of erythropoietin production in damaged kidneys is associated with profound anaemia. Until the production of genetically engineered erythropoietin many patients with ESRD were severely anaemic and suffered symptoms including marked lethargy and reduced exercise tolerance. The only treatment available until erythropoietin became commercially available was blood transfusion, which offers only short-term relief. Genetically engineered erythropoietin is now available and this can be given to patients, usually subcutaneously, with good results. Many patients with CRF have near normal haemoglobins and good exercise tolerance. Unfortunately, the majority of patients with sickle cell anaemia, who are already markedly anaemic, are resistant to erythropoietin. Resistance to erythropoietin in SCD is probably the result of up-regulation of pro-inflammatory cytokines that inhibit the effect of erythropoietin on red cell precursors. The combined effect of CRF and sickle cell anaemia resistant to injected exogenous erythropoietin is often extreme anaemia. Haemoglobin concentrations of 4 g/dL are not uncommon in this situation.

Such a low haemoglobin level is often associated with marked exercise intolerance and such patients require transfusions. In SCN patients who do respond to erythropoietin, a high haemoglobin level could precipitate painful crises. Therefore, a haemoglobin concentration of 6–9 g/dL is recommended [24].

Blood transfusions, although now considered safe with respect to the transmission of viruses, have a number of potential adverse affects. The most important of these is the production of antibodies directed against human leucocyte antigens (HLA). Anti-HLA antibodies accumulate following repeat transfusions and this can lead to difficulty in finding a suitable kidney when the patient ultimately requires transplantation. This may delay the offer of a suitable kidney, leading to a long waiting time on the transplant list.

The kidney is the site of activation, by 1 alpha hydroxylation, of vitamin D. Activated vitamin D plays a central role in calcium homeostasis and in bone metabolism. Renal failure is also complicated by phosphate retention. Defective vitamin D activation and phosphate retention promote hyperparathyroidism that, ultimately, leads to demineralization of bone and other adverse effects. Untreated hyperparathyroidism is associated with marked bone weakness and an increased fracture risk. To avoid these complications, patients with CRF and ESRD are required to take supplements of activated vitamin D (usually as 1-alpha calcidol) and dietary phosphate binders.

Survival of patients with ESRD and SCD on dialysis

Information on overall survival of patients with ESRD and SCD on dialysis is limited. Powars and colleagues [25], in a prospective 25-year cohort study, reviewed chronic renal failure in SCD and detailed the risk factors for renal disease, the clinical course of the disease and the effect of renal disease on mortality. Survival time for patients with sickle cell anaemia after the diagnosis of sickle renal failure was reduced despite dialysis. With improvement in dialysis and supportive treatment one would hope that the survival may improve but more

data are needed from further series to support this assumption.

Kidney transplantation in SCD

Transplantation is the treatment of choice for patients with end-stage renal failure. Patients may receive a suitable kidney from a living relative or, more commonly, a cadaver kidney from the national waiting list. Renal transplantation in patients with SCD is more complex than for a standard waiting list patient. SCD patients, for example, may require exchange transfusion before transplantation to prevent sickling in the transplanted organ that would have a deleterious effect on early graft survival.

Reports of transplant outcome in patients with sickle cell anaemia are limited. One series reported graft survival of 82% in living donor grafts and 62% in cadaveric graft recipients at 1 year post-transplantation [26]. Ojo and colleagues reported patient and allograft outcomes among 82 age-matched African-American kidney transplant recipients with ESRD as a result of SCN and 22 565 with ESRD due to all other causes. The incidence of delayed graft function and pre-discharge acute rejection in the SCN group (24% and 26%, respectively) was similar to that observed in the Other-ESRD group (29% and 27%, respectively). The mean discharge serum creatinine was 2.7 mg/dL in the SCN recipients compared to 3.0 mg/dL in the Other-ESRD recipients (p = 0.42). There was no difference in the 1-year cadaveric graft survival (SCN 78% vs Other-ESRD 77%), and the multivariable adjusted 1-year risk of graft loss indicated no significant effect of SCN (relative risk [RR] = 1.39, p = 0.149). However, the 3-year cadaveric graft survival tended to be lower in the SCN group (48% vs 60%, p = 0.055) and their adjusted 3-year risk of graft loss was significantly greater (RR = 1.60, p = 0.003) [27]. These results are inferior to registry reports of living donor and cadaveric graft survival in patients without sickle cell anaemia and are supported by the analysis of United Network for Organ Sharing (UNOS) registry reported in 2001 [28]. However, other authors have analysed ESRD data from the USA and suggested that transplanted SCD patient survival was similar to that of patients with other causes of renal diseases [29]. Transplantation in a small series of children with SCN has been described, suggesting acceptable results with graft survival at 12 and 24 months post-transplant of 89% and 71%, respectively [30]. The effect of transplantation on patient survival in ESRD due to sickle cell anaemia is not clear from the available literature. Graft failure would require a return to dialysis with an average patient survival time as outlined above.

Post-transplant polycythaemia

Renal transplantation in patients with SCD may improve anaemia [31] but, paradoxically, in addition to the complications of transplantation faced by many patients, sickle cell anaemia patients may become polycythaemic and this is a common cause of sickle crises in patients post-transplantation. The mechanism of this syndrome is unclear.

References

1. Herrick JB. Peculiar elongated and sickle-shaped red blood cells in a case of severe anaemia. *Arch Intern Med* 1910; **6**: 517–20.
2. Pham PT, Pham PC, Wilkinson AH, Lew SQ. Renal abnormalities in sickle cell disease. *Kidney Int* 2000; **57**: 1–8.
3. Scheinman JI. Sickle cell disease and the kidney. *Semin Nephrol* 2003; **23**: 66–76.
4. Ataga KI, Orringer EP. Renal abnormalities in sickle cell disease. *Am J Hematol* 2000; **63**: 205–11.
5. Osarogiagbon UR, Choong S, Belcher JD *et al*. Reperfusion injury pathophysiology in sickle transgenic mice. *Blood* 2000; **96**: 314–20.
6. Nath KA, Grande JP, Haggard JJ *et al*. Oxidative stress and induction of heme oxygenase-1 in the kidney in sickle cell disease. *Am J Pathol* 2001; **158**: 893–903.
7. Bank N, Kiroycheva M, Singhal PC *et al*. Inhibition of nitric oxide synthase ameliorates cellular injury in sickle cell mouse kidneys. *Kidney Int* 2000; **58**: 82–9.
8. Pawliuk R, Westerman KA, Fabry ME *et al*. Correction of sickle cell disease in transgenic mouse models by gene therapy. *Science* 2001; **294**: 2368–71.
9. Okpala I, Daniel Y, Haynes R, Odoemene D, Goldman J. Relationship between the clinical manifestations of sickle cell disease and the expression of adhesion molecules on white blood cells. *Eur J Haematol* 2002; **69**: 135–44.
10. Belcher JD, Marker PH, Weber JP, Hebbel RP, Vercellotti GM. Activated monocytes in sickle cell disease: potential role in the activation of vascular endothelium and vaso-occlusion. *Blood* 2000; **96**: 2451–9.
11. Hatch FE, Culbertson JW, Diggs LW. Nature of the renal concentrating defect in sickle cell disease. *J Clin Invest* 1967; **46**: 336.
12. Batlle D, Itsarayoungyuen K, Arruda JAL, Kurtzman NA. Hyperkalemic hyperchloremic metabolic acidosis in sickle cell hemoglobinopathies. *Am J Med* 1982; **72**: 188.
13. Dimashkieh H, Choe J, Mutema G. Renal medullary carcinoma: a report of 2 cases and review of the literature. *Arch Pathol Lab Med* 2003; **127**: 135–8.
14. Wesson DE. The initiation and progression of sickle cell nephropathy. *Kidney Int* 2002; **61**: 2277–86.
15. Falk RJ, Scheinman J, Phillips G *et al*. Prevalence and pathologic features of sickle cell nephropathy and response to inhibition of angiotensin-converting enzyme. *N Engl J Med* 1992; **326**: 910.
16. Guasch A, Zayas CF, Muralidharan K, Zhang W, Elsas LJ. Evidence that microdeletions in the alpha globin gene protect against the development of sickle cell glomerulopathy in humans. *J Am Soc Nephrol* 1999; **10**: 1014–19.
17. Dharnidharka VR, Dabbagh S, Atiyeh B, Simpson P, Sarnaik S. Prevalence of microalbuminuria in children with sickle cell disease. *Pediatr Nephrol* 1998; **12**: 475–8.
18. Bank N, Aynedjian HS, Qui JH *et al*. Renal nitric oxide synthases in transgenic sickle cell mice. *Kidney Int* 1996; **49**: 184.
19. Sklar AH, Campbell H, Caruana RJ *et al*. A population study of renal function in sickle cell anaemia. *Int J Artif Organs* 1990; **13**: 231–6.
20. Powars DR, Elliot-Mills DD, Chan L *et al*. Chronic renal failure in sickle cell disease: risk factors, clinical course, and mortality. *Ann Intern Med* 1991; **115**: 614.
21. Platt OS, Bramble DT, Rosse WF *et al*. Mortality in sickle cell disease. Life expectancy and risk factors for early death. *N Engl J Med* 1994; **330**: 1639–44.
22. Okpala I, Thomas V, Westerdale N *et al*. The comprehensive care of SCD. *Eur J Haematol* 2002; **68**: 157–62.
23. Abbott KC, Hypolite IO, Agodoa LY. Sickle cell nephropathy at end-stage renal disease in the United States: patient characteristics and survival. *Clin Nephrol* 2002; **58**: 9–15.
24. van Ypersele de Strihou C. Should anaemia in subtypes of CRF patients be managed differently? *Nephrol Dial Transplant* 1999; **14** (Suppl 2): 37–45.
25. Powars DR, Elliott-Mills DD, Chan L *et al*. Chronic renal failure in sickle cell disease: risk factors, clinical course and mortality. *Ann Intern Med* 1991; **115**: 614–20.

26. Chaterjee SM. National Study of natural history of renal allografts in sickle cell disease or trait: a second report. *Transplant Proc* 1987; **19**: 33–5.

27. Ojo AO, Govaerts TC, Schmouder RL *et al*. Renal transplantation in end-stage sickle cell nephropathy. *Transplantation* 1999; **67**: 291–5.

28. Bleyer AJ, Donaldson LA, McIntosh M, Adams PL. Relationship between underlying renal disease and renal transplantation outcome. *Am J Kidney Dis* 2001; **37**: 1152–61.

29. Abbott KC, Hypolite IO, Agodoa LY. Sickle cell nephropathy at end-stage renal disease in the United States: patient characteristics and survival. *Clin Nephrol* 2002; **58**: 9–15.

30. Warady BA, Sullivan EK. Renal transplantation in children with SCD: a report of the North American Pediatric Renal Transplant Cooperative Study (NAPRTCS). *Pediatr Transplant* 1998; **2**: 130–3.

31. Breen CP, Macdougall IC. Improvement of erythropoietin-resistant anaemia after renal transplantation in patients with homozygous sickle-cell disease. *Nephrol Dial Transplant* 1998; **13**: 2949–52.

Chapter 18

Assessment of severity and hydroxyurea therapy in sickle cell disease

Iheanyi E Okpala

Introduction

A striking variation in clinical severity occurs between individuals who have sickle cell disease (SCD). Marked differences in disease manifestation occur even among people who have the same haemoglobin genotype, such as SS [1]. Some HbSS individuals have very mild SCD [2]. They live virtually normal lives and are seldom in crisis. Others need frequent hospital treatment for debilitating and life-threatening manifestations of the haemoglobinopathy. They suffer from recurrent painful episodes and damage to vital organ systems. One of the most important challenges of SCD is to understand the biological and environmental basis of individual differences in disease severity, and to apply the knowledge in the medical treatment of affected people. In this context it is appropriate that medical treatment is tailored to suit the degree of clinical severity in a particular individual. For example, a conservative management policy could be adopted for mild SCD, with the affected person followed-up as an outpatient, and medical treatment given only when required. In contrast, a more pro-active approach would be appropriate in patients who have very severe disease and potentially fatal complications such as cerebrovascular accidents and the acute chest syndrome [3]. Individuals who have markedly severe disease could be considered for relatively intensive medical treatment such as hydroxyurea administration, haemopoietic stem cell transplantation or, in the future, gene therapy [4].

To attain this goal, it is necessary to be able to identify individuals who will have mild, moderate or severe SCD; and to do so before irreversible tissue damage and organ failure occur. If, as is currently the case, markedly severe SCD is identifiable only when major manifestations or the failure of vital organs have developed, the patient may not be medically fit for intensive but potentially curative therapy. Various genetic, cellular, humoral and environmental factors are known to influence the natural history of SCD. These include beta globin gene haplotype and HbF level [5], co-inheritance of the genes for other globin disorders such as alpha thalassaemia [6], steady-state neutrophil count and function [7], the level of expression of adhesion molecules on white blood cells [8], activity of the alternative pathway of complement and the level of circulating immune complexes [9], the plasma concentration of immunoglobulin G and the subtype IgG3 [10], the iron-binding protein transferrin and C-reactive protein [11], intercurrent infections and socio-economic status [3].

However, the relative contribution of each of these factors is yet to be determined. It is currently not possible to predict that a particular individual who has inherited the haemoglobinopathy will have very severe disease. The clinical decision to adopt a pro-active treatment policy cannot therefore be made when it is most timely. Notwithstanding this handicap, it is often necessary to assess the severity of SCD in an individual to help decide whether hydroxyurea therapy is appropriate. Considering that cytotoxic therapy could have irreversible side-effects that impact on the patient's quality of life, this decision should not be taken lightly – particularly because, currently, the long-term effects of hydroxyurea therapy are neither established nor well understood.

Determinants of severity in SCD

Haemoglobin genotype

In decreasing order of associated clinical severity, the common Hb genotypes in SCD are SS, $S\beta^0$thal, SC, $S\beta^+$thal, and S/HPFH or HbS with hereditary persistence of fetal haemoglobin. Of course, this order of severity usually observed in general does not always hold because other factors modulate the manifestations of SCD. However, by and large, haemoglobin genotype is one of the most important determinants of clinical severity in SCD, and HbSS individuals generally have more severe manifestations than people with $S\beta^+$thal. The latter may have normal adult haemoglobin (HbA) up to 20% in the blood, and this appears to make a clinically significant difference in disease severity. The general order of severity stated above should not be considered from only one perspective. For example, sickle retinopathy is more common in HbSC than HbSS individuals, although the latter generally have more severe anaemia with a higher incidence of cerebrovascular accidents [12, 13]. In this context, the retina can be regarded as part of the brain from the anatomical point of view, and loss of vision may affect quality of life as much as paralysis from stroke.

Beta globin gene haplotype

Although the genetic mutation that causes sickle cell anaemia (GAG → GTG) is identical in all individuals studied to date, the sequence of nucleotides in the genomic material flanking the β^s gene varies [5]. Different nucleotide sequences or haplotypes are associated with particular degrees of clinical severity in SCD. Severe SCD is associated with Bantu and Benin haplotypes, moderate disease with Senegalese haplotype and mild disease with Arab-Indian haplotype [5]. The differences in clinical severity reflect varying levels of fetal haemoglobin generally observed in adults who have particular haplotypes. So, low levels of HbF are found in people homozygous for Bantu or Benin haplotypes, and higher levels in homozygotes for the Senegalese and Arab-Indian haplotypes. A high level of HbF ameliorates SCD, and contributes to the clinically mild nature of the haemoglobinopathy in people homozygous for the Arab-Indian and Senegalese haplotypes.

The various nucleotide sequences in different haplotypes give rise to polymorphic endonuclease restriction sites. Detection of these sites is used in the laboratory to identify people with different haplotypes. Although most of these restriction sites have no proven role in expression of gamma globin genes (and HbF levels), the *Xmn*1 site located upstream (5′) to the $^G\gamma$ globin gene in the Arab–Indian and Senegalese haplotypes is associated with increased expression of $^G\gamma$ globin gene in comparison with the gene for $^A\gamma$ globin [14–16]. This DNA restriction enzyme site is associated with increased production of gamma globin chain and HbF even in people who do not have the sickle beta globin gene. Studies of twins also indicate that the nucleotide sequence recognized by *Xmn*1 influences HbF level [17]. The Arab–Indian, Bantu, Benin, Cameroon and Senegalese beta globin gene haplotypes probably reflect different genetic backgrounds in which the mutation that causes SCD occurred. This is because it is far less likely that five (or possibly more) successive mutations occurred in a single chromosome; considering the rarity of genetic mutation as a random event. Thus the implication is that the sickle gene mutation occurred in at least five separate locations and instances in the past.

HbF level

It is well known that SCD does not usually manifest clinically in babies born with the condition until the age of about 6 months, when the level of fetal haemoglobin in the blood has reduced considerably. This is because HbF does not crystallize like HbS in the presence of hypoxia to cause sickling of red blood cells [18]. Therefore, the higher the proportion of fetal haemoglobin in the blood, the lower the risk of sickling. This translates into a clinically milder SCD in people with high levels of HbF. While the total amount of HbF in the blood is clearly important in this context, its distribution among the red cell population is probably more relevant. That a red blood cell contains sufficient HbF to prevent it from sickling would be more beneficial than having a much smaller amount that is not enough to inhibit the process. If the HbF is distributed in such a way that all the red cells contain enough to prevent sickling, this would be better than concentrating the HbF in a few while the rest have so little that they can sickle. A red blood cell that contains a detectable amount of fetal haemoglobin is called an F cell. The higher the number of F cells, the higher the number of erythrocytes that may contain the critical amount of HbF required to prevent sickling. The clinical severity of SCD shows better correlation with number of F cells than %HbF, both in patients on hydroxyurea and those not on the therapy [19].

As stated previously, differences in beta globin gene haplotype contribute to variation in HbF level among people with SCD. In addition, HbF level is modulated by other genetic loci outside chromosome 11 which bears the non-alpha globin genes. Such trans-acting genetic loci are found in chromosomes Xp22.3–22.20, 6q23 and 8q [20–22]. The locus in chromosome X may partly explain why HbF level is higher in females than males. It is estimated from studies in identical twins that gender, age and the thymidine to cytidine (T → C) mutation found in nucleotide −158 upstream (5′) to the $^{G}\gamma$ globin gene together account for about 40% of the variation in HbF level between individuals [20].

Co-inheritance of the gene for alpha thalassaemia

People with SCD who also inherited alpha thalassaemia trait have a lower mean cell haemoglobin (MCV) and mean cell haemoglobin concentration (MCHC) than those who have the normal four alpha globin genes. This reduces the rate of polymerization of HbS, which depends on its concentration inside the erythrocyte. As a result, there is less sickling of red cells and their destruction in the body (haemolysis). Therefore, the haemoglobin level is higher in SCD patients with alpha thalassaemia trait relative to those without. So they have less symptoms of anaemia, a lower prevalence of leg ulcers and reduced incidence of stroke, the risk of which varies inversely with Hb level [23]. Paradoxically, the higher red cell count increases blood viscosity and, theoretically, the risk of micro-vascular occlusion. However, it is not generally accepted that vaso-occlusive crisis is more frequent. What is more clearly established is that avascular necrosis of the femoral head has a higher prevalence in SCD

patients with lower MCV and higher haematocrit, which may be due to co-inheritance of alpha thalassaemia trait [24, 25]. Deletion of one or two of the four alpha globin genes is common in people of African ancestry, especially descendants of West Africans of whom up to 30% have alpha thalassaemia trait. As a result, co-existence of SCD and alpha thalassaemia trait is common in people of West African ancestry.

Blood cell counts

The clinical severity of homozygous (HbSS) SCD has a direct correlation with steady-state neutrophil count [7], and leucocytosis is a risk factor for early disease-related death [26]. The importance of neutrophil count in assessing the severity of SCD and deciding whether an affected individual will benefit from hydroxyurea therapy is underlined by the observation that good clinical response to the medication coincides with a fall in neutrophil count, even in patients who have no increase in HbF [19]. Whereas there is no detectable rise in HbF in some individuals who have good clinical response to hydroxyurea, a drop in neutrophil count occurs in all patients who respond well to treatment. Also, multivariate analysis of data from the trial of hydroxyurea therapy in SCD identified high neutrophil count as a powerful predictor of good response [19]. In a very informative case report, an individual in steady-state SCD developed severe vaso-occlusive crisis and life-threatening acute chest syndrome following a rise in neutrophil count induced by granulocyte-colony stimulating factor (G-CSF) given to mobilize haemopoietic stem cells [27]. The chest syndrome and crisis quickly resolved as the neutrophil count fell in response to administration of hydroxyurea and withdrawal of G-CSF.

A high red cell count as reflected by the haematocrit is also associated with increased blood viscosity and prevalence of avascular necrosis of the femoral head [24, 25]. The relationship between Hb level and the clinical severity of SCD is not linear. Above 11 g/dL, the risks of sickle retinopathy and avascular necrosis are increased, probably because of higher blood viscosity. Below 6 g/dL, the risks of cerebrovascular accidents and anaemic heart failure increase. It appears that the optimal Hb level in SCD is 7–9 g/dL, and that in each individual the body strikes a compromise between high and very low values to avoid severe clinical manifestations. It is interesting that steady-state Hb level ranges from 7 to 9 g/dL in the majority of people with SCD. In contrast to the proven deleterious effects of high erythrocyte or leucocyte counts on the severity of SCD, the effects of high platelet count are not well established. One study noted increased risk of stroke in children with platelet count above 450×10^9/L [28]. However, adults of African ancestry for whom normal platelet counts range from 100 to 300×10^9/L [29], showed no significant differences in the prevalence of stroke and other complications of SCD when HbSS people with normal or high platelet counts were compared [30].

Expression of adhesion molecules on blood cells and vascular endothelium

Adhesive interactions between blood and vascular endothelial cells have a role in the genesis of vaso-occlusion – a fundamental pathological process in SCD [31]. Compared with age-matched HbSS adults who have no complications of SCD, those with complications showed significantly higher baseline (steady-state) expression of the adhesion molecules $\alpha M\beta 2$ integrin and L-selectin by leucocytes [8]. Leucocyte adhesion molecule expression was increased during sickle cell crisis relative to steady-state values. Moreover, reduced steady-state expression of these adhesion molecules coincided with clinical improvement during hydroxyurea therapy, before any significant rise in HbF level. It is probable that people with high constitutional expression of $\alpha M\beta 2$ integrin and L-selectin by leucocytes have severe manifestations of SCD.

As a ribonucleotide reductase inhibitor, hydroxyurea blocks the conversion of ribonucleoside to deoxyribonucleotides and reduces DNA synthesis. By so affecting DNA production, hydroxyurea reduces gene transcription and, ultimately, diminishes protein synthesis in a non-specific manner. This general effect on protein synthesis would account for observations that hydroxyurea therapy causes a global reduction in the expression of vari-

ous adhesion molecules by leucocytes [8], and down-regulates expression of the erythrocyte adhesive proteins $\alpha_4\beta_1$ integrin and CD36 [32], thereby reducing adherence of sickle erythrocytes to thrombospondin, the ligand for CD36 [33]. By a similar mechanism, hydroxyurea may reduce the synthesis of the protein components of the ligands for blood cell adhesion molecules expressed by vascular endothelium, such as intercellular adhesion molecules (ICAMs) -1, -2, -3, and vascular cell adhesion molecule-1 (VCAM-1). That the constitutional level or function of adhesive proteins expressed by vascular endothelium may be clinically important determinants of severity is suggested by the finding that a single nucleotide polymorphism (SNP) in the gene for VICAM-1 (G1238C) may protect SCD patients from symptomatic stroke [34].

Immune status

Impaired ability to fight pathogenic organisms increases the clinical severity of SCD because infection has a dominant role in the precipitation of sickle cell crisis and the pathogenesis of vaso-occlusion. The clinical severity of SCD correlates with a number of immunological parameters. The frequency of sickle cell crisis increases with the degree of the well-known complement defect in SCD [8]. The ability of neutrophils to kill candida has an inverse relationship with the severity of SCD [7].

To give or not give hydroxyurea?

It is apparent from the above that SCD is not a single gene disorder. Whereas HbS is the product of a point mutation in the beta globin gene, the clinical expression of this haemoglobinopathy (or SCD) is determined by a complex interaction of several genes with the internal and external environments. The decision to treat a particular patient with hydroxyurea should be based on the individual's profile of the known determinants of disease severity, and a careful balance of the desired benefits against potential side-effects of therapy; in other words, the risk:benefit ratio. The clinical efficacy of hydroxyurea is not in doubt, and has been repeatedly demonstrated in randomized, placebo-controlled, multicentre trials [19, 35, 36]. It is the potential long-term effects of this cytotoxic drug – teratogenicity, carcinogenesis, and impaired neurodevelopment in children – that call for caution in its administration to people with SCD who do not have a malignant condition. It is more so because the risks of these long-term effects are currently unknown, and the situations are not reversible; unlike the immediate side-effects such as blood cytopenias.

How much is known about the risks of irreversible effects of hydroxyurea therapy? Up to 15 women, 6 of whom had SCD, have had successful pregnancies with delivery of normal children while taking hydroxyurea. The majority of the women had myeloproliferative disorders (MPDs), another group of blood conditions that have been treated with hydroxyurea for a much longer time than SCD. No adverse effects on the growth and neurodevelopment of the children have been reported. Reassuring as this is, it is still advisable not to offer expectant mothers hydroxyurea therapy. This is standard practice among physicians attending to people with SCD. As an additional safeguard, an effective method of contraception should be used by all sexually mature men and women on hydroxyurea. Sperm banking is recommended before commencing hydroxyurea therapy in men who plan to have children at a later time. Up to three children taking hydroxyurea for SCD have developed leukaemia. In two of the children, this occurred after 6 and 8 years, respectively, of hydroxyurea therapy. A study of acquired DNA mutations during hydroxyurea therapy found that children with SCD treated for up to 30 months had more mutations in re-arranged T-lymphocyte receptor genes than normal controls and children who had 7 months' treatment [37]. The numbers of mutations in adults with SCD or MPDs were comparable to those of normal controls. Although the number of T-cell receptor gene mutations does not correlate directly with the incidence of leukaemia, it was recommended that young SCD patients on hydroxyurea be monitored serially for cellular changes that may precede malignant disease, such as acquired DNA mutations and chromosome breakage. Hydroxyurea has been used for a longer time to treat children with non-malignant blood conditions, such as erythrocytosis secondary to congenital heart disease. Of more than 60 such children treated with hydroxyurea for a mean duration of 5 years, none has developed leukaemia or other malignant disease. On the whole, the subject of long-term effects of hydroxyurea requires further studies.

So, until the harmful long-term effects are certain, which SCD patients should be treated with hydroxyurea? Essentially, people with markedly severe SCD who are likely to benefit, considering their individual combination of severity determinants, and the known mechanisms of action of hydroxyurea: increased HbF production, reduced blood cell counts and reduced adhesion of blood cells to blood vessel walls. Patients with markedly severe SCD are probably < 5% of the entire population of affected persons, although their frequent use of hospital-based health services may give an exaggerated impression of their proportion. No sweeping guideline can be used to identify these individuals. Hydroxyurea is yet to be licensed for treatment of SCD in practically all countries except the USA. This makes it the responsibility of the physician prescribing it on 'a named patient basis' to decide on the criteria for hydroxyurea therapy. In recognition of this, the criteria stated below are those applied in the author's institution.

1 Up to six sickle cell crises a year.

2 More than three crises per year with steady-state neutrophil $\geq 10 \times 10^9$/L.

3 More than three crises per year with steady-state platelet count $\geq 500 \times 10^9$/L.

Any one of the three criteria qualifies a person for hydroxyurea therapy. In people of black African ancestry, the reference ranges for neutrophil count ($1-3 \times 10^9$/L) and platelets count ($100-300 \times 10^9$/L) are lower than in Caucasians. The corresponding values are $2.5-7.5 \times 10^9$/L and $150-400 \times 10^9$/L, respectively. For patients of black African ancestry, the neutrophil count used to decide on hydroxyurea therapy is more than three times the upper limit of normal. The majority of patients with such a high steady-state neutrophil count have severe SCD. The clinical decision to treat with hydroxyurea is favoured if the patient has completed their family, or does not want to have children. Hydroxyurea is contraindicated if the individual is pregnant, has liver disease, platelet count $< 100 \times 10^9$/L, reticulocyte count $< 80 \times 10^9$/L or neutrophil count $< 1 \times 10^9$/L.

The dose of hydroxyurea given is the minimum required to achieve significant clinical benefit (minimum effective dose), rather than the maximum tolerable dose. This policy is adopted because, presumably, the lower the dose given to the patient, the lower the incidence and severity of side-effects. Treatment is started with 0.5 g (one capsule) per day in adults, and increased every 2 weeks by 0.5 g until good clinical response is obtained. With this approach, our adult patients are on 1–2 g/day. To monitor the toxicity of hydroxyurea, full blood count, liver function tests and kidney function tests are done every fortnight initially. The interval is increased to a month after 6 weeks of therapy, and to 2–3 months after 6 months. Treatment is suspended if the count of any blood cell falls into the range within which hydroxyurea therapy is contraindicated, and resumed with a lower dose of hydroxyurea when blood cell counts return to normal.

Benefits of hydroxyurea therapy

Treatment with hydroxyurea reduces the number of crises and painful episodes in SCD [28, 35, 36]. People on the medication need less hospital admissions and less blood transfusion. Acute chest syndrome, a life-threatening complication that is the most common cause of death in adults with SCD, is reduced in frequency. Haemolysis is reduced, steady-state haemoglobin level rises and the symptoms of anaemia improve. As a result, the person is more physically fit. It appears that the medication increases survival in people who have severe SCD. Hydroxyurea slows down the development of functional asplenia in children with SCD. It does not appear to prevent stroke in people with the haemoglobinopathy. However, children with moderate to severe SCD treated with hydroxyurea had cognitive function comparable to that of their brothers or sisters who did not have the condition. Children with equally severe SCD not treated with hydroxyurea had a lower mental ability than their siblings not affected by the disorder.

References

1. Serjeant GR. Sickle cell disease. *Lancet* 1997; **350**: 725–30.
2. Steinberg MH, Hebbel RP. Clinical diversity of sickle cell anemia: genetic and cellular modulation of disease severity. *Am J Haematol* 1983; **14**: 405–16.
3. Okpala IE. The management of crisis in sickle cell disease [review]. *Eur J Haematol* 1998; **60**: 1–6.
4. Charache S. Experimental therapy (of sickle cell disease). *Hematol Oncol Clin North Am* 1996; **10**: 1373–82.
5. Powars DR, Meiselman HJ, Fisher TC, Hiti A, Johnson C. Beta-S gene cluster haplotypes modulate haematologic and haemorheologic expression in sickle cell anemia. *Am J Pediatr Hematol Oncol* 1994; **16**: 55–61.
6. Embury SH, Dozy AM, Miller J *et al.* Concurrent sickle cell anaemia and alpha-thalassaemia. Effect on severity of anemia. *N Engl J Med* 1982; **306**: 270–4.
7. Anyaegbu CC, Okpala IE, Aken'Ova AY, Salimonu LS. Peripheral blood neutrophil count and candidacidal activity correlate with the clinical severity of sickle cell anaemia. *Eur J Haematol* 1998; **60**: 267–8.
8. Okpala IE, Daniel Y, Haynes R, Odoemene D, Goldman JM. Relationship between the clinical manifestations of sickle cell disease and the expression of adhesion molecules on white blood cells. *Eur J Haematol* 2002; **69**: 135–44.
9. Anyaegbu CC, Okpala IE, Aken'Ova AY, Salimonu LS. Complement haemolytic activity, circulating immune complexes and the morbidity of sickle cell anaemia. *APMIS* 1999; **107**: 699–702.
10. Hedo CC, Okpala IE, Aken'Ova AY, Salimonu LS. Correlates of severity in sickle cell anaemia. *Blood* 1996; **88** (Suppl): 17b.
11. Hedo CC, Aken'Ova AY, Okpala IE, Durojaiye AO, Salimonu LS. Acute phase reactants and the severity of homozygous sickle cell anaemia. *J Intern Med* 1993; **233**: 467–70.
12. Clarkson JG. The ocular manifestations of sickle cell disease: a prevalence and natural history study. *Trans Am Ophthalmol Soc* 1992; **90**: 481–504.
13. Charache S. Eye disease in sickling disorders. *Hematol Oncol Clin North Am* 1996; **10**: 1357–62.
14. Gilman JG, Huisman TH. DNA sequence variation associated with elevated fetal $^G\gamma$-globin production. *Blood* 1985; **66**: 783–7.

15. Nagel RL, Fabry ME, Pagnier J et al. Haematologically and genetically distinct forms of sickle cell anemia in Africa. The Senegalese and the Benin type. *N Engl J Med* 1984; **312**: 880–4.

16. Labie D, Srinavas R, Duanda O et al. Haplotypes in tribal Indians bearing the sickle gene: evidence for the unicentric origin of the beta S mutation and the unicentric origin of the tribal populations of India. *Hum Biol* 1989; **61**: 479–91.

17. Thein SL, Craig JE. Genetics of HbF/F cell variance in adults and heterocellular hereditary persistence of fetal hemoglobin. *Haemoglobin* 1998; **22**: 401–14.

18. Steinberg MH, Rodgers GP. Pathophysiology of sickle cell disease: role of genetic and cellular modifiers. *Semin Hematol* 2001; **38**: 229–306.

19. Charache S. Mechanism of action of hydroxyurea in the management of sickle cell anemia in adults. *Semin Hematol* 1997; **34** (Suppl 3): 15–21.

20. Garner C, Tatu T, Reittie JE et al. Genetic influences on F cells and other hematologic variables: a twin heritability study. *Blood* 2000; **95**: 342–6.

21. Game L, Close J, Stephens P et al. An integrated map of human 6q22.3-q24 including a 3 Mb high-resolution BAC/PAC contig encompassing a QTL for for fetal hemoglobin. *Genomics* 2000; **64**: 264–76.

22. Dover GJ, Smith KD, Chang YC et al. Fetal hemoglobin levels in sickle cell disease and normal individuals are partially controlled by an X-linked gene located at Xp22.2. *Blood* 1992; **80**: 816–24.

23. Ohene-Frempong K, Weiner SJ, Sleeper LA et al. Cerebrovascular accidents in sickle cell disease: rates and risk factors. *Blood* 1998; **91**: 288–94.

24. Milner PF, Kraus AP, Sebes JI et al. Sickle cell disease as a cause of osteonecrosis of the femoral head. *N Engl J Med* 1991; **21**: 1476–81.

25. Moran MC. Osteonecrosis of the hip in sickle cell hemoglobinopathy (review). *Am J Orthop* 1995; **24**: 18–24.

26. Platt OS, Brambilla DJ, Rosse WF et al. Mortality in sickle cell disease – life expectancy and risk factors for early death. *N Engl J Med* 1994; **330**: 1639–43.

27. Abboud MR, Laver J, Blau CA. Elevation of neutrophil count after G-CSF therapy leads to vaso-occlusive crisis and acute chest syndrome in a patient with sickle cell anaemia. *Blood* 1996; **88** (Suppl): 15b.

28. Miller ST, Sleeper LA, Pegalow CH et al. Prediction of adverse outcomes in children with sickle cell disease: a report from the cooperative study (CSSCD). *N Engl J Med* 2000; **342**: 83–9.

29. Essien EM. Platelets and platelet disorders in Africa (review). *Baillieres Clin Haematol* 1992; **5**: 441–56.

30. Okpala IE. Steady-state platelet count and complications of sickle cell disease. *Hematol J* 2002; **3**: 214–15.

31. Frenette PS. Sickle cell vaso-occlusion: multistep and multicellular paradigm. *Curr Opin Hematol* 2002; **9**: 101–6.

32. Styles LA, Lubin B, Vichinsky E et al. Decrease of very late activation antigen-4 and CD36 expression on reticulocytes in sickle cell patients treated with hydroxyurea. *Blood* 1997; **89**: 2554–9.

33. Hillery CA, Du MC, Wang WC, Scott JP. Hydroxyurea therapy decreases in vitro adhesion of sickle erythrocytes to thrombospondin and laminin. *Br J Haematol* 2000; **109**: 322–7.

34. Taylor JG 6th, Tang DC, Savage SA et al. Variants in the VICAM-1 gene and risk for symptomatic stroke in sickle cell disease. *Blood* 2002; **100**: 4303–9.

35. Ferster A, Vermylen C, Cornu G et al. Hydroxyurea for treatment of severe sickle cell anemia: a pediatric clinical trial. *Blood* 1996; **88**:1960–4.

36. Kinney TR, Helms RW, O'Branski EE et al. Pediatric Hydroxyurea Group: safety of hydroxyurea in children with sickle cell anemia: results of the HUG-KIDS study, a phase I/II trial. *Blood* 1999; **94**: 1550–4.

37. Hanft VN, Fruchtman SR, Pickens CV et al. Acquired DNA mutations associated with *in vivo* hydroxyurea exposure. *Blood* 2000; **95**: 3589–93.

Chapter 19

Haemopoietic stem cell transplantation for thalassaemia and sickle cell disease

Christina M Halsey and Irene AG Roberts

Introduction

Despite major advances in supportive care for thalassaemia and sickle cell disease (SCD), patients continue to suffer disabling symptoms and die prematurely. Stem cell transplantation (SCT) offers the only chance of cure for these patients. The replacement of the patient's bone marrow by haemopoietic stem cells from the bone marrow (or blood) of a healthy donor results in production of normal haemoglobin and resolution of the symptoms of disease. However, as SCT is a major procedure with significant risks both in the first few months after transplant and in the long-term, it is important to weigh up all potential risks and benefits of the procedure for each individual patient and their family.

In this chapter we will start with a brief guide to SCT for readers not familiar with the procedure. We will then present the most important issues that need to be considered in each case and summarize the evidence available to help patients and their health-care teams decide whether to proceed. There is wider experience of transplantation for thalassaemia than for SCD and considerably more published data. Indeed, successful transplantation in thalassaemia helped to provide 'proof of principle' that transplantation for SCD would be curative. Many of the issues facing both sets of patients are similar but we have highlighted differences where they occur. Transplantation for haemoglobinopathies remains a very specialized field and we feel that patients being considered for transplant should be referred to a centre with expertise. This allows adequate counselling and pre-transplant assessment and also facilitates collection of data

to continually refine the procedure and improve outcomes.

Brief guide to SCT

Source of stem cells for SCT: bone marrow versus peripheral blood or cord blood

The normal donor haemopoietic stem cells used in SCT may be collected from three potential sites: the bone marrow (by a bone marrow harvest), from the peripheral blood (by leucapheresis) or from umbilical cord blood at the time of birth of an unaffected baby. Where cells are collected from the bone marrow of the donor, the procedure is referred to as a bone marrow transplant (BMT) and the vast majority of SCTs for haemoglobinopathies are of this type. Small numbers of patients with thalassaemia and SCD have received one of the other two types of SCT using peripheral blood stem cells (PBSCT) or cord blood stem cells (CBT). As the principles of patient selection, the chemotherapy used, the results and the complications are similar in all types of SCT for haemoglobinopathies we have used the term SCT throughout this chapter except where there have been specific studies that highlight any differences between bone marrow, peripheral blood or cord blood.

Selecting a stem cell donor

SCT involves destruction of the patient's own bone marrow cells using chemotherapy and then replacement with haemopoietic stem cells from a suitable healthy donor. It relies on the presence of specialized stem cells in the marrow or blood, which are long-lived cells able to regenerate as well as mature to produce all blood components – red cells, white cells and platelets. The donor and recipient must be matched for cell surface proteins that are important in immune responses known as histocompatibility antigens (HLAs). The pattern of expression of histocompatibility antigens for each individual is inherited and is known as their 'tissue type', it is readily determined on a peripheral blood sample. There is a 1 in 4 chance that siblings will share the same HLA-type and therefore an approximately 1 in 4 chance that a child with thalassaemia or SCD will have an HLA-identical sibling donor. Because of the pattern of inheritance of the HLA-type, family members other than siblings (e.g. parents) will *not* be HLA-identical. The only exception to this is where there is parental consanguinity which may lead to the parents, or other members of the extended family, being HLA-identical. The importance of a full HLA-match between the donor and patient cannot be over-emphasized: if the patient and their stem cell donor are not HLA-matched then the transplanted cells will be seen as foreign and destroyed ('graft' rejection) or the donor cells will recognize the patient's normal tissue cells as 'foreign' and attack them to cause the complication known as graft-versus-host disease (GvHD).

Conditioning regimens for SCT: eradicating the patient's bone marrow

To allow engraftment of the donor haemopoietic stem cells the patient has to first receive chemotherapy to eradicate their own haemopoietic stem cells which are largely found in the bone marrow. In fact the chemotherapy is essential, not only to create enough space for the donor haemopoietic stem cells, but also to immunosuppress the patient sufficiently to prevent rejection of the donor cells. The chemotherapy used for SCT is referred to as 'conditioning'. Conditioning therapy normally takes 10–12 days to administer and must be completed before the donor stem cells are transfused. Many of the chemotherapeutic agents used produce side-effects such as nausea, vomiting, inflammation of the gut (mucositis) and hair loss; fortunately, most

of these can be well controlled with good symptomatic care.

Collecting ('harvesting') and transfusing the donor haemopoietic stem cells

Donor stem cells are normally harvested only after the conditioning therapy has been completed. The exception is where cord blood stem cells are used – in this situation the cells will have been frozen on the day of the birth of the baby donor and stored until they are needed. However, the vast majority of SCT for haemoglobinopathies use donor marrow and this is collected from the donor on the day of transplant from the posterior iliac spines of the pelvis under general anaesthetic. The procedure generally takes about an hour. The bone marrow is aspirated using a special needle and collected into a sterile bag for processing by a stem cell laboratory before transfusion into the patient. The volume of donor marrow collected varies (range 200–1000 ml) depending on the cell count of the marrow and the body weight of the patient. The best outcome is achieved with a cell dose of at least 3×10^8 nucleated donor cells/kg of the patient's weight. Where the blood group of the donor and recipient are different either red cells or plasma (depending on the nature of the blood group difference) are removed from the donor marrow in the stem cell laboratory to reduce the risk of transfusion reactions. The marrow is then transfused into the patient via a central line in the same way as a blood transfusion.

Engraftment of donor haemopoietic stem cells

Specialized receptors on the surface of the donor haemopoietic cells facilitate their engraftment in the patient's bone marrow, where they begin to multiply and mature. After 2–3 weeks mature donor haemopoietic cells appear in the peripheral blood. The first cells to be produced are neutrophils and monocytes, followed a week or two later by platelets and red cells. The chemotherapy administered before the SCT will have reduced the neutrophil count to undetectable levels by the time of the SCT and until the neutrophils reach at least 0.5×10^9/L the patient will be very vulnerable to infection. At this stage most of the infections are bacterial or fungal; for this reason the patient is kept in strict isolation and any fevers are promptly treated with broad-spectrum intravenous antibiotics. At the same time the patient will be dependent upon platelet and red cell transfusions until platelet and red cell production are fully established (usually by 4 weeks and 6 weeks, respectively, after the transplant).

GvHD

Around the time donor cells start appearing in the circulation the patient may develop signs of acute GvHD. This occurs in one-third of patients receiving stem cells from an HLA-identical sibling, although in the majority of cases it is mild. Acute GvHD particularly affects the skin, gut and liver and is caused by donor T lymphocytes reacting against patient-specific antigens on the surface of cells in these tissues. The clinical signs are an erythematous skin rash, which may be bullous in severe cases, vomiting and abdominal pain with copious, sometimes bloody, diarrhoea where the lower gut is involved, and progressive cholestatic jaundice. Many patients have GvHD affecting only one or two of these sites and < 10% of haemoglobinopathy patients have involvement of all three sites. Moderate or severe acute GvHD is usually treated with steroids, which may be required in high doses. Fortunately most patients respond well to treatment, however, acute GvHD is one of the commonest causes of transplant-related mortality. Chronic GvHD is also caused by donor T lymphocytes but has a different natural history to the acute disease. It develops 3–6 months after SCT and is usually indolent with chronic relapsing involvement, most often of the skin and gut. Most cases of chronic GvHD resolve within 1–2 years but for a small proportion of patients chronic GvHD is extensive and causes severe and long-term adverse effects on their quality of life.

Discharge from hospital and complications during the first year after SCT

If the transplant proceeds without complications patients are normally in hospital for 4–6 weeks after SCT. They then require intensive outpatient follow-up once to twice weekly and then monthly until a year post-transplant at which time visits can be spaced out. Return to school or nursery depends on how smoothly the procedure has gone but is generally possible 6–9 months post-transplant. Patients remain vulnerable to infection, especially measles and chickenpox and, unless immune suppression is severe, routine childhood vaccinations are repeated 1–2 years post-transplant.

SCT for thalassaemia major

Background

Thalassaemia major is a considerable public health problem affecting about 60 000 children worldwide [1]. Treatment with blood transfusion ameliorates symptoms but the resulting iron overload leads to multi-organ failure in the second and third decades. This can be partially prevented by additional use of iron chelation but this is expensive, difficult to administer and not without its own toxicity [2]. In Asia, where the majority of cases occur, lack of chelation therapy and a safe blood supply leads to considerable morbidity and death in childhood. In the UK, the recent establishment of a national thalassaemia register shows that about 50% of patients still die before the age of 35 years [3]. The majority of preventable deaths are due to poor compliance with chelation therapy, but even in well-treated patients, studies show only an 85% probability of survival to age 24 [4].

SCT offers the chance of cure. In successful cases it not only improves survival but also has considerable impact on quality of life by abolishing the need for lifelong transfusions and daily chelation therapy [5–7]. However, there remains a risk of transplant-related mortality and long-term effects from the transplant itself. This means that the decision to proceed to transplant is often difficult and needs to be tailored to the individual family. Informed consent is vital and it is critical that the family understands all the potential risks and benefits of the procedure. In the next sections we discuss the factors that affect the decision to transplant (see Table 19.1), review the available evidence for each and

Table 19.1 Factors affecting the decision to transplant a patient with thalassaemia major or SCD

Expected outcome of transplantation:
  cure rates
  transplant-related mortality
  risk of chronic GvHD
Long-term effects of transplantation
Age of the patient
Availability of a donor
Expected long-term survival without SCT based on:
  transfusion and compliance history
  clinical manifestations of the disease and its treatment
  impact of medical treatment on quality of life
Prospects for improved management in the future

Table 19.2 Outcome of BMT for thalassaemia major according to the Pesaro risk classification*

Parameter	Class 1	Class 2	Class 3
Survival (%)	94	84	80
Thalassaemia-free survival (%)	87	81	56
Transplant-related mortality (%)	6	15	18
Graft rejection (%)	7	4	33

*Patients were classified as class 3 if they had all three of the following risk factors: hepatomegaly (> 2 cm below costal margin), portal fibrosis on liver biopsy and a history of irregular chelation (desferrioxamine initiated > 18 months after the first transfusion or administered < 8 hours continuously on at least 5 days per week). Patients were identified as class 2 if they had any one or two of these risk factors and class 1 if they had none of these risk factors. These data are summarized from Angelucci et al. [5].

summarize the current indications for SCT for thalassaemia.

Outcome of SCT for thalassaemia major

Survival and thalassaemia-free survival

The largest series of patients treated in a single centre comes from the Pesaro group in Italy. They recently published data from 785 HLA-identical marrow transplants (761 siblings, 24 parents) [5, 6, 8]. The mean age of the patients was 10 years (range 1–35 years). Their overall survival was 78% but some patients had graft failure with return of transfusion dependence so thalassaemia-free survival was 71%. Data from elsewhere are broadly equivalent to the Pesaro group [9–16]. In the UK, early results were associated with lower overall and thalassaemia-free survival but included a number of poor risk patients [17]. Since then the outcome has improved with overall survival of 90% and thalassaemia-free survival of 76% reported from the main UK centres in 1996 [18]. A more recent update showed continued progress with a 92% overall survival and 82% thalassaemia-free survival among 57 consecutive transplants, despite > 50% of children having a poor chelation history [10].

Prognostic factors for survival and cure after SCT

After detailed analysis of their data the Pesaro group identified only three factors which predicted

transplant outcome: the presence or absence of hepatomegaly, portal fibrosis (on liver biopsy) and a history of poor compliance with chelation [6, 8]. These three factors can be used to classify an individual as good, intermediate or poor risk (class 1, 2 or 3, respectively). Table 19.2 shows how these risk groups predicted transplant outcomes in the Pesaro patients [5, 6]. Poor risk patients do particularly badly, probably because pre-existing organ damage makes them less able to tolerate chemotherapy. More recent data show that using lower doses of cyclophosphamide leads to improved survival; however, this approach is also associated with an increase in graft failure leading to a disappointing thalassaemia-free survival of 56% [5]. The Pesaro classification has not yet been shown to predict outcome in other centres. This may reflect the smaller numbers of patients involved and, in the UK, the low overall mortality rate [10].

Conditioning regimens

Most conditioning regimens employ a combination of chemotherapy, with busulphan and cyclophosphamide, and immunosuppression with cyclosporin and methotrexate [7, 8, 13]. Several groups have added anti-lymphocyte antibodies such as anti-lymphocyte globulin (ALG) or Campath® (Alemtuzumab) to reduce the risk of graft rejection by eradicating the patient's lymphocytes before infusion of donor stem cells. The optimum chemotherapy doses are difficult to ascertain, as there is considerable inter-individual variation in metabolism of busulphan [19–21]. Doses of > 16 mg/kg are toxic but lower doses are associated with increased graft rejection [6, 8, 22]. The most widely used regimen is a total busulphan dose of 14 mg/kg given over 4 days followed by cyclophosphamide 200 mg/kg over the next 4 days [7, 11]. This regimen is generally well tolerated. The low rates of mucositis mean that opiates and total parenteral nutrition are usually unnecessary. Some groups measure blood busulphan levels to help optimize the dose [13, 21, 23]. These problems with dosing are one of the reasons it is generally not recommended to transplant children under the age of 18 months. As previously mentioned, reduced conditioning (120–140 mg/kg cyclophosphamide) is recommended for Pesaro class 3 patients to avoid the high transplant-related mortality [8].

Transplant-related mortality and complications of SCT

Acute GvHD and infections are the two commonest causes of mortality, accounting for 32% and 24% of deaths, respectively, in the recent Pesaro series [5]. Other important causes of mortality after SCT for thalassaemia are chronic GvHD, marrow aplasia, hepatic disease and cardiac disease. Cardiac tamponade appears to be unexpectedly common and was reported in 8 cases/400 transplants from the Pesaro group, of which 6 were fatal [24]. Hepatitis B or C infection does not increase transplant-related mortality [25].

Graft rejection and mixed chimerism

Graft rejection is more common after SCT for haemoglobinopathies than SCT for most other disorders, particularly in poor risk patients. The reasons for this are not clear. There are three possible outcomes following rejection: marrow aplasia, return of thalassaemic haemopoiesis or mixed haemopoietic chimerism (a mixture of donor and patient haemopoietic cells are produced). Aplasia is rare but is often fatal unless a successful second transplant can be performed. Complete rejection of donor cells with return of thalassaemic

haemopoiesis leads to recurrence of transfusion-dependent anaemia and occurs in around 10% of patients [5, 6, 10]. The third scenario, mixed haemopoietic chimerism, is relatively common, occurring in up to 20% of patients [26, 27]. A review of 295 patients showed that in the first 2 months post-transplant 95 (32%) had mixed chimerism, by the second year 42 of these had become fully donor, 33 had progressed to rejection and 20 remained mixed [27]. The level of mixed chimerism varied from 30% to 90% donor cells but despite this range, all patients remained well, off transfusions, with a stable haemoglobin > 8 g/dL at 2–11 years post-transplant [28]. These findings imply that complete ablation of donor haemopoiesis is not necessary for long-term cure. Therefore considerable interest surrounds the possible use of non-myeloablative (i.e. doses too small to completely destroy host bone marrow) conditioning regimens to reduce toxicity. Preliminary attempts at such regimes confirm a low mortality but are associated with a high risk of graft rejection [29]. Current research is focusing on achieving the best balance between toxicity and rejection by manipulating immunosuppression [30] and giving further doses of donor lymphocytes or stem cells post-transplant [31].

Chronic GvHD

Severe chronic GvHD is a devastating complication for patients with thalassaemia, replacing one chronic disease with another. This is therefore a very important topic to discuss with patients and families before making a decision regarding transplant. The risk of severe chronic GvHD in thalassaemic patients undergoing SCT from an HLA-identical sibling is 2–5% [32]. Treatment is the same as for chronic GvHD after other forms of SCT.

Impact of age

The best results are seen in children aged < 17 years [33]. Nevertheless, using the protocol developed for poor risk children (Pesaro class 3) about two-thirds of young adults with thalassaemia are cured: of 107 patients aged 17–35 years transplanted by the Pesaro group, 69 survived (64%) of whom 66 are thalassaemia-free [34]. The high transplant-related mortality confirms that in older patients transplantation should be reserved for highly motivated individuals, with limited organ damage, who are aware of the risks involved.

Long-term effects of SCT for thalassaemia major

The long-term effects of SCT are influenced by the conditioning regimen used, the peri-transplant complications and pre-existing damage due to thalassaemia and its treatment, in particular the severity of iron overload.

Iron overload

Almost all patients with thalassaemia undergoing SCT have iron overload. This improves slowly post-transplant but can be accelerated by regular phlebotomy or chelation with desferrioxamine [35, 36]. This usually begins 1–2 years post-BMT and continues until the total iron burden is approaching normal (i.e. liver iron < 7 mg/g dry liver weight or serum ferritin < 300 ng/mL). Recent evidence confirms the particular importance of reducing iron overload post-SCT in patients infected with hepatitis B/C who otherwise have a high risk of progression to severe liver fibrosis [37].

Growth and development

This is one of the most difficult areas in which to disentangle effects of transplant from those of the underlying disease and pre-transplant treatment. Failure of growth and sexual development occurs in up to two-thirds of thalassaemics treated by blood transfusion [2]. For children transplanted early (< 8 years old) growth after transplant is normal. Older children and those in Pesaro class 3 often have severely impaired growth [38, 39]. Growth hormone is effective in some, but usually only the milder cases [40, 41]. About 37% of boys and 60% of girls fail to enter puberty spontaneously if transplanted, a proportion similar to those treated medically [42]. The majority of girls transplanted after puberty develop secondary amenorrhoea. There are few data on

fertility post-SCT for thalassaemia, and although successful pregnancy has been reported [43], experience of fertility after busulphan/cyclophosphamide conditioning in other disorders suggests that infertility is likely to be common [44, 45].

Non-sibling family donors

Where there is consanguinity, close relatives can sometimes provide an HLA-identical match. Data from these transplants are limited but no significant difference in outcome has been reported. In contrast, using mismatched relatives leads to disappointing results. A small series showed 6 successful outcomes, 10 transplant-related deaths and 13 graft failures [46].

Cord blood

The use of cord blood from a sibling overcomes the need to wait until the donor is 2 years old and avoids the need for a bone marrow harvest under general anaesthetic. In addition, some studies suggest that the use of cord blood reduces the incidence of GvHD [47, 48]. Despite these advantages, cord blood provides only limited numbers of stem cells, which is especially problematic where there is a large discrepancy in size between donor and recipient. There is also an increased rate of graft rejection unless increased intensity conditioning is used [48, 49]. The European database for cord blood transplants 'Eurocord' reported the results of 33, mainly good risk, patients. There was 100% overall survival but a thalassaemia-free survival of only 79% [48]. For this reason marrow stem cells have an advantage over cord blood unless the transplant is considered urgent.

Volunteer unrelated donors

Experience of unrelated donor SCT for thalassaemia is extremely limited. The only published series recently updated their experience in 32 patients, 17 of which were Pesaro class 3 [50]. Their overall survival was 81% but thalassaemia-free survival was only 69%. Rates of chronic GvHD are also higher (25%). At present we would not recommend the use of unrelated donors in any but the most exceptional circumstances.

Survival and quality of life in transplanted versus non-transplanted patients

The key question when considering an individual for transplant is: will it improve their prospects for survival and/or increase their quality of life? There are no controlled trials of transplant versus medical therapy and no quality of life studies to help answer this question. However, extrapolation from other data allows some conclusions to be drawn. These data indicate that for patients who comply well with iron chelation treatment and have no evidence of liver fibrosis their predicted long-term survival (until or beyond the fourth decade of life) is likely to be equivalent with medical treatment compared to SCT because such patients have a 90–95% of survival into their mid-thirties with either therapeutic approach. For such patients the decision to proceed to SCT will be based on quality of life – the perceived benefit of being free from lifelong transfusions, chelation therapy and, eventually, their long-term complications. In contrast, for patients with a history of poor compliance it is clear that very few survive into their mid-thirties and for these patients SCT offers not only an improved quality of life but also a much greater chance of long-term survival [51].

Prospects for improved management of thalassaemia major in the future

Advances in medical treatment and in prevention of transplant-related complications over the next decade are likely to influence the decisions of both physicians and their patients about the best options for individual patients. The main advances in medical treatment are likely to come from 'tailored' chelation regimes based on accurate magnetic resonance imaging (MRI) assessment of iron deposition in the liver and heart [52] and development of safe and effective oral iron chelators [53] In SCT the main advances may lie with development of effective non-myeloablative conditioning to reduce transplant-related toxicity without the currently

observed high risk of graft rejection and possibly with the use of 'molecularly' matched volunteer unrelated donor haemopoietic stem cells for selected patients failing medical treatment. Finally, as cure rather than palliation should remain a crucial goal, gene therapy continues to be developed and animal models are now providing useful data [54, 55], although human trials remain several years away.

Indications for SCT in thalassaemia major

The issues discussed above summarize the most important factors affecting the decision to proceed to SCT. Given recent data which clearly show that the outcome of SCT is good even in those children with liver damage and a poor chelation history, SCT should be *offered* to all families of children with thalassaemia major where there is an HLA-identical family donor. The majority of families will choose SCT because of the perceived improvement in quality of life and the removal of much of the uncertainty about future health once the first few months after SCT have passed. For children without HLA-identical family donors, SCT using unrelated donors may be an option in experienced centres if all approaches to medical treatment fail. The role of SCT for adults with thalassaemia major is unclear. For some well-motivated individuals 17–35 years of age the benefits of SCT may just exceed the risks using current conditioning regimens and it is reasonable to consider SCT if there is an HLA-identical sibling or extended haplotype-matched unrelated donor.

SCT for SCD

Background

Approximately 250 000 children are born worldwide with homozygous SCD every year. Their median survival is 45 years [56]. The clinical course of the disease is very variable both between patients and in a single patient over time. Recent advances in supportive care have improved mortality and morbidity for the majority of patients. None the less, disabling complications are inevitable for the vast majority. While hydroxyurea has improved the outlook for many of the most severely affected patients [57, 58], SCT offers the only available cure.

The factors influencing the decision to transplant a patient with SCD share many similarities with thalassaemia (Table 19.1). However, there are also crucial differences. Firstly, identifying those patients most likely to benefit from transplantation is more difficult, as the disease is so heterogeneous. Secondly, the timing of the transplant is more critical as it is usually necessary to wait until after major complications have manifest themselves in order to identify those patients most likely to benefit, while remaining aware that SCT should also be carried out before organ damage makes the procedure too hazardous. The criteria used to select those patients with SCD most likely to benefit from SCT and the factors which individual families and their healthcare teams need to consider in reaching a decision whether or not to proceed to transplant are summarized in Tables 19.1 and 19.3 and are discussed in detail below.

Table 19.3 Indications for BMT in SCD: British Paediatric Haematology Forum Criteria

Criteria for inclusion
1. Age < 16 years and HLA-matched sibling donor
2. One or more of the following:
    (a) SCD-related neurological deficit, stroke or subarachnoid haemorrhage
    (b) More than two episodes of acute sickle chest syndrome* and stage 1 chronic sickle lung disease
    (c) Recurrent, severe debilitating pain due to vaso-occlusive crises
    (d) Problems relating to future medical care, e.g. unavailability of adequately screened blood products
Exclusions
1. Donor with major haemoglobinopathy
2. One or more of the following:
    (a) Karnofsky performance score < 70%
    (b) Major intellectual impairment
    (c) Moderate/severe portal fibrosis
    (d) Glomerular filtration rate < 30% predicted
    (e) Stage III and IV sickle lung disease
    (f) Cardiomyopathy
    (g) HIV infection

*In view of recent data about the efficacy and safety of hydroxyurea we would now recommend a trial of hydroxyurea before SCT.

Selection of patients with SCD for SCT

Table 19.3 lists the current consensus criteria for patient selection devised in 1993 by the British Paediatric Haematology Forum, the paediatric group of the British Society for Haematology [59]. American guidelines from the Seattle collaborative study are similar but include sickle nephropathy with a glomerular filtration rate of 30–50%, bilateral proliferative retinopathy, osteonecrosis of multiple joints and red cell allo-immunization [60, 61]. In the UK, SCT as a recommended option has been limited to patients with homozygous SCD (HbSS) or $S\beta^0$ thalassaemia. The commonest indications for transplant are firstly, central nervous system (CNS) disease (stroke or recurrent transient ischaemic attacks), where transfusion with its inherent complications and limitations is the only alternative treatment [62, 63], and secondly, recurrent acute chest syndrome, the leading cause of death in SCD in the developed world [64]. Hydroxyurea has been shown to reduce the incidence and severity of acute chest syndrome and should therefore be tried first, with SCT offered where hydroxyurea fails [58, 65]. Patients identified by transcranial Doppler studies as being at increased risk of stroke, but who have not yet had a cerebrovascular accident, are not currently considered eligible for transplant, as blood transfusion has been shown to be protective in this setting [66, 67].

A rigorous pre-transplant work-up at the transplant centre is essential. It should include pulmonary, cardiac, hepatic, renal and neurological assessment (Table 19.4) both to help decide suitability for transplant and to help post-transplant monitoring for long-term effects. It is estimated that < 10% of children with SCD fulfil the criteria for transplant, only one in five of whom will have an HLA-identical sibling donor [68, 69].

Outcome of SCT for SCD

Survival and disease-free survival

Approximately 200 patients with SCD have been transplanted worldwide. Due to excellent multicentre collaboration, data on transplant outcomes is available for the majority of these. There are three

Table 19.4 Recommended pre-transplant investigations in patients with SCD

Full blood count and reticulocyte count
Hb electrophoresis including HbF, HbS and HbA2
Coagulation screen
G6PD assay
Full red cell phenotype and antibody screen
Biochemical profile including liver function tests, calcium, phosphate, magnesium, blood glucose, ferritin
Endocrine function including thyroid function, gonadotrophins, oestradiol or testosterone
HLA typing – class I and II
Blood for storage to enable later measurement of chimerism
Viral screen for CMV, HSV, VZV, hepatitis B and C, HIV1 and HIV2
Malaria screen if from an endemic area
Chest X-ray
High resolution computerized tomography of chest if previous lung disease
Lung function tests if > 8 years or any child with a history of acute chest syndrome
ECG
Left ventricular ejection fraction by MUGA scan, echo or MRI
Abdominal ultrasound to assess spleen size and presence/absence of gallstones
MRI of liver and heart to assess haemosiderosis
Liver biopsy if indicated by MRI
Ophthalmological assessment/audiometry if on desferrioxamine
MRI and MRA of brain
Neuropsychological assessment
Dental assessment

G6PD, glucose-6-phosphate dehydrogenase; CMV, cytomegalovirus; HSV, herpes simplex virus; VZV, varicella zoster virus; HIV, human immunodeficiency virus.

major series from France [13], Belgium [70] and a multicentre group comprising 27 American and European countries [61]. Their results are summarized in Table 19.5. The multicentre and French results are from children transplanted for symptomatic SCD. In contrast, the Belgian data comprise 36 patients transplanted because of previous morbidity but also 14 asymptomatic patients transplanted at a young age because they were going to return to countries where medical care was suboptimal. The results of these three series are largely concordant, with a projected overall survival of 92–94% and event-free survival of 75–84% at 6–11 years. The asymptomatic patients in the Belgian group did particularly well with an overall survival of 100% and event-free survival of 96%. Patients with stable engraftment no longer had clinical manifestations of SCD.

Conditioning regimens

The reported series used similar conditioning to that used for thalassaemia major. The principal chemotherapeutic agents are oral busulphan (14–16 mg/kg) and intravenous cyclophosphamide (200 mg/kg), some studies have added thiotepa with the aim of reducing graft rejection but its role is not yet clear. Other groups, including ours, have added ALG [13] or Campath® (Alemtuzumab) [51] to pre-SCT conditioning to reduce the rate of graft rejection with encouraging results, although it is

Table 19.5 Results of major published series of BMT for SCD

Parameter	Walters et al. [60, 61]	Bernaudin et al. [13]	Vermylen et al. [70]
Number of patients	50	26	50
Median follow-up (months)	39	55	60
Overall survival	94% (6 years)	92% (8 years)	93% (11 years)
Event-free survival	84% (6 years)	75% (8 years)	82% (11 years)
Graft rejection/ autologous reconstitution (%)	10	18	10
Stable mixed chimerism (%)	8.5	0	12.5
Acute GvHD > grade 2 (%)	7.7	23	20
Acute GvHD > grade 3 (%)	3.8	Not available	2
Chronic GvHD – limited (%)	Not available	7.7	14
Chronic GvHD – extensive (%)	3.8	7.7	6

important not to employ the high doses used by others to prevent GvHD.

Transplant-related mortality and other complications

With the exception of neurological complications, the spectrum and incidence of post-transplant adverse events are similar to those seen with thalassaemia. The commonest causes of death are GvHD and infections. Acute GvHD occurs in 20–30% of transplants but is seldom severe [13, 70]. Haemorrhagic cystitis, pneumococcal sepsis, veno-occlusive disease and aseptic necrosis have all been described but there are insufficient data to determine whether these occur at increased incidence in sickle transplants [70]. Patients with SCD are at increased risk of neurological complications post-transplant, particularly seizures and intracranial haemorrhage. Initial results from the multicentre study reported neurological complications in a third of their 21 patients [71]. Intracranial haemorrhage was associated with a prior history of stroke. This led to the use of prophylactic measures, namely maintenance of platelet counts $> 50 \times 10^9$/L and haemoglobin levels between 9 and 11 g/dL along with anticonvulsant prophylaxis, rigorous control of cyclosporin levels, magnesium levels and blood pressure. Since then no further cases of haemorrhage have occurred, although there continues to be a high incidence of seizures (20%) [70].

Graft rejection and mixed haemopoietic chimerism

The incidence of graft failure with return of host haemopoiesis is relatively high at 10–18% [60, 70]. Marrow aplasia is relatively rare (3%). No clear risk factors have been identified, but in the French series the addition of ALG to pre-transplant conditioning decreased the incidence of these events from 25% to 7%. As seen in thalassaemia, the presence of stable mixed chimerism is compatible with resolution of sickle-related symptoms and occurred in 8.5% of the multicentre and 12.5% of Belgian patients [72]. In addition, an unstable case of increasing host haemopoiesis has been restored to 100% donor haemopoiesis by the use of donor lymphocyte infusions [73]. These observations suggest that non-myeloablative regimens with subsequent manipulation of the graft using immunosuppression and donor lymphocyte infusions may be successful in future, although disappointingly the first such study in 10 patients with SCD recently found an 80% rate of graft rejection [29]. Clearly further work is needed to understand the mechanisms of engraftment and rejection of allogeneic haemopoietic stem cells in SCD and to use this information to develop new protocols.

Chronic GvHD

This has been reported in 15–20% of patients. It has been extensive in 6–8% and has been responsible for four of the seven deaths [13, 61, 70].

Impact of age

The vast majority of SCTs for SCD have been carried out in children < 16 years of age. A small number of adults have been transplanted with generally disappointing results – perhaps because the toxicity of conditioning regimens is too great for older patients with multi-organ damage [74]. Certainly the Belgian data, with 100% survival in their very young cohort of asymptomatic patients, suggest that transplantation is much better tolerated when performed early.

Long-term effects of SCT in SCD

Impact of SCT on pre-existing organ dysfunction

There is good evidence that at least some of the end-organ damage associated with SCD can be stabilized and even reversed post-transplant. A recent evaluation of CNS disease in 26 patients with at least 2 years of post-transplant follow-up showed that 19 of 26 had evidence of CNS abnormalities pre-transplant but none had neurological events post-transplant [61]. The majority had stabilization or improvement of vasculopathy as assessed by magnetic resonance angiography (MRA) scanning. In a separate study complete reversal of severe stenosis on MRA was demonstrated in two patients post-transplant [75]. In addition, pulmonary function stabilizes [61] and one study has shown an increase in the splenic red cell pool, suggesting that there may be improvement in splenic reticuloendothelial function post-transplant [76].

Growth and development

Most patients with SCD demonstrate improved growth post-SCT unless they remain on immunosuppression for chronic GvHD. Unfortunately, gonadal failure and delayed sexual development appear to be fairly common, although there are too few patients to assess this properly. In the reported series 11 of 13 girls had primary amenorrhoea. The majority of evaluable males have normal sexual development but follow-up remains short and many have not yet entered puberty. Gonadotrophin and testosterone levels are available for five boys, all under 8 years old; they show normal LH/FSH levels but low testosterone in some cases. Experience with busulphan and cyclophosphamide in other transplant settings suggests that infertility is likely to be common. Thyroid function is normal in almost all patients.

Secondary malignancy

It is too early to assess fully the secondary malignancy rate post-transplant. A case of myelodysplasia evolving into refractory acute myeloid leukaemia 4.5 years post-transplant has been reported, although this patient had intensive immunosuppression with azathiaprine and thalidomide for chronic GvHD [70].

Quality of life

There have been no detailed quality of life studies post-transplant. However, in the multicentre and Belgian series > 90% of engrafted patients had Karnofsky or Lansky scores of 100% with the lower scores seen in patients with chronic GvHD.

Source of donor cells

Unfortunately only one in five children who fulfil the criteria for transplant has a suitable HLA-identical sibling donor. The presence of sickle cell trait in the donor is not a contraindication to transplantation. Data about the use of cord blood from siblings too young to donate bone marrow (i.e. < 2 years old) are still very limited [48]. There may be an increased rate of graft rejection and thiotepa has been added to the conditioning regimen by some groups to reduce this risk [48]. However, cord blood should probably be reserved for patients where rapid transplantation is considered essential. The use of volunteer unrelated donors would considerably expand the availability of SCT for patients with SCD. However, to date the experience of this approach is limited to occasional case reports [77].

Prospects for improved management of SCD in the future

Hydroxyurea has greatly improved the quality of life for many patients with severe SCD disease [57]. It has already had an impact on the use of SCT in that its proven role in reducing recurrent acute chest syndrome means that transplant should now be reserved for patients failing to respond to hydroxyurea. A number of other advances may improve medical management, such as therapies targeting endothelial dysfunction, prevention of cellular dehydration and abnormal coagulation [78].

Novel SCT approaches are also likely to make an impact over the next few years, in particular the development of non-myeloablative (also known as 'reduced intensity') conditioning regimens. Their principal advantages would be the prospect for preserving fertility and of extending the role of SCT to adults with SCD where, arguably, there is a greater need for definitive therapy. Therefore, despite the recent disappointing results of this approach [29], it is important to note that non-myeloablative regimes are used successfuly for children with congenital immune deficiencies [79] and have been reported in a few cases for SCD [80, 81]. Further research is clearly needed. A mouse model of SCD has shown that it is possible to induce various levels of mixed haemopoietic chimerism ranging from 1% to 99% donor haemopoiesis to look at the effect on disease parameters [82, 83]. It appears that, although only 25% donor haemopoiesis is needed to achieve a normal haemoglobin, up to 80% donor haemopoiesis may be needed to prevent end-organ damage. This emphasizes the importance of collecting data on all new transplant procedures and looking at long-term as well as short-term outcomes.

Summary

SCT is currently the only cure for SCD and thalassaemia. When deciding whether or not to proceed with transplantation the risks of the procedure, including transplant-related mortality and graft failure, must be weighed against the expected survival and quality of life with medical treatment. In thalassaemia major the outcome of transplant is best in patients under 16 years old with a good chelation history and no evidence of liver dysfunction. These patients can expect a long-term survival of 95% and a thalassaemia-free survival of 90%. Patients with poor risk features may have a reduced chance of cure (56–82%) and a higher transplant-related mortality (up to 20%) but there is still a long-term survival advantage over conventional medical management. SCD is more heterogeneous and therefore selection of the patients most likely to benefit from SCT is more difficult. Advances in medical treatment, in particular the use of hydroxyurea, have narrowed the indications for transplant but it still has a valuable role, particularly in patients with CNS disease. Long-term survival after SCT for SCD in childhood is about 92–94% with a cure rate of 86%.

Transplantation techniques continue to evolve. Gene therapy remains a tantalizing prospect for the future. Investigation of innovative, less toxic non-myeloablative SCT protocols will be important if the role of SCT is to be successfully extended to adults, but should be carried out only in the context of careful clinical trials. The complexity of the decision-making process and the need to continually refine and improve outcomes mean that transplantation should only take place in tertiary centres with special expertise in haemoglobinopathy transplants. We hope that this chapter has provided the background information necessary to help patients, their families and health-care teams to decide whether referral to one of these centres for further assessment is appropriate.

References

1. WHO. Guidelines for control of haemoglobin disorders. Unpublished document of the WHO. Obtainable free of charge from the Hereditary Diseases Programme, WHO, Geneva, Switzerland. WHO/HDP/HB/GL/94.1. 1994.
2. Olivieri NF. The beta-thalassemias. *N Engl J Med* 1999, **341**: 99–109.
3. Modell B, Khan M, Darlison M. Survival in beta-thalassaemia major in the UK: data from the UK Thalassaemia Register. *Lancet* 2000, **355**: 2051–2.
4. Davis BA, O'Sullivan C, Eliahoo J, Porter JB. Survival in beta thalassaemia major: a single centre study. *Br J Haematol* 2001, **113** (Suppl 1): 53.
5. Angelucci E, Lucarelli G. Bone marrow transplantation in beta thalassaemia. In: Steinberg MH, Forget BG, Higgs DR, Nagel RL, eds. *Disorders of Hemoglobin: Genetics, Pathophysiology and Clinical Management.* Cambridge: Cambridge University Press, 2001: 1052–72.
6. Lucarelli G., Galimberti M, Polchi P *et al.* Bone marrow transplantation in patients with thalassemia. *N Engl J Med* 1990; **322**: 417–21.
7. Roberts I. Current status of allogeneic transplantation for haemoglobinopathies. *Br J Haematol* 1997; **98**: 1–7.
8. Lucarelli G, Clift RA, Galimberti M *et al.* Marrow transplantation for patients with thalassemia: results in class 3 patients. *Blood* 1996; **87**: 2082–8.
9. Mentzer WC, Cowan MJ. Bone marrow transplantation for beta-thalassemia: the University of California San Francisco experience. *J Pediatr Hematol Oncol* 2000; **22**: 598–601.
10. Lawson S, Amrolia PJ, Roberts I, Darbyshire P. Bone marrow transplantation for beta-thalassaemia: experience of two UK centres. *Br J Haematol* 2001; **113** (Suppl 1): 33.
11. Di Bartolomeo P, Di Girolamo G, Olioso P *et al.* The Pescara Experience. *Bone Marrow Transplant* 1997; **19** (Suppl 2): 48–53.
12. Ghavamzadeh A, Nasseri P, Eshraghian MR *et al.* Prognostic factors in bone marrow transplantation for beta thalassemia major: experiences from Iran. *Bone Marrow Transplant* 1998; **22**: 1167–9.
13. Bernaudin F, Souillet G, Vannier JP *et al.* Report of the French experience concerning 26 children transplanted for severe sickle cell disease. *Bone Marrow Transplant* 1997; **19** (Suppl 2): 112–15.
14. Li CK, Yuen PM, Shing MM *et al.* Stem cell transplantation for thalassaemia patients in Hong Kong. *Bone Marrow Transplant* 1997; **19** (Suppl 2): 62–4.
15. Peristeri J, Kitra V, Goussetis E *et al.* Haematopoietic stem cell transplantation for the management of haemo-

globinopathies in Greek patients. *Transfus Sci* 2000; **23**: 263–4.

16. Fang J, Huang S, Chen C, Zhou D, Wu Y, Bao R. Allogeneic peripheral blood stem cell transplantation in beta-thalassemia. *Pediatr Hematol Oncol* 2002; **19**: 453–8.

17. Vellodi A, Picton S, Downie CJ *et al.* Bone marrow transplantation for thalassaemia: experience of two British centres. *Bone Marrow Transplant* 1994; **13**: 559–62.

18. Roberts I, Darbyshire P, Will AM. BMT for children with beta-thalassaemia major in the UK. *Bone Marrow Transplant* 1997; **19** (Suppl 2): 60–1.

19. Vassal G, Deroussent A, Challine D *et al.* Is 600 Mg/M2 the appropriate dosage of busulfan in children undergoing bone marrow transplantation? *Blood* 1992; **79**: 2475–9.

20. Poonkuzhali B, Srivastava A, Quernin MH *et al.* Pharmacokinetics of oral busulphan in children with beta thalassaemia major undergoing allogeneic bone marrow transplantation. *Bone Marrow Transplant* 1999; **24**: 5–11.

21. Yeager AM, Wagner JE Jr, Graham ML *et al.* Optimization of busulfan dosage in children undergoing bone marrow transplantation: a pharmacokinetic study of dose escalation. *Blood* 1992; **80**: 2425–8.

22. Slattery JT, Sanders JE, Buckner CD *et al.* Graft-rejection and toxicity following bone marrow transplantation in relation to busulfan pharmacokinetics. *Bone Marrow Transplant* 1995; **16**: 31–42.

23. Balasubramanian P, Chandy M, Krishnamoorthy R, Srivastava, A. Evaluation of existing limited sampling models for busulfan kinetics in children with beta thalassaemia major undergoing bone marrow transplantation. *Bone Marrow Transplant* 2001; **28**: 821–5.

24. Angelucci E, Mariotti E, Lucarelli G *et al.* Sudden cardiac tamponade after chemotherapy for marrow transplantation in thalassaemia. *Lancet* 1992; **339**: 287–9.

25. Giardini C, Galimberti M, Lucarelli G *et al.* Bone marrow transplantation in class 2 thalassaemia patients. *Bone Marrow Transplant* 1997; **19** (Suppl 2): 59–62.

26. Amrolia PJ, Vulliamy T, Vassiliou G *et al.* Analysis of chimaerism in thalassaemic children undergoing stem cell transplantation. *Br J Haematol* 2001; **114**: 219–25.

27. Nesci S, Manna M, Lucarelli G *et al.* Mixed chimerism after bone marrow transplantation in thalassemia. *Ann N Y Acad Sci* 1998; **850**: 495–7.

28. Andreani M, Nesci S, Lucarelli G *et al.* Long-term survival of ex-thalassemic patients with persistent mixed chimerism after bone marrow transplantation. *Bone Marrow Transplant* 2000; **25**: 401–4.

29. Walters MC, Nienhuis AW, Vichinsky E. Novel therapeutic approaches in sickle cell disease. *Hematology (Am Soc Hematol Educ Program)* 2002; 10–34.

30. Adams AB, Durham MM, Kean L *et al.* Blockade, busulfan, and bone marrow promote titratable macrochimerism, induce transplantation tolerance, and correct genetic hemoglobinopathies with minimal myelosuppression. *J Immunol* 2001; **167**: 1103–11.

31. Aker M, Kapelushnik J, Pugatsch T *et al.* Donor lymphocyte infusions to displace residual host hematopoietic cells after allogeneic bone marrow transplantation for beta-thalassemia major. *J Pediatr Hematol Oncol* 1998; **20**: 145–8.

32. Gaziev D, Polchi P, Galimberti M *et al.* Graft-versus-host disease after bone marrow transplantation for thalassemia: an analysis of incidence and risk factors. *Transplantation* 1997; **63**: 854–60.

33. Baronciani D, Galimberti M, Lucarelli G *et al.* Bone marrow transplanatation in class 1 thalassaemia patients. *Bone Marrow Transplant* 1997; **19** (Suppl 2): 56–8.

34. Lucarelli G, Clift RA, Galimberti M *et al.* Bone marrow transplantation in adult thalassemic patients. *Blood* 1999; **93**: 1164–7.

35. Angelucci E, Muretto P, Lucarelli G *et al.* Phlebotomy to reduce iron overload in patients cured of thalassemia by bone marrow transplantation. Italian Cooperative Group for Phlebotomy Treatment of Transplanted Thalassemia Patients. *Blood* 1997; **90**: 994–8.

36. Giardini C, Galimberti M, Lucarelli G *et al.* Desferrioxamine therapy accelerates clearance of iron deposits after bone marrow transplantation for thalassaemia. *Br J Haematol* 1995; **89**: 868–73.

37. Angelucci E, Muretto P, Nicolucci A *et al.* Effects of iron overload and hepatitis C virus positivity in determining progression of liver fibrosis in thalassemia following bone marrow transplantation. *Blood* 2002; **100**: 17–21.

38. de Sanctis V, Galimberti, M, Lucarelli G *et al.* Growth and development in ex-thalassaemic patients. *Bone Marrow Transplant* 1997; **19** (Suppl 2): 48–53.

39. Gaziev J, Galimberti M, Giardini C, Baronciani D, Lucarelli G. Growth in children after bone marrow transplantation for thalassemia. *Bone Marrow Transplant* 1993; **12** (Suppl 1): 100–1.

40. Proceedings of the Ares-Serono Foundation 2nd International Workshop on Growth and Endocrine Complications and Reproduction in Thalassaemia. Ferrara, Italy. 2–4 April. *J Pediatr Endocrinol Metab* 1998; **11** (Suppl 3): 771–1008.

41. De Simone M, Olioso P, Di Bartolomeo P *et al.* Growth and endocrine function following bone marrow transplantation for thalassemia. *Bone Marrow Transplant* 1995; **15**: 227–33.

42. De Sanctis V, Galimberti M, Lucarelli G *et al.* Gonadal function in long term survivors with B thalassemia major following bone marrow transplantation. *Bone Marrow Transplant* 1993; **12** (Suppl 1): 104.

43. Borgna-Pignatti C, Marradi P, Rugolotto S, Marcolongo A. Successful pregnancy after bone marrow transplantation for thalassaemia. *Bone Marrow Transplant* 1996; **18**: 235–6.

44. Gulati SC, Van Poznak C. Pregnancy after bone marrow transplantation. *J Clin Oncol* 1998; **16**: 1978–85.

45. Sanders JE, Hawley J, Levy W *et al*. Pregnancies following high-dose cyclophosphamide with or without high-dose busulfan or total-body irradiation and bone marrow transplantation. *Blood* 1996; **87**: 3045–52.

46. Gaziev D, Galimberti M, Lucarelli G *et al*. Bone marrow transplantation from alternative donors for thalassemia: HLA-phenotypically identical relative and HLA-nonidentical sibling or parent transplants. *Bone Marrow Transplant* 2000; **25**: 815–21.

47. Rubinstein P, Carrier C, Scaradavou A *et al*. Outcomes among 562 recipients of placental-blood transplants from unrelated donors. *N Engl J Med* 1998; **339**: 1565–7.

48. Locatelli F, Rocha V, Reed W *et al*. Related umbilical cord blood transplant in patients with thalassemia and sickle cell disease. *Blood* 2003; **101**: 2137–43.

49. Chik KW, Shing MM, Li CK *et al*. Autologuous marrow recovery in a multitransfused beta-thalassemia major patient after umbilical cord blood transplantation. *Blood* 1996; **88**: 755.

50. La Nasa G, Giardini C, Argiolu F *et al*. Unrelated donor bone marrow transplantation for thalassemia: the effect of extended haplotypes. *Blood* 2002; **99**: 4350–6.

51. Vassiliou G, Amrolia P, Roberts IAG. Allogeneic transplantation for haemoglobinopathies. *Baillieres Best Pract Res Clin Haematol* 2001; **14**: 807–22.

52. Wonke B, Wright C, Hoffbrand AV. Combined therapy with deferiprone and desferrioxamine. *Br J Haematol* 1998; **103**: 361–4.

53. Galanello R. Iron chelation: new therapies. *Semin Hematol* 2001; **38**: 73–6.

54. Tisdale J, Sadelain M. Toward gene therapy for disorders of globin synthesis. *Semin Hematol* 2001; **38**: 382–92.

55. May C, Rivella S, Chadburn A, Sadelain M. Successful treatment of murine beta-thalassemia intermedia by transfer of the human beta-globin gene. *Blood* 2002; **99**: 1902–8.

56. Platt OS, Brambilla DJ, Rosse WF *et al*. Mortality in sickle cell disease. Life expectancy and risk factors for early death. *N Engl J Med* 1994; **330**: 1639–44.

57. Charache S, Terrin ML, Moore RD *et al*. Effect of hydroxyurea on the frequency of painful crises in sickle cell anemia. Investigators of the Multicenter Study of Hydroxyurea in Sickle Cell Anemia. *N Engl J Med* 1995; **332**: 1317–22.

58. Ferster A, Tahriri P, Vermylen C *et al*. Five years of experience with hydroxyurea in children and young adults with sickle cell disease. *Blood* 2001; **97**: 3628–32.

59. Davies SC. Bone marrow transplant for sickle cell disease – the dilemma. *Blood Rev* 1993; **7**: 4–9.

60. Walters MC, Patience M, Leisenring W *et al*. Bone marrow transplantation for sickle cell disease. *N Engl J Med* 1996; **335**: 369–76.

61. Walters MC, Storb R, Patience M *et al*. Impact of bone marrow transplantation for symptomatic sickle cell disease: an interim report. Multicenter Investigation of Bone Marrow Transplantation for Sickle Cell Disease. *Blood* 2000; **95**: 1918–24.

62. Powars D, Wilson B, Imbus C, Pegelow C, Allen J. The natural history of stroke in sickle cell disease. *Am J Med* 1978; **65**: 461–71.

63. Pegelow CH, Adams RJ, McKie V *et al*. Risk of recurrent stroke in patients with sickle cell disease treated with erythrocyte transfusions. *J Pediatr* 1995; **126**: 896–9.

64. Castro O, Brambilla DJ, Thorington B *et al*. The acute chest syndrome in sickle cell disease: incidence and risk factors. The Cooperative Study of Sickle Cell Disease. *Blood* 1994; **84**: 643–9.

65. Kinney TR, Helms RW, O'Branski E *et al*. Safety of hydroxyurea in children with sickle cell anemia: results of the HUG-KIDS Study, a phase I/II trial. Pediatric Hydroxyurea Group. *Blood* 1999; **94**: 1550–4.

66. Nietert PJ, Abboud MR, Silverstein MD, Jackson SM. Bone marrow transplantation versus periodic prophylactic blood transfusion in sickle cell patients at high risk of ischemic stroke: a decision analysis. *Blood* 2000; **95**: 3057–64.

67. Adams RJ, McKie VC, Hsu L *et al*. Prevention of a first stroke by transfusions in children with sickle cell anemia and abnormal results on transcranial Doppler ultrasonography. *N Engl J Med* 1998; **339**: 5–11.

68. Davies SC, Roberts IAG. Bone marrow transplant for sickle cell disease – an update. *Arch Dis Child* 1996; **75**: 3–6.

69. Walters MC, Patience M, Leisenring W *et al*. Barriers to bone marrow transplantation for sickle cell anemia. *Biol Blood Marrow Transplant* 1996; **2**: 100–4.

70. Vermylen C, Cornu G, Ferster A *et al*. Haematopoietic stem cell transplantation for sickle cell anaemia: the first 50 patients transplanted in Belgium. *Bone Marrow Transplant* 1998; **22**: 1–6.

71. Walters MC, Sullivan KM, Bernaudin F *et al*. Neurologic complications after allogeneic marrow transplantation for sickle cell anemia. *Blood* 1995; **85**: 879–84.

72. Walters MC, Patience M, Leisenring W *et al*. Stable mixed hematopoietic chimerism after bone marrow transplantation for sickle cell anemia. *Biol Blood Marrow Transplant* 2001; **7**: 665–73.

73. Baron F, Dresse MF, Beguin Y. Donor lymphocyte infusion to eradicate recurrent host hematopoiesis after allogeneic BMT for sickle cell disease. *Transfusion* 2000; **40**: 1071–3.

74. van Besien K, Bartholomew A, Stock W *et al*. Fludara-

bine-based conditioning for allogeneic transplantation in adults with sickle cell disease. *Bone Marrow Transplant* 2000; **26**: 445–9.

75. Steen RG, Helton KJ, Horwitz EM *et al.* Improved cerebrovascular patency following therapy in patients with sickle cell disease: initial results in 4 patients who received HLA-identical hematopoietic stem cell allografts. *Ann Neurol* 2001; **49**: 222–9.

76. Ferster A, Bujan W, Corazza F *et al.* Bone marrow transplantation corrects the splenic reticuloendothelial dysfunction in sickle cell anemia. *Blood* 1993; **81**: 1102–5.

77. Yeager AM, Mehta PS, Adamkiewicz T *et al.* Unrelated placental/umbilical cord blood cell (UCBC) transplantation in children with high-risk sickle cell disease. *Blood* 2000; **96**: 366b.

78. Bennekou P, de Franceschi L, Pedersen O *et al.* Treatment with NS3623, a novel Cl-conductance blocker, ameliorates erythrocyte dehydration in transgenic sad mice: a possible new therapeutic approach for sickle cell disease. *Blood* 2001; **97**: 1451–7.

79. Amrolia P, Gaspar HB, Hassan A *et al.* Nonmyeloablative stem cell transplantation for congenital immunodeficiencies. *Blood* 2000; **96**: 1239–46.

80. Krishnamurti L, Blazar BR, Wagner JE. Bone marrow transplantation without myeloablation for sickle cell disease. *N Engl J Med* 2001; **344**: 68.

81. Schleuning M, Stoetzer O, Waterhouse C *et al.* Hematopoietic stem cell transplantation after reduced-intensity conditioning as treatment of sickle cell disease. *Exp Hematol* 2002; **30**: 7–10.

82. Iannone R, Luznik L, Engstrom LW *et al.* Effects of mixed hematopoietic chimerism in a mouse model of bone marrow transplantation for sickle cell anemia. *Blood* 2001; **97**: 3960–5.

83. Kean LS, Durham MM, Adams AB *et al.* A cure for murine sickle cell disease through stable mixed chimerism and tolerance induction after nonmyeloablative conditioning and major histocompatibility complex-mismatched bone marrow transplantation. *Blood* 2002; **99**: 1840–9.

Chapter 20

Practical guidelines on antibiotic therapy, exchange blood transfusion and peri-operative management in sickle cell disease

Iheanyi E Okpala

Introduction

The clinical management of patients with sickle cell disease (SCD) and thalassaemia has become increasingly multidisciplinary and complex. This trend calls for the development of guidelines for the management of specific clinical problems and protocols for various therapeutic procedures, to facilitate uniformity and standardization of care across different disciplines. Such guidelines and protocols should be regularly revised and updated in line with developments in clinical practice and findings from scientific research. This chapter provides practical guidance on dealing with some frequently encountered issues in the management of SCD.

Antimicrobial agents for prophylaxis and treatment of infections in SCD

People with SCD are susceptible to infections because of hyposplenism, a defect in activation of the alternative pathway of complement, and possibly, reduced leucocyte function. Infection is the dominant predisposing factor to sickle cell crisis and the commonest cause of death related to the haemoglobinopathy. Therefore, prevention of infections and effective treatment of established episodes are very important aspects of the care of affected individuals.

Prophylactic antibiotics

A controlled clinical trial showed that penicillin V is effective in reducing mortality from pneumococcal septicaemia associated with SCD [1]. Prophylaxis is recommended from the age of 3 months, at a dose of 125 mg b.d. In adults, the dose is doubled to 250 mg b.d. Individuals allergic to penicillin could be given clarithromycin 250 mg b.d. For people who continue to have recurrent infections (especially of the urinary or respiratory tract) while on penicillin V or clarithromycin, ciprofloxacin 250 mg b.d may be used.

Therapeutic antibiotics

Once specimens have been taken for microbiology investigations, first-line medications should be chosen such as to cover for the common pathogens that cause infections in SCD. These are gram-positive organisms, especially staphylococci, and gram-negative organisms such as salmonella species. Examples of appropriate anti-staphylococcal agents are flucloxacillin, or sodium fusidate in patients allergic to penicillins. Effective gram-negative cover may be provided with oral ciprofloxacin at the therapeutic doses of 500 mg b.d, or 750 mg b.d for severe infections; intravenous cefuroxime 750 mg t.d.s; or cefadroxil 500 mg b.d orally. All three are effective against salmonella organisms, which are second to staphylococci as the aetiological agents of osteomyelitis in SCD. Anaerobes may cause infections in the mouth such as tooth abscess, or cholecystitis. Metronidazole is the drug of choice in treating anaerobic infections. Appropriate combinations of the above may be used as first-line antibiotics while microscopy, culture and sensitivity results are awaited. The definitive choice of drugs may be altered in the light of microbiology reports. Clarithromycin at therapeutic doses could be added to the antibiotic regimen if atypical bacteria are suspected as the cause of respiratory tract infection, or if the patient has a community-acquired chest infection.

Exchange blood transfusion

Venesection to reduce the proportion of HbS red cells with transfusion of normal HbA blood is often beneficial in the treatment or prevention of life-threatening and other manifestations of SCD [2]. The conventional aim in this process of exchange blood transfusion (EBT) is to reduce HbS to 30%; the mean proportion in carriers of sickle cell gene who usually do not have clinical illness due to the presence of this haemoglobin variant. The situations are not strictly identical because people with sickle cell trait have a mixture of HbA and HbS inside each erythrocyte, whereas HbSS patients who have undergone EBT still have 100% HbS in a proportion of their red cells. The environment inside erythrocytes of HbAS individuals is more protective against sickling than in post-transfusion HbSS patients who have a considerable number of red cells filled with HbS. This difference notwithstanding, clinical experience shows that HbSS patients on regular EBT not only have a lower incidence of vaso-occlusive events such as stroke and sickle cell crisis, but also have regeneration of the spleen with improved resistance to infections [2, 3]. EBT can be done manually, or automatically with a red cell apheresis machine. Whereas automated EBT is more effective in reducing the proportion of HbS, it requires trained staff with technical expertise, and is often not feasible to organize at short notice in emergency situations. In contrast, manual EBT involves no more than venesection and transfusion. The only practical skill required is the ability to perform venepuncture. This makes it more feasible when exchange transfusion is needed urgently. For example, although manual EBT may achieve only 50% reduction of HbS in a patient with acute chest syndrome, this confers significant clinical benefit and can save the life of a person who develops this severe complication, which is the leading cause of mortality in adults with SCD.

Indications for EBT

1 Cerebrovascular accidents
2 Acute chest syndrome
3 Prior to major surgery
4 Multi-organ failure, including systemic marrow fat embolism
5 Multiple pregnancy
6 Prevention of recurrent stroke.

Relative indications

1 Intractable or very frequent severe crises
2 Major priapism unresponsive to other therapy.

Preparation for EBT

1 Discuss objective of EBT with patient, obtain informed consent and body weight.
2 Coagulation screen to detect any bleeding tendency: thrombin time, prothrombin time, activated partial thromboplastin time and platelet count.
3 Blood chemistry, including calcium level. Full blood count and %HbS.
4 Cross-match and extended phenotyping of blood for C, E, S, Fy, K and Jk antigens.

For automated EBT further preparatory steps would be necessary, and vary according to the type of apheresis machine used.

Manual EBT

As a rough guide, 10–15 mL/kg of RBC concentrate, or 1 unit of blood per 10 kg body weight is required for adults with Hb level up to 6 g/dL, and transfusion or removal of 1 unit of blood changes the haemoglobin concentration by 1 g/dL in the average adult. Generally, a 6-unit exchange over 24 hours is well tolerated. If more units of blood need to be transfused, it is advisable to spread the manual exchange over 48 hours, and transfuse 3–4 units/day.

Procedure

1 Give 500 mL of dextrose saline intravenously over 30 minutes.
2 Remove 500 mL of blood over 30 minutes.

3 Give the second bag of 500 mL of dextrose saline over 30 minutes.

4 Remove the second unit (500 mL) of blood over 30 minutes.

5 Transfuse the first unit of red cell concentrate or blood over 1 hour.

6 Remove the third unit (500 mL) of blood over 30 minutes.

7 Transfuse 5 units of red cell concentrate at 1 unit/3 hours, over the next 15 hours.

The Hb level should not be increased above 11 g/dL (haematocrit > 0.33). One or two units of blood could be removed by venesection with fluid replacement if the Hb level after the exchange is > 11 g/dL. In patients with pre-transfusion Hb level of about 5 g/dL who need manual EBT, there is no need for steps 3–6 above. In such situations, after giving 500 mL of intravenous fluid and removing the first 500 mL of blood, 5 units of red cell concentrate could be transfused over the next 10 hours (step 7). If the patient's pre-transfusion Hb level is ≤ 4 g/dL, EBT is not necessary. Top-up transfusion of 6 units of red cell concentrate over 12 hours will achieve the same end.

Automated EBT

EBT with an erythrocytopheresis machine is more efficient than the manual procedure in that it exchanges a larger proportion of the blood volume, is less tedious for patients and staff, and takes far less time to complete. In addition to the general preparation noted previously, automated EBT requires:

1 Insertion of a double lumen femoral or central catheter big enough to accommodate the rate of blood flow needed to exchange 6–8 units over 3 hours. Catheterization is facilitated if done under radiological (e.g. ultrasound) guidance.

2 Prior priming of the apheresis machine and blood warmer.

3 A red cell exchange disposable set, compatible with the apheresis machine.

4 Citrate anticoagulant (1 litre).

5 Two vials of 10% calcium gluconate.

6 Dextrose saline or normal saline (1.5 litres).

7 Sterile packs containing forceps or haemostats, scissors, gloves, needles and syringes.

8 For computing the total volume of blood to be used in the procedure, a calculator!

Elective EBTs in steady-state patients for non-acute indications, such as prevention of recurrent stroke, could be done as day procedures. Admission into a high dependency unit is advisable for EBT done as treatment of acute illness, e.g. acute chest syndrome. A general medical examination is essential to ensure that the patient is fit for automated EBT. The actual procedure should be done following the manufacturer's operating instructions as detailed in the handbook of the particular apheresis machine used. It is advisable to programme the machine to perform the EBT over a minimum period of 3 hours, because the likelihood of an adverse event associated with the procedure, such as citrate toxicity, is higher if it is done too rapidly. For people who have fluid overload, as may occur in kidney disease, the procedure time should be a minimum of 4 hours, and excess body fluid could be reduced by setting the desired fluid balance below 100%, e.g. to 90%. To avoid possibly fatal air embolism, one should ensure there are no air bubbles in the access and return lines before connecting the patient to the apheresis machine. Vital signs should be measured within 15 minutes of starting EBT, and at 30-minute intervals. To prevent citrate toxicity, 5 mL of 10% calcium gluconate diluted to 15 mL with normal saline should be given slowly over 5 minutes via the return line when the fourth unit of blood is running through the machine.

Post-EBT care

Considering that adverse events associated with EBT can occur late, it is advisable to observe the vital signs at 15-minute intervals for a minimum of 30 minutes after the procedure. If a steady-state patient who was clinically stable before exchange is still unwell an hour after EBT performed as a day procedure, admission into the ward may be considered for further observation and possible treatment. In the absence of clinical problems, and if vital signs are satisfactory 30 minutes after EBT, the femoral catheter may be taken out. Blood samples for post-transfusion FBC, %HbS and chemistry should be taken from another (peripheral) vein to ensure more accurate results. In acutely ill patients exchanged in a high dependency unit, the catheter used for EBT may be left in place for up to 5 days if required for other intravenous therapy. Blood samples for post-transfusion haematology and chemistry should then be taken 24 hours later, to allow time for optimal equilibration.

Management of adverse events associated with EBT

Blood transfusion reactions and citrate toxicity are the usual complications.

Blood transfusion reactions

The features of a transfusion reaction include pain in the chest and back, rigors, skin rash, fever, bronchospasm, hypotension and shock with reduced urinary output. The causes are incompatible red cell transfusion, reaction to leucocyte, platelet and plasma protein antigens, and giving infected blood. The EBT should be suspended, 10 mg of piriton and 100 mg of hydrocortisone given intravenously, and vital signs closely monitored. If there is hypotension, intravenous fluids should be given, the patient kept in a head-down position, and urinary output monitored. Inotropes may be needed if the hypotension does not respond to the measures above. Disseminated intravascular clotting (DIC) can be triggered by immediate transfusion reaction. A coagulation screen and fibrinogen assay facilitate diagnosis. The renal physicians should be invited to participate in the management if DIC is associated with acute renal shutdown. If reaction against incompatible red cells is a differential, samples from the suspected units of blood (particularly the one being transfused when the adverse event started) should be sent to the laboratory with the patient's venous blood and urine samples for investigations.

Citrate toxicity

Without prophylactic administration of intravenous calcium gluconate, about 15% of automated blood apheresis procedures may be complicated by citrate toxicity [4]. The incidence rate depends on several factors: the duration or rapidity of apheresis, the concentration of citrate anticoagu-

lant used, the rate of infusion of citrate, and the patient's susceptibility – which is related to how quickly the infused citrate can be metabolized. Citrate acts by chelating calcium ions, which is the reason why administration of calcium gluconate during EBT reduces the risk of citrate toxicity. As would be expected, the features are those of hypocalcaemia – circumoral muscle twitching and paraesthesia, nausea, vomiting, chills, cardiac arrhythmias and syncope. Full-blown tetany is rare. If the patient is not kept warm during the procedure, or the transfused blood is not pre-warmed, this increases the severity or likelihood of citrate toxicity. It is pertinent to bear in mind that severe hypo-calcaemia may occur without forewarning by the symptoms above.

It is therefore important to prevent citrate toxicity. The patient should be informed about the symptoms and advised to immediately call the attention of hospital staff if they occur. It is unusual for citrate toxicity to develop during EBT if calcium gluconate is given in the middle of the procedure as stated previously. Should it occur before the calcium gluconate is given, or despite doing so halfway through the EBT, the exchange should be discontinued. Calcium gluconate (2 ml of 10% solution) should be given over 5 minutes. The procedure can be resumed when the clinical and ECG features of hypocalcaemia have resolved. Increasing the total procedure time should be considered when the EBT is resumed, and on subsequent exchanges in the same person.

Peri-operative management of patients with SCD

Surgery requiring general anaesthesia may increase the risk of vaso-occlusive events in SCD. Surgical trauma and the inflammatory response to tissue injury, hypoxia associated with general anaesthesia and dehydration from reduced oral fluid intake; all are recognized precipitating factors for sickle cell crisis and other vaso-occlusive manifestations of the haemoglobinopathy. It is therefore necessary to take appropriate preventive or therapeutic measures in SCD patients and individuals at risk of carrying the gene for HbS.

Determination of haemoglobin genotype

The majority of known SCD patients would have had their Hb genotype ascertained prior to an elective or emergency surgery requiring general anaesthesia. However, people with previously undiagnosed SCD or sickle cell trait need to have their Hb genotype determined not only to ensure appropriate peri-operative management, but also for medicolegal reasons. In this context, people who had previous blood transfusion within the lifespan of normal red cells (up to 4 months) may have misleading Hb genotype results, if this is not taken into account when interpreting the laboratory data. Various procedures are used to determine Hb genotype, depending on local circumstances and the preference of the haematology laboratory. Methods that give accurate results include electrophoresis, high-performance liquid chromatography (HPLC), iso-electric focusing and mass spectrometry. It is essential to counsel people who are found to have SCD or sickle cell trait and explain the significance of the result. If surgery is not urgently needed, it is advisable to defer the operation until the patient's Hb genotype is known.

When it is not feasible to determine Hb genotype before surgery

Pre-operative determination of Hb genotype may not be feasible in emergency situations. If deferring the surgery will put the patient's life in danger, practical guidance on immediate clinical management may be provided from the results of the following investigations, which should be requested urgently:

1 Full blood count
2 Sickle solubility test
3 Peripheral blood film.

If the Hb level and blood film are normal, and the sickle solubility test is negative in a patient older than 6 months who was not transfused in the previous 4 months, SCD or trait is unlikely. Peri-operative management could be carried out as for HbAA individuals. Sickle cells in the peripheral blood film, low Hb level and positive sickle solubility test are highly suggestive of SCD, and the patient should be treated accordingly. A positive sickle solubility test with normal Hb level and normal blood film may be found in sickle cell trait. In emergency situations when the Hb genotype cannot be confirmed, it is recommended that peri-operative management is carried out as if the patient had SCD. This recommendation also applies to situations in which the patient had blood transfusion in the previous 4 months, and the sickle solubility test is negative with normal blood film and Hb level. However, the %HbS needs to be < 20% for the sickle solubility test to be negative, and peri-operative clinical problems related to HbS are unlikely to arise in such situations. The situation is similar to that of SCD patients with HbS maintained below 30% by regular exchange blood transfusions, who seldom develop new vaso-occlusive clinical problems.

It is necessary to determine the Hb genotype as soon as it is possible in all patients for whom this could not done before emergency surgery. The low probability of HbS-related clinical problems notwithstanding, it is important to bear in mind that false negative results of the sickle solubility test may be obtained in HbSS infants aged < 6 months before HbF is substantially replaced by HbS, and in HbAS or HbSS adults following blood transfusion. In previously transfused patients, accurate Hb genotype may not be obtainable from blood tests until 4 months after transfusion. DNA analysis can provide reliable results of Hb genotype within 4 months of blood transfusion. Patients who were not transfused, including infants aged < 6 months, can still have accurate determination of Hb genotype on blood samples. If an individual was transfused peri-operatively, a pre-transfusion blood sample taken during the episode of illness can be used for haemoglobin genotyping.

Peri-operative management of SCD patients

Blood transfusion

Exchange blood transfusion to achieve HbS below 30% and Hb level 10–11 g/dL is recommended before major surgery such as hip replacement, complex neurosurgical, abdominal or thoracic operations, and tonsillectomy. For not so major surgery such as caesarian section and cataract removal, top-up blood transfusion to a haemoglobin level

10–11 g/dL will suffice [5]. SCD patients are prone to red cell antibody formation [6]; it is therefore important to request blood a minimum of 1 day before the planned transfusion so that there is ample time to obtain compatible units of blood.

Oxygen therapy

Hypoxaemia predisposes to sickling, and its prevention by oxygen administration is of paramount importance in the peri-operative management of SCD patients. Oxygen may be required from the time of pre-medication, especially if respiratory depressant drugs have been given. Pre-oxygenation is essential before the induction of anaesthesia. A higher than standard oxygen concentration in the anaesthetic gases is used during surgery. Oxygen administration is continued postoperatively until the patient starts to mobilize, or through the first day. In view of the usual drop in oxygen saturation during sleep, the inhibition of respiratory (breathing) movements because of postoperative pain in the thorax or abdomen, and the tendency of vaso-occlusive events in SCD to develop at night, it is advisable to administer oxygen during the 2nd to 4th nights after surgery in the thorax or abdomen. Monitoring the blood oxygen saturation peri-operatively with a pulse oximeter, or by measuring arterial blood gases, helps to ensure that hypoxia is prevented, or detected and treated.

Hydration

SCD is associated with hyposthenuria – the inability to concentrate urine – a result of recurrent infarction and loss of functional kidney tissue. The obligatory passage of large volumes of urine makes SCD patients prone to dehydration. This pre-existing tendency to dehydration is exacerbated by the reduction in oral fluid and food intake associated with surgery. Dehydration increases the intracellular concentration of HbS in erythrocytes, the risk of sickling and of peri-operative occurrence of vaso-occlusive events. Therefore, the prevention of dehydration is of paramount importance in the management of SCD patients undergoing surgery. Sufficient intravenous fluid administration is essential to maintain adequate hydration. In view of the reduced ability of SCD patients to excrete sodium, 5% dextrose solution or dextrose in saline (but not 0.9% sodium chloride solution) is preferred.

Normothermia

Exposure to cold frequently precipitates sickle cell crisis [7]. Hypothermia during surgery may stimulate reflex shivering early in the postoperative period, peripheral vaso-constriction, increased oxygen consumption by skeletal muscles, tissue hypoxia, sickling and vaso-occlusive crisis. To prevent these, it is crucial to ensure that the body temperature is maintained at normal values during surgery in SCD patients.

Other conditions that predispose to vaso-occlusion (such as infection, circulatory stasis, and respiratory or metabolic acidosis) need to be prevented or treated. The existence of organ disease previously caused by SCD calls for specific preventive or treatment measures during the period around surgery. Kidney failure from sickle nephropathy implies closer attention to fluid balance and hydration, chronic sickle lung may impair gaseous exchange and blood oxygen saturation, and previous stroke associated with damage to the vasomotor centre might make the control of blood pressure and circulation more difficult during the period of general anaesthesia. SCD does not cause thrombocytopenia, and is uncommonly associated with clinically significant derangement of coagulation because of hepatic dysfunction. Therefore, the majority of affected individuals can safely have epidural anaesthesia. If a coagulation screen detects a clinically significant impairment of haemostasis, appropriate clotting factor replacement therapy should be given. In SCD patients with low platelet counts due other co-existent conditions, platelet transfusion may be needed before epidural anaesthesia. SCD per se is not a contraindication to the procedure.

Sickle cell trait

There is no evidence of a clinically significant increase in the risk of general anaesthesia to HbAS individuals. Therefore, their peri-operative management should be same as for HbAA people. There is a possibility of red cell sickling and vaso-occlusion if severe hypoxaemia occurs in HbAS patients under general anaesthesia. The issue may arise as to whether local hypoxia caused by orthopaedic tourniquet could lead to sickling in people who have sickle cell trait. Clinical experience has been that the use of orthopaedic tourniquet does not lead to HbS-related problems in HbAS patients.

References

1. Gaston MH, Verter JI, Woods G *et al.* for the Prophylactic Penicillin Group. Prophylaxis with oral penicillin in children with sickle cell anaemia: a randomized trial. *N Engl J Med* 1986; **314**: 1593–9.

2. Ohene-Frempong K. Indications for red cell transfusion in sickle cell disease. *Semin Hematol* 2001; **38** (Suppl 1): 5–13.

3. Campbell PJ, Ryan KE, Davies SC. Splenic re-growth in sickle cell disease following hypertransfusion. *Br J Haematol* 1994; **86** (Suppl): 4.

4. British Society of Haematology. Guidelines for the clinical use of blood cell separators. *Clin Lab Haematol* 1998; **20**: 265–78.

5. Vichinsky EP, Neumayr LD, Haberkern C *et al.* A comparison of conservative and aggressive transfusion regimens in perioperative management of sickle cell disease. The Perioperative Transfusion in Sickle Cell Disease Group. *N Engl J Med* 1995; **333**: 206–13.

6. Cox JV, Steane E, Cunningham G, Frenkel EP. Risk of alloimmunization and delayed hemolytic transfusion reactions in patients with sickle cell disease. *Arch Intern Med* 1988; **148**: 2485–9.

7. Serjeant GR. Sickle cell disease. *Lancet* 1997; **350**: 725–30.

Chapter 21
Opiate dependence in sickle cell disease

Ikechukwu Obialo Azuonye

Introduction

It is thought that sickle cell disease (SCD) is a balanced polymorphism, put simply, a condition resulting from Nature's attempt to solve a problem. The problem in question is that of malaria. Confronted with a devastating situation with the *Plasmodium* organism, the human body worked out a solution: when the *Plasmodium* organism infects a red cell, let the shape and structure of the cell change such that the cell is preferentially selected for destruction, along with the parasite, by the spleen.

This works very well in the heterozygote, who is relatively immune to malaria. Unfortunately, the homozygote is left with a serious disease which causes considerable distress and limits life expectancy: sickle cell disease. The problem arises because when HbSS is deoxygenated, the erythrocyte undergoes a characteristic change in shape, becoming 'sickled', less elastic, and much more likely – as semi-solid masses – to stick to the walls of blood vessels. HbSS is initially able to return to its original soluble form, but with repeated deformations, the red cell is permanently damaged.

These polymerized, semi-solid masses of deformed red blood cells block small blood vessels everywhere in the body. It is this vaso-occlusion which is responsible for virtually all the manifestations of SCD. The manifestations of SCD include pain, cerebrovascular accidents, pulmonary complications, vulnerability to infections, acute splenic sequestration, impairment of hearing in children, and chronic damage and failure of the various organs of the body. Of these, pain accounts for > 90% of admissions for treatment in hospital.

Pain

The pain experienced in SCD can be extremely severe. In fact, the severity of pain, and the number of episodes of pain per year, constitute one of the principal markers of the severity of the condition, and this is a dependable predictor of early death in patients under the age of 20 years. This pain is caused by oxygen deprivation of the tissues, as well as avascular necrosis of the bone marrow: these two factors bring about inflammation, and the body's attempt to repair the damage causes an increase in intramedullary pressure which is experienced as pain of varying severity.

Management of pain

Pain crises can be managed in the community or in hospital, depending on the severity of the attack. Less severe crises respond to simple analgesia given by mouth, and further help may be obtained by giving the patient fluids, rest, massage and warmth.

For more severe pain, the so-called 'analgesic ladder' tends to be used: start with, for example, paracetamol; if that proves insufficient, try one of the non-steroidal anti-inflammatory drugs (NSAIDs); if more is needed, try codeine phosphate; if, at this point, there is no obvious relief of pain – and/or the patient's joints are swollen, there is evidence of central nervous system (CNS) involvement or acute chest syndrome – admit the patient to hospital and give opioids.

It is worth bearing in mind that opiates are the first-line treatment for severe acute pain. The opiates in question are pethidine, morphine and diamorphine (also known as heroin). There is, however, some dispute about which opiates to use in severe pain in SCD. Current thinking is that morphine is the opiate of choice. There have been concerns about a by-product of pethidine known as norpethadinic acid, which can accumulate to toxic levels in the patient and cause epileptiform seizures.

Concerns about addiction

It is well known that the opiates can be addictive drugs. There are also 'rumours' about the relationship between SCD and opiate addiction. Suffice it to say that SCD does not protect the sufferer from opiate addiction, and also does not predispose the sufferer to this form of addiction.

Worries about opiate addiction are a common cause of distress, with parents expressing anxiety about their children being given heroin for the control of pain.

These concerns are actually not justified. The risk of a SCD sufferer developing opiate addiction is very low, for an obvious reason: the acute severe bone pain crisis lasts only a few days, so if opioid analgesics are administered during these brief periods and withdrawn, the patient would not be at any greater risk of developing an addiction than any member of the general public. In fact, the prevalence of opiate addiction in SCD is the same as the prevalence for the general population.

SCD and opiate dependence

What this means is that while the risk of developing dependence on opiates is not any higher in SCD than in the general population, this risk is not zero. Opiate dependence does occur in a small proportion of people with SCD.

It is important to be able to recognize opiate dependence, for the following important reasons:
1 Opiate dependence makes it more difficult to treat the symptoms of the SCD, and
2 SCD, for its part, makes it difficult to manage the dependence syndrome successfully.

We must distinguish between tolerance, physical dependence and psychological dependence.
- *Tolerance* is the phenomenon in which a patient requires larger doses of the drug to achieve the same degree of pain relief, generally without an increase in adverse effects.
- *Physical dependence* results from the pharmacological effects of the drug, the effect of which is that the patient experiences withdrawal symptoms when the drug is discontinued too rapidly.
- *Psychological dependence* ('addiction') is characterized by an abnormal use of the drug, craving for it for purposes other than the relief of pain, sometimes going to extraordinary lengths to acquire the drug, and reverting to using it again after a period of apparently successful detoxification.

Psychological dependence on opioid analgesics does occur in SCD, but is fortunately only an occasional observation. However, when it does occur it needs to be taken seriously because of the adverse interplay between SCD and opiate addiction.

Management of opiate addiction in SCD

The most important first step in the management of opiate addiction is to recognize it. Recognition of opiate addiction is achieved by reference, for example, to the diagnostic criteria under the DSM-IV (*Diagnostic and Statistical Manual of Mental Disorders*, 4th edn of the American Psychiatric Association, or the ICD-10 (*International Classification of Diseases*, 10th revision, World Health Organization).

The addiction syndrome is likely if you observe three or more of the following in the patient during a 12-month period:
- The substance is often taken in larger amounts or over longer periods than intended.
- Persistent desire or unsuccessful efforts to cut down or control the use of the substance.
- A great deal of time is spent in activities necessary to obtain the substance, (e.g. visiting multiple doctors or driving long distances), use the substance (e.g. chain-smoking) or recover from its effects.
- Important social, occupational or recreational

activities are given up or reduced because of substance abuse.

• Continued substance use despite the knowledge of having a persistent or recurrent psychological or physical problem that is caused or exacerbated by the use of the substance.

• Tolerance, as defined by: need for larger amounts of the substance in order to achieve intoxification or desired effect; or markedly diminished effect with continued use of the same amount.

• Withdrawal, as manifested by either: characteristic withdrawal syndrome for the substance; or the same (or closely related) substance is taken to relieve or avoid withdrawal symptoms.

What can cause confusion is that SCD itself can cause similar experiences, so it is important to establish that what is observed has been caused by the use of the drug for purposes other than the relief of pain. The point is that while it is true that the bone pain crises in SCD tend to last only a few days, it is also known that bone infarction, joint disease caused by SCD and/or aseptic necrosis of bones can produce *chronic* severe pain and hence the need for long-term medication with opiates – and the likelihood of the emergence of phenomena which may be mistaken for addiction to opiates.

Individual treatment plan

In order to limit the room for such doubt, it is very useful for have an individual treatment plan for the patient, and to begin by documenting at least the following through the course of assessments:

• The year and age at which the patient was first exposed to opiates

• Types of analgesia used to treat acute pain crises

• Allergic reactions observed

• Reactions to the patient's drug of choice

• Evidence of tolerance and/or physical dependence

• Evidence of craving for the drug, going to great lengths to obtain it, or using it other than for pain relief

• The longest time without opiates

• Disruption of normal daily life because of the drug

• Presence of underlying psychological or psychiatric problems

• The patient's strategies for coping with the demands and challenges of everyday life

• The support mechanisms available to the patient.

The individual treatment plan also incorporates appropriate physical examinations and laboratory tests.

Once the diagnosis of opiate dependence is made, the patient should be offered the opportunity of detoxification in a specialist unit. If the patient happens to be one of those who require long-term treatment with opiates, such treatment should involve a dedicated specialist drug dependency service. The patient should aim to be opiate-free as an outpatient, and should be encouraged to agree to random urine and blood tests to check that they are still abstinent.

Prevention

While it is helpful to try to offer effective detoxification to the addicted patient, it is better to try to prevent the emergence of opiate addiction in the first place.

The commonest causes of dependence are:

1 inappropriate use of the stronger opiates for the relief of any pain, and

2 use of opiates for purposes other than pain relief.

The graded approach (analgesic ladder) to pain treatment should always be borne in mind. Less potent opioids should be tried first. When opiates are used, they should be tapered off and stopped as soon as the patient shows a significant degree of improvement. If a patient has shown dependence on a particular opiate in the past, that drug should not be used for the treatment of future pain crises, even if the patient requests it.

Last but not least, psychological approaches should always be part of the patient's overall support: relaxation, behavioural therapy (including cognitive behaviour therapy, CBT) where appropriate, general supportive psychotherapy (counselling) and continuing advice and education about the illness and its treatment.

Further reading

Anon. Sickle cell anaemia. In: *Encyclopaedia Britannica*. London: Encyclopoedia Britannica UK, 2002.

Davies S, Oni L. Fortnightly review: management of patients with sickle cell disease. *BMJ* 1997; **315**: 656–60.

Eckman J, Platt A. *Substance Abuse and Addiction*. Atlanta, GA: Georgia Sickle Cell Center, 1997.

McQuay H, Moore A, Justins D. Fortnightly review: treating acute pain in hospital. *BMJ* 1997; **314**: 1531

NIH. *Management and Therapy of Sickle Cell Disease*, 3rd edn. NIH Publication No. 95–2117. Revised December 1995. National Institutes of Health.

Pegelow C. Sickle cell anaemia. *eMedicine Journal* 2002; **3**: 23 July.

Chapter 22

The roles and functions of a community sickle cell and thalassaemia centre

C Rochester-Peart

Introduction

As the title suggests, this chapter is concerned with the roles and functions of *community*-based sickle cell and thalassaemia services. This chapter presents the reader with a range of activities that can be carried out from a community-based entity, and the benefits and challenges of delivering such services.

Being mindful of the title of the text, this chapter will offer the reader information for practical application, particularly for those who might be considering setting up similar services.

Given the very many possible meanings, it is contextually useful to clarify the meaning of the term 'community' and the term 'centre' as used in the title.

Firstly, taking the word *community,* it has many and varied meanings. *Collins Family English Dictionary* [1] states that it is a plural noun meaning: '1 all the people living in one district; 2 a group of people with shared origins or interests; 3 a group of countries with certain interest in common; 4 the public, society; 5 a group of interdependent plants and animals inhabiting the same region . . .'

The concepts of community are very many. It is a place, a physical location; a group, a sociological location; a certain structure, a cultural or environmental location.

All these meanings alluded to the notion of the plurality of the term giving a sense of shared and single or common interest to all concerned.

In health and social care parlance, the term refers to the setting in which health care is provided away from the busy hospital or acute environment. Non-hospital settings are generally the place in which patients or users reside, resulting in acute settings as distinct to community setting, hence the existence of two diverse but linked environments in which health care can be delivered. In this text the meaning most applicable is that which lends itself to the perception of the community as an area or locus away from the busy, overtly clinical hospital environment.

Turning to the term *centre, Collins Family English Dictionary* [1] gave different explanations to describe the meanings of the word 'centre' and stating its contextual meaning. It offered the following: '1 the middle point or part of something. 2 a place where a specified activity takes place. 3 a person or thing that is a focus of interest. 4 a place of activity or influence. 5 a political party or group that favours moderation. 6 a player who plays in the middle of the field rather than on a wing'. These descriptions point to the meaning as that which pertains to being the central focus. The most suitable meaning applicable to this text is the one given as 'a place where a specified activity takes place'.

Historical context

Screening for beta thalassaemia in the Mediterranean Basin is recognized as the initial experience of population screening for thalassaemia [2]. Population screening was achieved through the Greek Orthodox Church. As part of pre-marriage counselling and preparation the Church raised with the couples the issue of beta thalassaemia and directed them to undertake the necessary blood tests. The genetic significance of the couple's thalassaemic status was fully explained, alerting them to the physical, financial and emotional demands of caring for children with beta thalassaemia major. In particular, the issues of availability of blood for regular transfusion and the inherent costs of such vital, life-saving treatment were presented to couples. Here, we observe matters of physical health being addressed by a body that does not include matters of physical health as its prime duties.

Sickle cell centres emerged from the middle to the late 1970s in the USA [3]. They were the result of political legislation in the aftermath of racial unrest in the 1970s when charges of widespread racial discrimination extended to include the health of black people in the USA. The early centres existed to provide the African-American population with information on and opportunities for screening for sickle cell disease (SCD). The outcome of these centres was not as favourable as intended because of the mishandling of the screening programme. Namely, screening was not backed up by the provision of genetic counselling; without the provision of genetic counselling the success of the programmes was thwarted. Lessons learnt from this early mistake were applied in the establishment of subsequent centres and screening programmes. Such centres, located in hospitals as well as in the community, were mainly concerned with SCD. Increasingly as these centres developed, they not only addressed issues of SCD or thalassaemia, but also of all clinically important haemoglobin variants. In the UK, these centres have always provided services for all the haemoglobinopathies. As screening programmes continue to be implemented more clinically important haemoglobin variants are being described; thus adding to the work of the centres. In this text all references to sickle cell and thalassaemia centres include other haemoglobin variants that cause disease.

Setting, staffing and design

The rationale for the delivery of community-based health-care services for SCD, thalassaemia and other haemoglobinopathies is similar to that for other medical conditions, and includes the following:

1 Local or disease-needs driven
2 Government directives
3 Health promotion issues.

Most people in a community will not be in need of acute medical interventions; however, a significant number will have need for some interaction with health-care facilities. This point is demonstrated in some of the health awareness campaigns such as anti-smoking, breast and prostate cancer screening, healthy heart, diabetes and other high profile health drives. Health interventions in the primary care settings are aimed at reducing the populations' dependency on acute care. The old adage 'prevention is better than cure' is very true of the principles of community-based health services. There is continual change in the relationship between individuals in the community as a whole and the care settings. The change pertains to the increasing proportion of health-care activities delivered in the community environment. Sickle cell and thalassaemia centres are sited in various locations in the community; some are within existing health-care buildings, others are free-standing entities. Many centres evolved from short-term funded projects; some services survived and became part of the National Health Service (NHS), others were deemed to be non-viable and did not receive further financial support.

Today in the UK, sickle cell and thalassaemia centres are largely mainstream-funded, as part of the NHS. Initially most were funded as projects with limitations on their operational status in terms of their capacity as well as the length of time for which the services were guaranteed. The design and staffing of these services are interdependent and usually rely on the local needs and funding arrangements. Centres that started as NHS-supported projects have tended to become established core services. These centres are mainly staffed by specialist nurses and managed as nurse-led services within the NHS organizational structures. The more comprehensive services are staffed by multidisciplinary teams, including nurses, doctors, psychologists, counsellors and social workers. These disciplines form various models of service design, some involving partnerships with government and non-government agencies. The centres provide a range of services, with some services being more comprehensive than others. The range of service provision is determined primarily by the local demography and includes haemoglobinopathy screening, genetic counselling, psychological support, facilitation and co-ordination of community care.

Roles and functions of a sickle cell and thalassaemia centre

In the community, the multifaceted roles of the sickle cell and thalassaemia centres can be accounted for as: an identifiable local resource for information; a one-stop shop for the specialism, linking with key personnel in the field; a means of bridging the interface between acute care centres and the community. The activities of centres are concerned with haemoglobinopathy screening and genetic counselling, psychological support, facilitation and co-ordination of community care, health advice and support, user involvement, health promotion, and training and collaborative research.

Haemoglobinopathy screening and genetic counselling

Sickle cell and thalassaemia centres take blood samples, or arrange for such sampling, from individuals who need to be tested for haemoglobin variants and thalassaemia. The blood samples are sent to haematology laboratories for testing. Screening must be appreciated as a method of identifying most clinically important haemoglobin variants and thalassaemias, with diagnostic limitation. Therefore requests for further blood samples could be made if definitive diagnosis is required. Genetic counselling is described by Clarke [4] as 'what happens when an individual, a couple or family asks questions of a health professional (the genetic counsellor) about a medical condition or disease that is or may be of genetic origin'. It is good practice to conduct pre-screening genetic counselling as well as post-screening counselling, which includes offering written information for later reference. A core factor in this process is the provision of specific details about the condition and the genetic significance of the identified variant; exploring the various reproductive options. Genetic counselling sessions are conducted in a non-directive manner, helping individuals or couples to make the best possible decisions suitable for them.

In the UK, the pending NHS Haemoglobinopathy Screening Programme acts as a lever for awareness among health professionals. Sickle cell and thalassaemia centres have played and will continue to play a significant role as a resource in the planning and implementation of this programme.

Health promotion

The health promotion function of the sickle cell and thalassaemia centres has been a core activity since their emergence in the medical field; indeed for some centres health promotion backed up by screening and counselling is their only function.

Generally nurses have always held pivotal roles in health education and health promotion; they are key promoters of health. Health promotion has been the source of much debate. The World Health Organization (WHO) Constitution states that 'Health is a state of complete physical, mental and social well being; and not merely the absence of disease or infirmity' [5, 6]. Despite criticism of this definition [7, 8], it is accepted that health promotion involves the actions taken to prevent the population from becoming unnecessary users of acute care facilities. The WHO has expounded the ideals and principles of health promotion, and outlined strategies to attain this goal [9]. Community-based multidisciplinary entities such as sickle cell and thalassaemia centres are well placed to perform this function through joint initiatives between health and non-health professionals.

Health advice

The varied functions of sickle cell and thalassaemia centres allow the staff to gain a broad knowledge base of the possible clinical and social impact of these conditions. Services designed to interface with acute and primary care permit the staff to offer seamless care to individuals and families affected by SCD and thalassaemia. This arrangement provides grounding opportunities for staff, making them ideally positioned to act as advocates for individuals and their families. Contacts can be made either at the centres or in families' homes.

Psychological support

The need for psychological care in chronic illness has long been established. Psychological care can be delivered in different forms. Clients with sickling and thalassaemic conditions receive psychological input largely from specialist nurse counsellors and clinical psychologists with special interest in the field. This type of support seems to have the most effect on people's lives if provided from an early age.

Facilitation and co-ordination of community care

The multidisciplinary environment of a sickle cell and thalassaemia centre creates the opportunity for marshalling innovative care packages. The close proximity of the various disciplines enables traditional barriers to be broken down more easily. Health and social care delivery needs to reflect the constant changes occurring in today's communities and demands that professionals work closer together to provide services that put patients'/clients' needs at the heart of planning. Community-based nurses have a significant influence in this process.

User involvement

The involvement of users has gradually evolved into formal health service care structures. Currently there is a great push to establish firm systems and initiatives to better engage users in the provision of health and social care. There is a host of illness-related user groups and these are commonly employed to represent themselves and issues relating to their care, or range of their care, or about the quality of the services in general, or to assist in training of health and non-health professionals. Recently the NHS has been engaging users to inform the planning process in service developments. This particular approach in user involvement represents a cultural shift for health-care providers. It recognizes that active participation of users can lead to a better understanding of not only their needs but those of others. Increased

patient satisfaction and better compliance are other positive outcomes of this new relationship between providers and users of health services. A number of support groups for SCD and thalassaemia exist as single bodies in isolation. Others have close relationships with sickle cell and thalassaemia centres, while some have formal affiliation with larger, more recognized, non-governmental organizations.

Research and training

The UK Department of Health (1993) document *Research for Health* summarized the benefits of its research and development strategy [10]. The document promoted and demonstrated the value of an integrated approach in forming alliances in health research. In the UK, unlike the USA, there is no accountability for research attached to funding allocations. Therefore, researchers have been restricted in the number of funded projects they can undertake. Sickle cell and thalassaemia centres are well placed to participate in collaborative research. In the UK, in particular, there is a dearth of nurse-led research projects in this field. The staff of sickle cell and thalassaemia centres have a wealth of knowledge gained from their close working with the 'at-risk' and affected population, and therefore constitute a valuable teaching and training resource. They are able to offer training sessions to health and non-health professionals, as well as the lay public. A number of the present academically accredited haemoglobinopathy courses in the UK originated from the initial courses run by sickle cell and thalassaemia centres.

A model of a local comprehensive sickle cell and thalassaemia centre

There are various models of service design for sickle cell and thalassaemia centres (Fig. 22.1). An example is the local model of service delivery based at the South East London Sickle Cell and Thalassaemia Centre in Kennington, London. The centre is part of Lambeth Primary Care Trust and hosts this specialist service for the residents of Lambeth, Southwark and Lewisham (LSL). Due to local

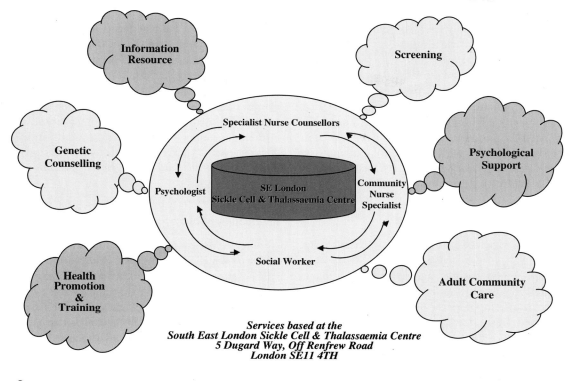

Fig. 22.1 The functions of a sickle cell and thalassaemia centre.

demographics these three boroughs collectively have the largest population of people with SCD in the UK [11], and small numbers of individuals with thalassaemia. The services (as listed above) provided in the centre are detailed below.

Haemoglobinopathy screening and genetic counselling

This is available either though direct referrals or the antenatal, neonatal and opportunist screening programmes. The genetic counselling to support these programmes for local residents is provided by specialist nurse counsellors (SNCs) based at the centre.

Antenatal screening programme:

• Women are screened comprehensively with their consent by midwives or practice nurses as part of antenatal booking sessions.

• The centre receives copies of all the results requiring counselling and follow-up.

• Women's addresses are received from GP surgeries and antenatal clinics in the local hospitals.

• Women are sent their results and invited for genetic counselling, with date and time of appointment sent at the same time as their results.

• Women who attend are counselled accordingly, partner screening is carried out or arranged for as soon as possible.

• Couples who have been confirmed as at risk of having children affected by sickling and thalassaemic conditions are asked to return for follow-up counselling.

• Women or couples requesting prenatal diagnosis are referred to their local Fetal Medicine Unit according to agreed local guidelines.

• GPs and midwives are sent reports of the outcome of each woman's appointment; this is particularly important for those who did not attend for counselling, as they need to be alerted to the genetic importance of the results.

Neonatal screening programme:
- All babies are screened using dried blood samples taken from the Guthrie card or 'heel spot tests' taken approximately 1 week after birth.
- The screening laboratory sends all results which have been confirmed as normal, sickle cell trait and haemoglobin C trait with the relevant explanatory leaflets, directly to mothers, GPs, the local community Child Health Register and the nursing staff at the centre.
- All results requiring follow-up are sent to the nursing staff at the centre.
- All repeat testings are initiated by the nursing staff (i.e. SNCs).
- Babies whose results suggest that they have inherited sickling or thalassaemic disorders are followed-up at home by the SNCs.
- Genetic and supportive counselling will be given to the parents of these children.
- Supportive counselling and health advice will be given continuously at their homes, at the outpatient clinics or at the centre.

These screening programmes are key core activities of the centre. Approximately 30 women are invited for genetic counselling each week. About 50 babies newly diagnosed as having SCD are followed up by the SNCs each year. Rochester-Peart [12] outlined the role of the specialist nurse in the community setting in providing support for clients with SCD and thalassaemia.

The opportunistic screening programme:
- Individuals may self-refer or may be referred by other health professionals including GPs, practice nurses, health visitors.
- Blood testing (venepuncture) is available with pre- and post-screening counselling conducted as an integral part of the process. Written evidence of clients' results is given to clients and with their approval to their GP.

Health promotion and training

Awareness of the haemoglobinopathies is promoted in various ways in the community. These include setting up manned and unmanned stalls at various locations, e.g. car parks of local markets and supermarkets, annual local county shows. Displays are set up at local libraries, schools and colleges (usually at their request) to link with their health promotion agenda. Talks are also given by centre staff to schools, colleges and various lay groups in the community. The annual Sickle Cell and Thalassaemia Awareness month occurs in July. This time of the year is a particularly busy period for centre staff as they fulfil their health promotional role.

Information resource

The centre holds information in various forms. There are leaflets containing information about carrier states, clinically important haemoglobin variants, and alpha and beta thalassaemia. There is a locally produced book prepared for parents caring for children with sickling conditions. Videos addressing both sickle cell and thalassaemia are available for viewing at the centre. The videos are also used by the SNCs as an additional tool for teaching parents spleen palpation.

Psychological care

Clients receive psychological care from the SNCs in the form of supportive counselling. Psychological counselling and other interventions are offered by psychologists based at the centre and in the local hospitals.

Adult community care

Co-ordination of community care for adults is provided by three community specialist nurses (CNS). Their roles are detailed in Chapter 23. In addition, the centre is involved with outreach work within primary care. A SNC currently conducts monthly genetic counselling sessions for patients screened by the practice nurse. The sessions are held at the GP's surgery, jointly with the practice nurse in attendance. Because of the geographical spread of the local area, through partnership arrangements the centre offers a satellite service at a health centre in the borough of Lewisham. The centre actively encourages the users to network through the formation of support groups. This is not core service activity but is an important aspect of supporting clients affected by these conditions. The centre works closely with voluntary organizations to ensure that clients receive appropriate support and assistance.

Benefits and challenges

There is much to gain from having a centre in the community serving the population at risk or affected by haemoglobinopathies. The design of the model described provides a seamless service between the neonatal screening programme and the paediatric follow-up and support by the SNCs. There is continuity of care and bridging of the hospital/community interface. The staff acquire a wealth of expertise. A multidisciplinary team approach aids in forging links and breaking down traditional professional barriers.

The challenges presented by providing services from sickle cell and thalassaemia centres broadly pertain to access and resources. The latter relates to funding, manpower and materials. Making the services accessible and appropriate in meeting the diverse needs of the client population is crucial. Improved accessibility will lead to improvement in health and reduces inequality. Access is not only concerned with the physical and geographical location of the actual building housing the services. Accessibility also encompasses clients' ability to read the necessary information related to their interaction with the service such as appointment letters, leaflets and interpreting. Other funding issues include salaries, materials, and 'tools of the trade', such as teaching and screening equipment. This has implications for the allocation of funds. Securing adequate funds could be difficult. Another challenge is staffing the service; determining the number of staff needed, their qualifications and grades.

Conclusions

This chapter provides some background information regarding the emergence of sickle cell and thalassaemia centres. In addition, the rationale for the various functions performed by the centres has been discussed. The expected increase in the number of births affected by haemoglobinopathies in the UK has implications for purchasers, providers and users of the health service. It behoves all care providers to maximize the use of available resources, and so provide appropriate care with utmost efficiency.

References

1. *Collins Family English Dictionary*. Glasgow: Harper Collins, 1999.
2. World Health Organization. *Guidelines for the Control of Haemoglobin Disorders*, Modell B, ed. WHO/HDP/GL/94.1, 1994
3. Anionwu EN, Atkin K. *History and Politics of Sickle Cell and Thalassaemia in the UK*. Buckingham: Open University Press, 2001.
4. Clarke A. *Genetic Counselling Practice and Principles*. London: Routledge, 1994.
5. World Health Organization. *Constitution*. Geneva: WHO, 1946.
6. Downie RS, Fyfe C, Tannahil A. *Health Promotion Models and Values*. Oxford: Oxford University Press, 1990.
7. Dubos R. *The Mirage of Health*. New York: Harper and Row, 1959.
8. Aggleton P. *Health*. London: Routledge, 1970.
9. World Health Organization. *Regional Strategy for Attaining Health for All by the Year 2000*. Copenhagen: WHO, 1981.
10. Department of Health. *Research for Health*. London: DOH, 1993.
11. Streetly A, Maxwell K, Mejia A. *Sickle Cell Disorders in Greater London – A Needs Assessment of Screening and Care Services*. The Fair Shares for London Report. Department of Public Health Medicine, United Medical and Dental Schools of Guy's & St Thomas' Hospitals, London, 1997.
12. Rochester-Peart C. Specialist nurse support for clients with blood disorders. *Nursing Times* 1997; **93**: 52–3.

Chapter 23

Community nursing care of adults with sickle cell disease and thalassaemia

Sadie Daley

Introduction

This chapter will provide an overview of community nursing care of adults with the sickle cell and thalassaemia disorders, from a community nurse specialist (CNS) approach. The CNS service is a recent addition to the services already provided for people who have sickle cell disease (SCD) and thalassaemia. The topics covered within this chapter are: looking at the creation of the CNS role; holistic nursing assessment; interprofessional working; the CNS as an educator; and achievements, benefits and lessons learnt.

The CNS team works across all sectors of the community, aiming to work closely with the key personnel who care for and support clients with haemoglobinopathies.

The role was developed following the outcome of the review *Beyond Crisis Management* [1], which looked at service provision for people with haemoglobinopathies living within the London boroughs of Lambeth, Southwark and Lewisham. The steering group consisted of representatives from service users and the acute, community and voluntary services, and the main findings were as follows:

- Underdevelopment of primary and community services for SCD and thalassaemia.
- Service provision focused on the acute sector.
- Minimal input/involvement from primary services.
- Disjointed services and poor community links between the acute sector and primary care (GPs, district nurses, practice nurses and midwives).
- Lack of awareness and knowledge of SCD and thalassaemia among local service providers (social services housing, health, voluntary sector).

- There were a small number of high service users (4+ admissions per year) from 3% of total affected population, but they accounted for 90% of hospital admissions within this client group.
- The adult population felt less supported.

These findings support the outcome of the Standing Medical Advisory Committee (SMAC) [2] and also the work of Maxwell and Streetly [3] in the study *Living with Sickle Pain*. As a result of the above findings the CNS service for adults and young people aged 16 years and over was created. For the service pathway see Fig. 23.1.

The CNS team works alongside the specialist nurse counsellors; there are clear boundaries between their roles and remit and these will be reviewed later in the chapter.

There are many definitions and titles for the role of specialist nurses. For the purposes of this chapter the author feels the following best illustrates our role.

CNSs are described as delivering expert patient care that is based on advanced nursing models with two main characteristics, clinical judgement and leadership [4].

The creation of the CNS service

Based at the South East London Sickle Cell and Thalassaemia centre (see Chapter 22) the CNS team provides a service to residents within the Lambeth, Southwark and Lewisham (LSL) boroughs. There are approximately 2500 people affected by sickle cell disorders and 100 people affected by thalassaemia living within these boroughs [1]. The boroughs have a rich cultural diversity, with one-third

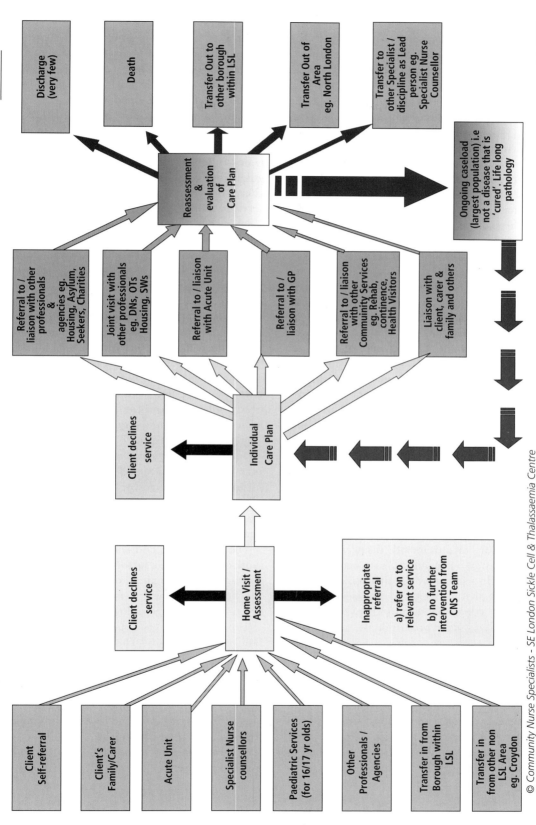

Enter Service

Exit Service

Client Self-referral

Client's Family/Carer

Acute Unit

Specialist Nurse counsellors

Paediatric Services (for 16/17 yr olds)

Other Professionals / Agencies

Transfer in from Borough within LSL

Transfer in from other non LSL Area eg. Croydon

Client declines service

Home Visit / Assessment

Inappropriate referral

a) refer on to relevant service

b) no further intervention from CNS Team

Client declines service

Individual Care Plan

Ongoing caseload (largest population) i.e not a disease that is 'cured'. Life long pathology

Referral to / liaison with other professionals & agencies eg. Housing, Asylum, Seekers, Charities

Joint visit with other professionals eg. DNs, OTs Housing, SWs

Referral to / liaison with Acute Unit

Referral to / liaison with GP

Referral to / liaison with other Community Services eg. Rehab, continence, Health Visitors

Liaison with client, carer & family and others

Reassessment & evaluation of Care Plan

Discharge (very few)

Death

Transfer Out to other borough within LSL

Transfer Out of Area eg. North London

Transfer to other Specialist / discipline as Lead person eg. Specialist Nurse Counsellor

© *Community Nurse Specialists - SE London Sickle Cell & Thalassaemia Centre*

July 2002

Fig. 23.1 Community Nurse Specialist team: sickle cell and thalassaemia service pathway. LSL: Lambeth, Southwark and Lewisham Boroughs; CNS: Community Nurse Specialist; Rehab: Rehabilitation; DN: District Nurse; OT: Occupational Therapist; SW: Social Worker; GP: General (Medical) Practitioner.

of the population of each borough made up of black and minority ethnic people [5].

Lambeth, Southwark and Lewisham have areas of affluence alongside pockets of deprivation, which the Health Authority has identified as being within the 20% most economically deprived nationally [5], it has identified sickle cell disorders and thalassaemia as a key health priority.

Interventions recommended by the Health Authority and the Local Modernisation Review in response to the NHS Plan (2000) [6] include reducing inequalities and improving access to service provision, through culturally appropriate primary care services and interpreting services, which are based on consistently high standards of care.

Haemoglobinopathies have for the first time been addressed by a government within the NHS Plan (2000) [6], with the rolling out of universal screening across the UK. These policies are driving our service delivery, along with clinical governance, which is now the foundation on which all NHS care is delivered. Elements such as the National Service Frameworks, benchmarking and lifelong learning are the strategies for improving client and service outcomes in the most cost-effective way. This can be seen through the development of national nursing guidelines for SCD and thalassaemia through the Haemoglobinopathy Association of Counsellors (THAC), a professional body for practitioners working within the haemoglobinopathy field.

There has been a growth of specialist nurses in most areas of health care within the NHS over the last decade. Various authors [7–9] have indicated that the reasons for this include the need to fill the gap between staff nurses and nurse managers with a highly skilled nurse; the reduction of junior doctors' hours alongside role extension of nurses and areas where role confusion occurs between nurses and other health-care professionals, particularly doctors.

As stated earlier in the chapter the CNSs have a different role to their colleagues, the specialist nurse counsellors (Chapter 24), CNSs do not carry out genetic screening or counselling. The premise of their referrals is that a physical nursing need has been identified, e.g. coping with complex pain, chronic leg ulcer management, complications of avascular necrosis of a joint (see section below on the holistic nursing assessment). If there are occasional instances where the roles overlap, liaison between the two nurses and, if needed a joint visit, is undertaken to establish which specialist is best placed to lead for that individual case.

Being based at the centre has afforded the CNS and SNC teams excellent channels of communication and involvement in the centre activities. Both teams collaborate on joint initiatives and referral guidelines were developed to prevent role confusion in the acute and primary sectors when the new service was introduced.

It was felt from the inception of these posts that the CNS service would be modelled on other CNS teams found within the mainstream health services, e.g. diabetic, multiple sclerosis and HIV teams. This approach was felt to be crucial for working towards inclusion into the mainstream services, as many clients or staff can feel marginalized [10].

There are aspects of care that can be managed within the mainstream services with the initial support of the CNS and the wider haemoglobinopathy team. This will have a twofold benefit; for example, clients with leg ulcers can attend leg ulcer or complex wound management clinics run by either district nurses or community tissue viability nurses. Health professionals can build up their knowledge and skill base of these disorders to achieve best practice and improved patient outcomes. Secondly, inclusion is promoted by the opportunity to link with organizations and voluntary bodies known to mainstream services, helping to reduce isolation and increase social contacts.

The CNS works and consults with a wide network of agencies and sectors within the community and acute sector to attain optimum quality of care for clients. This requires interprofessional working and finely tuned negotiating skills.

The CNS also serves as an advocate for the client, family or community. The main goals are to improve the quality of life for clients, identify gaps in service provision, help to implement government policies with the wider team in the most cost-effective way and to improve knowledge of these disorders through education and research programmes for all sectors of the community.

The nine sub-roles of the CNS are:

• Clinical expert

- Researcher
- Consultant
- Educator
- Change agent
- Staff advocate
- Collaborator
- Networker
- Organizational developer. (Adapted from Martin [11] and Miller [12].)

Liaising with the GP and primary services is an all-important role. The GP is ideally placed to manage the day-to-day care of these clients, collaborating with the acute sector as appropriate. The aim is to prevent reports by clients, for example, of being sent to the Accident and Emergency Department with urinary tract infections or attending outpatient departments for prophylactic immunizations. Many GPs welcome an expert resource to help them become more central in the day-to-day management of clients with these disorders [1]. The holistic nursing assessment and interprofessional sections of this chapter will demonstrate how the role of the GP and primary care services can best support these client groups.

Holistic nursing assessment

The CNS identifies issues for individual clients by undertaking a holistic needs assessment within the home environment. The holistic assessment comprises not just physical but emotional, social and pastoral aspects. In partnership they can plan what services are needed for this episode of care and how the client can develop effective coping strategies, with input from the relevant services.

This is a continuous process with actions and feedback between the CNS and the client [13]. The information obtained needs to be accurate and comprehensive, as this will have an important bearing on the decision-making process for the nurse and thus affect outcomes.

It is vital that the assessment process occurs from a non-judgemental approach [14]. For this to happen the CNS has to be aware of his or her own attitudes, beliefs and values. This is to ensure that the nurse does not impose their personal views on the client, otherwise important information or subtle behaviour from the client may be missed, losing the opportunity to identify issues or give much needed health-enhancing information.

Communication skills are essential for this part of the nurse's role. These include verbal and non-verbal skills and active listening based on empathy. This is necessary so that the client can see that the nurse understands their 'world'. Egan [15] suggests that the 'helper' needs to develop a warm relationship to enable the client to explore 'the problem' from the client's frame of reference and then to focus on specific concerns.

There is a different emphasis on the delivery of care in the hospital and within a client's home. The CNS has been invited into the client's personal space. The power base shifts and a partnership needs to occur. Failure to take these elements into consideration may prevent the nurse from engaging with the client or may limit subsequent nursing interventions.

The initial assessment/visit may reveal a range of issues or problems. Well-developed information collecting skills are needed to gradually build up a picture of the client's haemoglobinopathy disorder and the positive or negative impact this has had on their lives [16]. Some clients need time to build up a rapport with the CNS, which is based on trust. An explorative, empathetic and respectful approach will support this process.

For quality interaction to occur, the CNS's framework of practice needs to include a transcultural understanding of the client. Leininger [17] believed that nurses have a duty to gain knowledge about cultural care values, beliefs and practices and use this to provide culturally specific care for well and sick people.

Respect for different cultural practices is essential, indeed becoming aware of different cultural practices is an ideal time to enquire sensitively and openly to gain more understanding of a client and community group. This will lead to a store of rich information, which will improve the CNSs' approach to clients and therefore their practice.

Cultural, social, political and economic factors influence the impact of SCD and thalassaemia on clients' lives. Ignoring this context will lead to incomplete collection of information and therefore inappropriate care leading to increased stress, isolation and poorer access to health care for the client [18, 19].

Thus the nursing assessment is undertaken through a framework of eclectic nursing processes [20, 21]. This ensures a holistic plan of care for the clients, which is delivered in partnership within the context of their lives (see Table 23.1).

The nature of assessment is often complex; chronic conditions usually involve change at some stage. This affects not just the client but the family and/or caregiver. It is therefore important to assess the carer's needs alongside the client.

The important principles of a holistic nursing assessment are [22]:
• Sufficient time.
• Client-centred rather than professionally defined assessment process.
• Liaising with and obtaining relevant information from health professionals and other agencies with respect to confidentiality.
• A suitable balance of interprofessional team and specialist assessment.
• The significance of reflective practice within assessment.
• Promoting independence.
• The link between assessment, action, outcomes and evaluation.

There are clients who are well supported with good social networks. However, there are those for whom social isolation is the lived experience. In fact social isolation is one of the most important aspects of chronic illness that the CNS needs to address, as it not only impacts on the client's social network, but it can also lead to depression and even suicide [23].

We must not forget that the majority of clients with these disorders are living full and productive lives despite having an unpredictable and chronic illness, although health professionals continue to be confounded by the wide-ranging variation in the

Services involved with the client	Name, address, designation, department, telephone, email and fax details
Initial assessment	Brief medical history, review referral information, family history, social history and family support, emotional assessment, understanding of the disorder, accommodation, occupation
Medical history	Review systems and organs of the body – neurological, eyes, pulmonary, cardiac, liver/gall bladder, bones/joints, leg ulcers, priapism, renal, sexual development, genetic counselling referral needed? Transfusion programme, iron overloaded, nutritional problems. More than 4 admissions for painful crisis yearly
General health screen	Ophthalmology screen, dental check, breast and cervical screening, prophylactic immunization programme – Pneumovax, Hib, meningococcal, flu vaccine, hepatitis B
Nursing care plan	Date, problem/need, action/management plan, evaluation dates, date resolved, reviews, record keeping (Trust policy followed)
Pain assessment chart	May include verbal and numerical rating scales, body diagrams, list of medication (prescribed and over-the-counter), traditional cultural remedies, pattern of using these (analgesic ladder, pharmacological understanding), non-pharmacological strategies (e.g. aromatherapy, transcutaneous nerve stimulation (TENS), stress management)
Documentation from other agencies	Referrals, reports and investigations and correspondence

Table 23.1 Areas to include in a holistic nursing assessment

disease process between clients and siblings who have the same genotype.

Following the holistic nursing assessment, liaison and referrals to other services usually occurs. This will include social workers, physiotherapists and district nurses (see the section on interprofessional working).

Pain is one of the most under-treated symptoms in both primary care and the acute sector. Approximately 40% of clients present to their GP with unresolved pain [24, 25]. There are many elements to the experience of pain – physiological, psychological, behavioural, motivational, affective and environmental factors – which can make the assessment complex [26].

The role of the CNS is to assess the nature of the pain, ideally within the home environment. The fear of the unpredictable onset and severity of pain is understandably common with SCD clients and can lead to difficulties in coping [27, 28].

A pain assessment tool is crucial to measure and obtain quality information about the type of pain experienced and should include the:

- Site
- Intensity
- Aggravators
- Nature (acute or chronic)
- Frequency and duration
- Analgesia prescribed or purchased over the counter
- Alternative therapies used.

The advantage of undertaking this pain assessment in the home is that the CNS can see what could be contributing to the frequency and/or severity of painful episodes and how the client handles this within their own environment. Realistic suggestions and solutions can then be discussed with the client (see Chapter 8 for pain management).

It is vital to liaise with both the hospital haematology team and the GP to ensure that care, information and advice are consistent. A severe crisis will usually lead to hospitalization and either subcutaneous or intravenous opiates. This will require careful reduction back down the analgesic ladder, to prevent withdrawal symptoms, as a substantial number of clients return to A&E departments within 24–48 hours experiencing withdrawal pains, which have triggered another painful occlusive cri-

sis [29]. Involving the pain team, for expert advice and support for both client and staff for treating complex pain, is highly advantageous.

Discharge planning for clients with complex medical issues is vital from the day of admission to ensure that the necessary professionals or agencies are involved. This will ensure the client has the support and services needed to continue with recovery once home. Recuperation may take weeks following a severe painful crisis. Therefore when the client has been discharged, the GP and CNS can play a significant role in helping clients to cope within their homes, by ensuring that the most suitable analgesia is prescribed during uncomplicated mild to moderate painful crises. Also, conducting home visits and consultations in the GP surgery can prevent inappropriate visits to the hospital. This is of course, in addition to the numerous services available from within the GP practice, for example, the district nursing service. The CNS can provide the GP with specialist knowledge and support to help create that all-important seamless link between home, community and hospital services.

Interprofessional liaison

Interprofessional, teamwork and collaboration are terms used to explain professionals or agencies working together. There are many examples of this, from multidisciplinary clinical guidelines to child protection and elder abuse procedures/protocols. Ross and MacKenzie [22] looked at the link between developing policies for interprofessional work in primary health care and how these ideas were reflected in practice. They found confusion of the meaning and relationship between collaboration at an interagency, interprofessional and interpersonal level, and multidisciplinary working. The latter shows the range and quantity of different disciplines, whereas the former describes interactive working. The term collaboration allows for different levels of working together and does not exclude participation by the service user [30].

The CNS frequently collaborates with the following disciplines:

- Specialist nurse counsellors
- Primary health care team – GP, practice nurse,

nurse practitioner, district nurse, midwife and health visitor

- Community physiotherapists
- Community occupational therapists
- Acute sector
- Psychology services
- Adult disability teams
- Visual and hearing impairment teams
- Social workers
- Housing officers
- Local Authority workers – home helpers, advocates and meals-on-wheels service
- Voluntary services
- Professional bodies
- Colleges and universities
- Rehabilitation centres
- Alternative therapists.

Government policies place the client at the centre of care and services. This is vital to ensure that new ways of care provision are meaningful and inclusive. For interprofessional teams to work common organizational objectives are needed. Jones [31] suggests that the concept of interprofessional teams would be more understood in the context of the task it is performing. This will then define the outcome, for example, professionals providing terminal care at home would be able to define the objectives, individual roles and contribution and the agreed measure of outcomes. The CNS has a pivotal role in interprofessional working for this client group.

An understanding and respect of each discipline or team member's role and remit and contribution to the work of the team will have benefits for the client, professionals and their organizations [32]. Interprofessional working carries the risk of excluding the views of the service user. Brigewatt [33] stressed the need for teams to practise person-centred decision making to avoid this, believing the needs of clients with chronic condition to be fundamentally different from other clients. The range of services, systems and personnel delivering long-term care creates a complex support system. Therefore a person-centred decision-making approach means that the client is involved in all the decisions about their ongoing care. This is also likely to ensure the best possible outcome of interventions and to improve compliance with difficult or complex treatments.

Following the holistic nursing assessment the CNS needs to work collaboratively with other professionals, including:

- **The GP and primary services.** The CNS liaises to enable clear lines of communication to increase the knowledge base and provide specialist advice and information to support these services in caring for clients within the community. This includes attending primary health-care team meetings and offering training and information packs, ideally in conjunction with representatives from other teams within the haemoglobinopathy service. Regular meetings with the GP should take place to look at any issues for individual clients or to update their care plans.

- **Specialist social workers** for haemoglobinopathies have made significant improvements to the social and economic aspects of clients' lives. Duties include arranging for practical help to help maintain and run a home, and support for carrying out the activities of daily living. Shopping services and taxi schemes all contribute to a client being able to live independently. A social worker's depth of knowledge and links with government departments, and organizations in the statutory and voluntary sectors mean that the CNS can get the relevant advice and information when needed.

- **A psychologist/counsellor** can provide excellent support for clients coming to terms with unresolved issues around having a lifelong disorder. Living with a chronic condition, experiencing unpredictable episodes of pain and possible isolation can be daunting. Timely liaison and referral can have a positive life-changing effect. The CNS can support the psychologist by reinforcing positive attempts by the client to improve his or her coping strategies.

- **Housing officers.** Local Authority, Housing Association and private landlords need to be aware that inadequate housing can exacerbate the complications of these disorders. Centrally heated homes, with flats not above the first floor, are recommended. It may be necessary to provide a medical/nursing report from the community perspective to help secure appropriate accommodation.

- **Community physiotherapists** can visit homes, performing and teaching appropriate exercises to clients for reduction of chronic pain or to rehabilitate limbs or joints.

- **Community occupational therapists** within

Local Authority social services departments will undertake joint visits with the CNS to assess the client's home for safety and practical functions; indicating where equipment and adaptations should be installed. Providing information on the chronic progression of the disorders is usually extremely useful.

• **Speech and language therapists** (SALT) will assess and help the client to improve clarity of speech when dysphagia occurs as a result of stroke.
• **The community wheelchair and walking aid service** will provide a yearly check for safety and suitability of wheelchairs and walking aids. It has been known for wheelchair-bound clients not to receive this review for many years.

The acute sector has a small core of high service users inappropriately attending the Accident and Emergency Department. Maxwell and Streetly [3] have shown that adult coping strategies and locus of control are influenced by the parent/family's approach to painful occlusive crises during childhood. The amount of involvement the child had in decision-making is also important. The CNS can play an important role in working with the wider teams to help break the cycle of the largely psychological dependence on hospitals.

The follow-up of non-attenders at the outpatient department is useful. These clients may not be aware of the benefits of regular reviews and the detection of the silent sickling process, which results in damage to soft and bony tissue. By attending multidisciplinary team meetings within the haematology departments, pre-discharge planning meetings and ward rounds, the CNS will help to facilitate all-round quality care.

The CNS should endeavour to attend the relevant special interest groups, e.g. the Stroke group, which is open to all disciplines and where the latest research and government guidelines are discussed. Attendance also raises the awareness of these conditions when working parties are created to formulate Trust guidelines.

The community nurse as an educator

The CNS has education of both clients, health professionals and all sectors of the community as a fundamental role to enable clients to change lifestyle behaviours if needed, and to manage their chronic condition, leading ultimately to social change, improved health service provision and delivery of care.

Effective education can help to empower clients. Saarman *et al.* [34] believe that a behaviour change as a result of giving education on its own is not effective. Once the client is given health-enhancing information they need to act on this. Therefore learning about the need, becoming motivated and building effective coping strategies necessary to support the change needs to occur. The making and sustaining of that change should be the aim of the CNS.

Education should also target carriers of the disorders and the wider community. Dyson [35] looked at the knowledge level of sickle cell in a screened population. He found no significant differences in levels of sickle cell awareness between carriers and non-carriers. Inheritance patterns and the minority ethnic groups who carry the sickle cell trait were least understood. He stressed the considerable demand for written literature and further counselling but felt that screening on its own did not raise levels of knowledge.

There is a need to ascertain the gaps in knowledge and the type of information that clients want. Bird *et al.* [36] looked at education materials for clients through literature provided by health professionals working in the haematology field. The results showed that materials about client behaviour and psychosocial issues were often unavailable or unsatisfactory, compared with information about the disease process and treatment. They also found no published evaluation of client or parental education within this population. This suggests that there need to be regular reviews of health promotional content, methods, targeting, access and evaluation. Ideally this should occur in collaboration with the service users and agencies involved in client care. Access to health promotion literature is poor for clients or communities who are non-English speaking. Interpreting and translating services should be working with the haemoglobinopathy service to identify common local dialects and set up information sessions with an interpreter and language-appropriate literature with pictorial information for those who may speak several dialects but not read them.

Compliance with difficult treatments can be greatly improved through knowledge about the importance of the treatment. Atkin and Ahmad [18] studied teenagers who needed to use the Desferal pump. Many felt that knowledge about consequences of non-compliance instead of being told 'the treatment is important' would be much better understood and more effective. This is obviously just part of the multifactorial problem of compliance, particularly in this age group. Other chronic conditions such as diabetes and cystic fibrosis also face these challenges [37].

Educating health professionals and other agencies of care about sickle cell and thalassaemia is a massive task but needs to be consistently addressed. Apart from the core body of information, the level and content will be different for each agency. The CNS team provides education through seminars, lectures, conferences, workshops and in-house training and will be developing information packs for each local agency to support learning outcomes. This often occurs in partnership with the wider haemoglobinopathy team. Those health professionals practising within areas that have a higher incidence of sickle cell and thalassaemia disorders should have mandatory training. The SMAC report [2] showed that there was minimal information in the nursing and medical curricula. This is also supported by findings in a study by Thomas et al. [38] on health professionals' education needs in LSL.

Support groups and client forums provide support, advice and information about these conditions and often link up with their nearest sickle cell and thalassaemia centre staff, ensuring acceptance as well as empathy. Client forums are vital as a platform for clients to voice gaps in service provision or how services may be more effectively provided.

The Expert Patient Programme initiated by the Department of Health [39] is an exciting move towards a natural progression of roles that support groups and client forums undertake. The programme will enable patients to develop their knowledge of their chronic condition to a level that enables self-management within the medical regime. This means a fundamental shift in the way that chronic disorders are managed. Many com-

mon issues such as pain management, stress and the need to develop coping skills affect most chronically ill patients. In Coventry [39] the Multiple Sclerosis Self Management Programme run by tutors who have MS showed benefits of:

- Reduced severity of symptoms
- Significant decrease in pain
- Improved life control and activity
- Improved resourcefulness and life satisfaction.

Indeed, the task force set up to take this forward led by the government's Chief Medical Officer included the Director of the Sickle Cell Society.

Benefits, achievements and lessons learnt

The CNS service has received verbal and written anecdotal evidence from both clients and staff suggesting that effective practice is occurring, although an independent consultant will be evaluating the service in the very near future.

Being borough-focused has allowed the CNS to build up effective working relationships, knowledge of the area and maximum use of the local resources. Weekly contact with hospital staff provides clear lines of communication and support for ward personnel. This brings a much needed multidimensional view of the client.

A survey on the influence of health needs assessment on health-care decision making in London Health Authorities showed that a needs assessment was more likely to lead to policy action when the priority was revealed through the analysis of local data or through focusing the needs assessment on specific issues of local relevance [40].

The following case study illustrates the work of the CNS within SCD and thalassaemia.

Case study

Winston is a 33-year-old single man with homozygous (HbSS) SCD who was referred to the CNS service by hospital staff. His issues were as follows:

- Frequent episodes of acute painful occlusive sickle cell crises with monthly admissions to hospital
- Bilateral leg ulcers with chronic pain
- Past medical history of acute chest syndrome

- Anxiety attacks
- Isolation and depression
- Living in a cold flat with no seating
- Welfare benefit problems.

Following a holistic assessment within the home the CNS referred Winston to the district nursing service (DN) for leg ulcer dressings to be carried out at home (three times per week). The CNS and DN visited to review him together every 3 months. Winston was referred to the clinical psychologist for support and was offered a course of cognitive behavioural therapy (CBT), which he accepted. Another referral was made to the specialist social worker for sickle cell/thalassaemia. A care package was agreed which provided Winston with meals on wheels 3 days per week, and weekly attendance at a resource centre for learning computer skills. The welfare benefits were sorted out and funding was obtained through a charitable organization to purchase seating. Winston's housing needs were discussed with a social housing provider. A purpose-built groundfloor flat with central heating was identified. Winston was nominated and was successful. The CNS organizes 6-monthly planning meetings with Winston and key professionals, and multidisciplinary team meetings when appropriate, to review his care and discuss any further issues.

This case illustrates how complex the issues associated with SCD can be.

Conclusion

This chapter has given an overview of the way a CNS service can support clients alongside their colleagues within the haematology team. The focus is much more mainstream than a disease specialism, which has enabled a more inclusive service for an already marginalized group. It is accepted that there will be areas of care that will need to remain specialist; the key is to have that broad outlook so that these opportunities are not missed.

It is hoped that the areas of care described have also shown that the CNS service is ideally placed to help identify the gaps in care and bridge the gap between primary, community and acute sectors. Working within the community and clients' homes means being at the interface of care, a privileged po-

sition. Views 'on the ground' are often shared with the team and can contribute to possible solutions as stakeholders continue to work on improving patient care and outcomes.

The roles of the CNS as a change agent, educator, consultant, researcher, information resource and networker demonstrate the breadth of nursing care involved in working with client groups who have chronic disorders. Continuity of care occurs as the CNS acts as a pivotal point. It is hoped that this chapter has enabled other health and community personnel to look at the scope of practice, which is needed, and can be provided by a CNS.

Acknowledgements

My thanks go to Joan Walters, Marvelle Brown, and my colleagues Vivienne James and Ibrahim Momoh for their advice and support.

References

1. Lambeth, Southwark and Lewisham Sickle Cell Steering Group, Report 1. *Beyond Crisis Management: Living with Sickle Cell Disease in South East London*. London: LSLHA, 1999.
2. Standing Medical Advisory Committee (SMAC). *Report on Sickle Cell, Thalassaemia and other Haemoglobinopathies*. London: The Stationary Office, 1993.
3. Maxwell K, Streetly A. *Living with Sickle Pain*. London: Guy's King's & St Thomas' School of Medicine, Department of Public Health Sciences, 1999.
4. Spross JA, Baggerly J. Models of advanced nursing. In: Harnic AB, Spross JA, eds. *The Clinical Nurse Specialist in Theory and Practice*. Philadelphia, Saunders, 1989.
5. Lambeth, Southwark and Lewisham Health Authority. *Annual Report of the Director of Public Health*. London: LSLHA, 2001/2002.
6. Department of Health. *The NHS Plan*. London: The Stationary Office, 2000.
7. Felder L. Direct patient care and independent practice. In: Hamric A, Spross J, eds. *The Clinical Nurse Specialist in Theory and Practice*. Orlando, FL: Grune and Stratton, 1983.
8. Head S. Nurse practitioners: the new pioneers. *Nursing Times* 1988; **84**: 27–8.
9. Bowman G, Thompson D. When is a specialist not a specialist? *Nursing Times* 1990; **86**: 48.
10. Anionwu E, Atkin K. *The Politics of Sickle Cell and Thalassaemia*. Buckingham: Open University Press, 2001.

11. Martin P. An exploration of the services provided by the CNS within one NHS Trust. *J Nurs Manage* 1999; 7: 149–56.

12. Miller L. The clinical nurse specialist: a way forward? *J Adv Nurs* 1995; 22: 494–501.

13. Cowley S, Bergan A, Young K, Kavanagh A. The changing nature of needs assessment in primary health care; cited in Bryans A, McIntosh J. *J Adv Nurs* 1996; 24: 24–30.

14. Nursing and Midwifery Council (2002) *Code of Professional Conduct*. London, NMC.

15. Egan G. *The Skilled Helper: A Systematic Approach to Effective Helping*, 4th edn. Brookes/Cole Publishing, 1992.

16. Kleinmuntz D. Cognitive heuristics and feedback in a dynamic decision environment. *Management Sci* 1985; 31: 680–702.

17. Leininger M. Culture Care Theory: a major contribution to advance transcultural nursing knowledge and practices. *J Transcultural Nurs* 2002; 13: 189–92.

18. Atkin K, Ahmad WIU. Pumping iron: compliance with chelation therapy among young people who have thalassaemia major. *Sociol Health Illness* 2000; 22: 500–24.

19. Ahmad WIU. *Race and Health in Contemporary Britain*. Buckingham: Open University Press, 1993.

20. Roper N, Logan W, Tierney A. *The Elements of Nursing*. Edinburgh: Churchill Livingstone, 1980.

21. Orem D. *Nursing Concepts of Practice*, New York: McGraw-Hill, 1985.

22. Ross F, Mackenzie A. *Nursing in Primary Health Care: Policy into Practice*. New York: Routledge, 1996.

23. Lubkin IM, Larsen PD. *Chronic Illness: Impact and Interventions*, 5th edn. Massachuetts: Jones & Bartlett Publishers, 2002.

24. Manytyselka P, Kumpusalo E, Ahonen R. Pain as a reason to visit the doctor. A Finnish study in primary health care. *Pain* 2001; 89: 175–80.

25. McHugh J, Thomas J. Patient satisfaction with chronic pain management. *Nurs Standard* 2001; 51: 33–8.

26. Woods S. Pain. [Special Focus.] *Nurs Times* 2002; 98: 41–4.

27. Glenview I. *APS Clinical Guideline Practice no 1*. American Pain Society (APS), 1999.

28. Ballas S. Treatment of pain in adults with sickle cell disease. *Am J Hematol* 1990; 34: 49–54.

29. Thomas V, Westerdale N. *Br J Commun Health Nurs* 1996; 1: 466–71.

30. Gregson B, Cartlidge A, Bond J. Interprofessional collaboration in primary health care organizations. Occasional paper no. 52. In: Owens P, Carrier J, Horder J. *Interprofessional Issues in Community and Primary Health Care*. Wiltshire: MacMillan, 1995.

31. Jones R. Teamwork in primary care: how much do we know about it? *J Interprof Care* 1992; 6: 24–9.

32. Hennermann E, Lee J, Cohen J. Collaboration: a concept analysis. *J Adv Nurs* 1995; 21: 103–9.

33. Bringewatt R. Integrating care for people with chronic conditions. *Creative Nurs* 1996; 2: 7–9.

34. Saarmann L, Daugherty J, Reigel B. Patient teaching to promote behavioural change. *Nurs Outlook* 2000; 48: 281–7.

35. Dyson S. Knowledge of sickle-cell in a screened population. *Health Social Care Commun* 1997; 5: 84–93.

36. Bird S, Earp J, Drezner S, Cooper H. Patient education for sickle cell disease: a national survey of health care professionals. *Health Educ Res* 1994; 9: 235–42.

37. Geiss S, Hobbs S, Hammersley-Maercklein G, Kramer J, Henley M. Pyschosocial factors related to perceived compliance with cystic fibrosis treatment. *J Clin Psychol* 1992; 48: 99–103.

38. Thomas NV, Cohn PJ, Wilson Barnett J *et al*. *Lambeth, Southwark & Lewisham Health Authority review of haemoglobinopathy training among professionals working in acute care, primary care, education, social services, housing and voluntary sector*. Internal Report. London: LSLHA, 2001.

39. Department of Health. *The Expert Patient: A New Approach to Chronic Disease Management for the 21st Century*. London: The Stationary Office, 2001.

40. Hensher M, Fulop N. The influence of health needs assessment on healthcare decision-making in London health authorities. *J Health Serv Res Unit* 1999; 4: 90–5.

Further reading

Atkin K, Waqar I, Anionwu A. Service support to families caring for a child with a sickle cell disorder or beta thalassaemia major: parents' perspectives. In: Ahmad W, ed. *Ethnicity, Disability and Chronic illness*. Buckingham: Open University Press, 2000.

Erickson E; cited in Sugarman L. *Life-Span Development, Concepts, Theories and Interventions*. Routledge, 1986: 84–93.

Khamisha C. Cultural diversity in Glasgow, part 1: are we meeting the challenge? *Br J Occup Ther* 1997; 60: 17–22.

Pritchard P. Learning to work effectively in teams. In: Ownes P, Carrier J, Horder J, eds. *Interprofessional Issues in Community & Primary Care*. MacMillan Press, 1995.

United Kingdom Central Council. *Standards for Specialist Education and Practice*. London: UKCC, 2001.

Chapter 24

Counselling people affected by sickle cell disease and thalassaemia

C Onyedinma-Ndubueze

Introduction

Sickle cell disease (SCD) and thalassaemia are genetic conditions that have tremendous physical, psychological, emotional and social implications for both the client and the families, albeit with differing severity and urgency. It is important also to recognize the psychological and emotional implications for individuals found to be carriers of these conditions. In view of the above implications, it is imperative that if a comprehensive service for these client groups is advocated by health-care providers, counselling should be a major component of such service [1]. There is also evidence in the literature suggesting that counselling services for haemoglobinopathies for both disease diagnosis and carrier identification has been *ad hoc* and patchy and occasionally not related to client needs [2]. This could be related to lack of understanding and/or non-appreciation of the magnitude of the problems related to haemoglobinopathies by health-care professionals, as well as the lack of adequate preparation of these health-care professionals to deal with these problems and challenges. Midwives, nurses, health visitors, practice nurses and doctors are often the first point of contact for affected families and so are in positions which automatically place them in a counselling role. Furthermore, as primary health care is at the forefront of the new NHS in the UK, the role of primary health-care professionals in providing haemoglobinopathy screening and counselling is recognized in various government policy documents [1, 3].

This chapter aims to equip practitioners in the field of haemoglobinopathies to begin to fulfil this privileged role confidently and with expertise. All health professionals involved with the care of clients and families with SCD and thalassaemia need to be made aware of the challenging manifestations, life-threatening complications and the optimal management, as well as the attendant treatment challenges of these conditions.

Definition of counselling

'Counselling is a process through which one person helps another by purposeful conversation in an understanding atmosphere; seeking to establish a helping relationship in which the counsellee can express his thoughts and feelings in such a way as to clarify his own situation, come to terms with some new experiences, see his difficulty more objectively, and so face his problem with less anxiety and tension. Its basic purpose being to assist the individual to make his own decision from among choices available to him' (British Association of Counselling, BAC [4].)

If the goal of counselling as suggested by the BAC [4] is to ensure that the client is provided with an opportunity to work towards living in a more satisfying and resourceful way, then the counsellor must possess certain skills and adopt specific strategies that will enhance this dynamic and enabling interaction between the client and the counsellor. In order to tailor the discussion of these skills to haemoglobinopathy a brief overview of the cultural implications of haemoglobinopathies will follow.

Cultural implications of haemoglobinopathies

Cultural variations and practices are rife among the affected client groups and these tend to colour almost every aspect of interaction with these clients and their families. If the role of the counsellor as stated by the BAC [4] is to facilitate the client to function in ways which respect the client's values, personal resources and capacity for self-determination, it is incumbent on practitioners to have and to demonstrate an understanding of the richness of the cultural diversity of the client groups and their implications for counselling. Haemoglobinopathy counsellors have the responsibility to educate themselves about the cultural beliefs of individuals they care for. These cultural variations include the following.

Differing customs and values systems

The fact that the racial group affected with SCD is predominantly black should not lead to a blanket approach to cultural identification. Africans have different customs and value system from Caribbeans but quite often practitioners fail to make this distinction. On the other hand, Greeks, Italians and Asians, groups where thalassaemia is prevalent, also have rich cultural beliefs and practices that influence their acceptance, access and management modalities for haemoglobinopathies.

Differing religious affiliations

Muslim, Pentecostal Christians, Jehovah's Witnesses, Adventists and Orthodox Christians are among the religious beliefs and practices prevalent among haemoglobinopathy client groups. An understanding of the basic tenets of each of the religious backgrounds of clients by practitioners is likely to enhance the helping interaction. Hopes for miracles, divine intervention and avoidance of some therapeutic intervention such as blood transfusion due to some strong religious convictions may prevent individuals or families from accepting treatment options and modalities. Care must be taken to avoid over-generalization and stereotyping of clients due to ignorance on the part of the practitioner. Religious inclinations should be sensitively explored with clients/families for confirmation, because in some cases, commitment of the client may not be commensurate with that generally upheld by members of the same religious affiliation. There is evidence in the literature suggesting that religious affiliation greatly influences response to genetic counselling and reactions to genetic diagnosis, as well as acceptance of prenatal diagnosis and termination of affected pregnancy [5].

Differing ways of viewing illness, health and cures

There is evidence in the literature suggesting that clients function within their cultural context when it comes to health and illness beliefs [6–8]. Konotey-Ahulu [9] gives account of the myths and misconceptions that coloured SCD in Ghana before it became a Western medicalized condition related to blood. For instance, in some parts of West Africa, there are many superstitious beliefs about SCD. Because of the familial connection of SCD, it is sometimes seen as a generational curse with tremendous cultural implications for affected families. Such illnesses are thought to bring shame to the family hence the non-disclosure, denial and blame that are frequently seen in SCD. Cure is sometimes attempted by scarification and tattooing over the heart, spleen and some bones in patients who have been treated by a traditional tribal medicine man as an attempt to 'drain out the bad blood of sickle cell disease'. A male child with SCD in some West African groups is expected to be strong and not show he is in pain, unlike a female child with the same condition. This has implications for family counselling.

Differing ways of organizing marriages and socially acceptable customs connected with procreation

Among some of the ethnic groups at risk of haemoglobinopathy, marriages are conducted according to cultural practices and customs. It is not unusual to find an increased frequency of arranged marriages and close relative marriages among Asians. This is socially acceptable to this group but it does have genetic implications in terms consanguinity and frequency of inherited conditions [10, 11].

Differing ways of assessing descent

There are patrilineal and matrilineal customs among the at-risk groups with haemoglobinopathies. The sex of a child carries significant connotation for the family and the birth of an affected male child may be a dent to the image of the family, affecting their prospects of marriage and procreation. This is yet another reason for non-disclosure of the condition.

Skills essential for haemoglobinopathy counselling

Communication skills

In the course of their everyday practice, healthcare professionals are expected to be versed in the process of basic communication. For a therapeutic interaction such as haemoglobinopathy counselling, this cannot be over-emphasized. The skills of observing, listening, questioning, silence, proxemics, use of body language, touch, language and paralanguage are all essential and should be put to optimal use if both the client and the counsellor are to benefit from this interaction [12, 13]. It is important at this point to further explain some of the communication skills particularly pertinent to haemoglobinopathy counselling in view of the cultural implications of haemoglobinopathies, because people's background informs their norms and actions as they interpret their world and what is going on around them.

Language and paralanguage

The client comes into a haemoglobinopathy counselling relationship through various avenues. It may well be that the client had no prior knowledge of the need for counselling, as is quite often the case with the concept of universal neonatal screening and carrier identification whereby the client responds to an appointment sent through the post or made over the phone. It could also be that the client had prior knowledge of the condition or his/her risk status; in which case he approaches the interaction with a readiness to learn and gain further insight into the diagnosis that has been made. It is important that

counsellors appreciate that understanding of the information they give to clients may be limited if there is a language or cultural gap between the practitioner and the client. This can be compounded when medical/technical jargon is unwittingly used to explain a condition. Choice of words is very important in a counselling interaction. The aim is to provide information with minimal jargon to enhance a client's understanding. Terms should be simplified as much as possible without loss of meaning. Jargon and technical language may exclude clients from meaningful communication [12].

Practitioners should also be aware of the impact of the lexical content of the communication such as accent, tone of voice, pitch, volume and emphasis. There are tremendous transcultural connotations to paralanguage, especially among these client groups, because they provide meaning to the spoken words. It is very easy to convey contrasting messages if the correct lexical content is not chosen.

Touch

The use of touch in a counselling interaction can be therapeutic but it is one that should be used judiciously. Touch, according to Watson [14], can serve the purpose of connecting people, provide affirmation and reassurance, share warmth, provide reassurance and possibly improve self-esteem. It is advised that practitioners should be aware of the cultural interpretation of touch, which varies among ethnic groups [14–16]. A gentle touch on a distressed client's hand or a tender hold on the shoulder of a distressed client may be reassuring, supportive and therapeutic.

Silence

It is important that the haemoglobinopathy counsellor has the capacity to be comfortable with silence, as this can often be a good indication of possession of reflective listening skills. It enables the counsellor to concentrate on the client and to pace the information appropriately. It allows the client opportunity to assimilate information. The counsellor should also be able to accept silence from the client as a legitimate response in the interaction process.

Proxemics

The spatial distance between the counsellor and the client can either enhance or impede the interaction, an observation made by Hall (cited in Kenworthy *et al.* [12]). Ideally, a quiet environment is needed for counselling. However, some features of a setting and seating arrangement may militate against effective communication. Counsellors are advised to be sensitive to the ways in which a setting affects any interaction and endeavour to make the most strategic use of the far from ideal settings in which many practitioners may find themselves. A notice on the door ('Do Not Disturb, Counselling In Progress') would minimize or possibly avoid interruption. A drawn curtain or one-way screen may be used to ensure a client's privacy and dignity, for distance and interpersonal space to be favourably assured.

Kinesics

Gestures and body movements play an important role in the counselling process and have significant implications because of the differing connotations ascribed to them by clients from differing cultural background. The experienced counsellor aims to use these judiciously and sensitively to convey positive messages during the counselling process.

Gaze

The use of eye contact in communication has tremendous cultural connotations and varies among cultural groups. The haemoglobinopathy counsellor must tactfully use gaze to attract and maintain the client's attention, being constantly aware of the possibility of staring. Use of eye contact by clients is also fraught with misinterpretations of disinterest, disrespect or deception. For instance, in some African cultures it is not the norm to look speakers in the eyes for fear of being disrespectful.

Counselling skills

Counselling skills are essential in the interaction with the haemoglobinopathy client to enable the practitioner to acquire an in-depth awareness and appreciation of the client's problems. This will enable the counsellor to adopt the helping role in this interaction. The skills include: reflective questioning and listening, paraphrasing and clarifying, empathy, genuineness, supporting, facilitating client's self-disclosure, sensitivity, and being non-judgemental. It also includes the skills of self-awareness, and use of self (presence).

Empathy

Heron [17] describes true empathy as 'a participative communion with the other – a feeling with'. Empathy could also be defined as 'the ability to sense the client's world as if it were your own but without losing the "as if" quality'. Although seen as the most essential ingredient of a helping interaction, the haemoglobinopathy counsellor must use their person and self-awareness to enhance this skill while at the same time maintaining some objectivity to minimize the danger of becoming overwhelmed by the client's situation, thereby rendering them less effective and not in control. Language can be the channel of empathy where both the counsellor and the client discover that their ability to establish rapport is enhanced by the use of a common language. In fact one can best identify with another through a common language [18]. I have been privileged in my counselling role to share similar African language and dialect (being multilingual) with my clients. My experience proves that language has a magnificent impact on the counselling relationship. The client instantly warms to the counselling process and understanding is further enhanced.

Supporting

According to Heron [21], a supportive intervention is essential to a counselling relationship because it affirms the client's worth and value in an unqualified manner. Byrne and Sebastian [19] summarize the supportive aspect of counselling as involving three facets: an attitude of mind which respects and values humanism; an intervention involving interpersonal and physical interaction; and a role dimension involving the counsellor as a practitioner, an educator and an advocate for the client. The counsellor must respond to patient's cues of distress by her reassuring presence, which may take the form of simply being there for the client, holding hands or providing factual information. Effective reassurance may relieve a patient's anxiety so that energy can be used for dealing with the health problem at hand. Merely being present with the client in a qualitative way as they experience their situation may be more supportive than verbal communication. The haemoglobinopathy client should be accepted as a person with unique characteristics and qualities, including the beliefs, values and norms they hold. The chosen actions and decisions of the client must be accepted unconditionally. This involves adopting a non-judgemental stance.

Sensitivity

According to Rollo May [18], the distinguishing mark of the counsellor is that special sensitivity to people. The counsellor should be particularly sensitive to subtle expressions of character such as paralinguistic phenomena as previously discussed, as well as kinesics, posture, facial expression and appearance. It is also important that the counsellor is sensitive to the client's anxiety, fears, hopes and personality tensions. In view of the particular client groups affected by haemoglobinopathies, cultural sensitivity is vital to the success of any counselling interaction. It is important to learn what the client 'thinks' and 'feels' about the information being shared.

Genuineness

Anyone who undertakes to be a counsellor must be prepared to interact with the client as a real person, while striving towards awareness and understanding of the factors involved in the process of counselling. Corey [20] describes the authentic helper as one without false fronts whose outer expression is congruent with their inner experiences. Genuineness is essential for the building of a trusting and confidential relationship with the client. It enhances the client's self-disclosure as the client readily establishes rapport with the counsellor. This authentic presence of the practitioner is essential in haemoglobinopathy coun-

selling because of the multidimensional implications of SCD and thalassaemia.

Helping strategies

Counselling should enable the client and families to develop and adopt coping strategies that will result in the resolution of discomforting feelings such as anxiety, fear, guilt, shame and denial, to mention but a few. It should also lead to enhanced self-esteem, improved relationships with others and improvement and maintenance of a state of wellness, in spite of the chronic and unpredictable nature of haemoglobinopathies, particularly SCD. Miller [21] has developed a model that clients use to cope with chronic illness. The counsellor must adopt helping strategies that will enable and empower the client to make informed decisions and choices. Macleod-Clarke *et al.* [13] stipulate that the strategies must include giving information, giving advice, teaching, taking action, changing system and counselling.

The above discussions of the communication skills and strategies required for effective counselling are not exhaustive. It is strongly advocated that reference be made to some specific texts on the practicalities of counselling and therapeutic communication for further details. In view of the nature of SCD and thalassaemia, the counselling process will be discussed according to client categories and needs:

• Genetic counselling for sickle cell disease and thalassaemia.
• Counselling parents of a newborn with haemoglobinopathy.
• Counselling the young adult with SCD or thalassaemia.

The aim is to make the psychological, physiological, genetic and social discussion pertinent to the specific client group in recognition of the overt and covert needs of the client. The key is to adopt a holistic approach to the client's needs.

Genetic counselling in haemoglobinopathies

Genetic counselling is the clear communication

of all medical, psychological, social and genetic factors related to the condition under discussion. It has been defined by Murray [22] as 'the process of communicating all the factors that relate to the disease or the condition in question including the manifestations of the disease, the prognosis of the disease, the genetics of the disease and the alternatives of one or another course of action'. He added that the information to be provided should include:

- Genetic and pathological mechanisms of the condition
- Natural history of the condition
- Prognosis and/or treatment
- Reproductive options and consequences.

Having previously mentioned that a comprehensive approach should be adopted in haemoglobinopathy counselling, it is pertinent to add that the social, emotional and psychological aspects of the condition must be included in genetic counselling.

Aims of genetic counselling

The WHO Advisory Group [23] recommended that the 'objective of medical genetics is to help people with a genetic disadvantage to live and reproduce as normally as possible'. To achieve this objective, genetic counselling should aim to:

- Provide a clear understanding of the natural history and genetics of the condition.
- Dispel any myths and misconceptions the client may have about the condition.
- Relieve any anxiety by creating an atmosphere where clients experience respect, warmth and a caring attitude.
- Offer meaningful and continued support.

Because of the genetic implications of the condition, there are specific implications that should be addressed when offering genetic counselling. This would differentiate it from any other type of counselling. Genetics refer to the very blueprint, the fundamental make up of an individual and as such any helping interaction that aims to discuss this must appreciate the impact on the recipient of such information. Procter [24] states that genetic counselling should offer individuals or couples the opportunity to confront the many

complex physical, social and psychological implications of the condition and to use this experience/information to enhance their decision making. It is therefore important that genetic counselling should have specific characteristics to enable both the counsellor and the client to gain from the interaction.

Characteristics of genetic counselling

Non-directive

Genetic counselling is not an advice-giving process. It is an interactive process whereby the counsellor exposes the client to all the relevant information that will enable the client to make informed choices. The genetic counsellor must always refrain from allowing their own feelings and opinions to be transmitted to the client or offering their own direct opinion about what decision the client should make regarding their reproductive options. It may be necessary to add a note of caution here. It is not unusual for clients to ask for the counsellor's opinion. Every experienced counsellor must have heard this said to them many times – 'What would you do if you were in my shoes?'. Never hesitate to respond that you are not in their shoes even if you have faced a similar genetic challenge before. No two situations are exactly the same when it comes to such complex discussions as genetics. Genetic counselling has a characteristic of a non-directive ethos.

Supportive

To be effective, genetic counselling must not only concentrate on giving risk explanations but should include a variety of other supportive actions. A trusting relationship needs to be established with the client from the onset of the encounter, with the counsellor employing all the essential communication and counselling skills discussed earlier in this chapter. Rogers [25] describes a purely supportive interaction as a way of being present with another person in a qualitative way as they experience their particular situation. Skills of empathic understanding, reflective listening and responding, as well as accepting the client unconditionally whatever views and beliefs they may hold, will all come into play to ensure that this characteristic is evident in the counselling process.

Informative

The accuracy of the information to be given to the client is very important in the discussion. The genetic counsellor needs the following information.

- An accurate and precise diagnosis from the laboratory verified with the client.
- Up-to-date information on the genetics of SCD or thalassaemia.
- An adequate family history obtained from the client.

This characteristic implies that the genetic counsellor must constantly keep abreast with the increasing knowledge in the new genetics as they affect haemoglobinopathies. If there is any doubt about the diagnostic result, one should consider postponing the counselling session until this is resolved.

Explaining the inheritance pattern of SCD or thalassaemia needs to be done with clarity to avoid any misunderstanding. Richards [8], in his research on the relevant issues for social scientists in the new genetics, discovered that clients already have beliefs about inheritance and proneness to particular diseases and suggests that these must be explored and understood in order to assist the client to make sense of the clinical genetics. For instance, the notion of 1 in 4 probability must be carefully explained by the counsellor to ensure that the client/couple fully assimilate the correct meaning of this. Use of dice or coin games may help facilitate this understanding. Getting the client to repeat what has been said in their own words can be helpful. A simple illustration using a Punnett square or the Mendelian graph is important (Fig. 24.1). The chance implication of the inheritance pattern has to be emphasized (chance has no memory!).

Simple, user-friendly, information materials (leaflets and posters) that are translated into various ethnic languages need to be made available for genetic counsellors to use in addition to the verbal information. However, these should be given out in tune with the discussion and not just

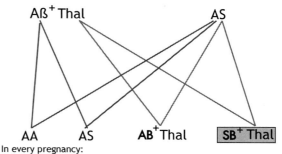

In every pregnancy:

Hb AA - Normal 1:4 (25%)

Hb AS - Sickle Cell Trait 1:4 (25%)

AB$^+$ thal — Beta Thalassaemia Trait 1:4 (25%)

SB$^+$ thal — Sickle Beta$^+$ Thalassaemia Disease 1:4 (25%)

Fig. 24.1 Possible Hb genotypes in the offspring if one parent has sickle cell trait and one has beta thalassaemia trait. In every pregnancy there is a 1 in 4 chance, respectively, that the offspring will have genotype HbAA, HbAS, HbAB$^+$thal or HbSB$^+$thal.

as a matter of routine. Wonke and Modell [26] produced a list of useful information materials that should be made available for some aspects of haemoglobinopathy service provision. Information to be imparted should also include the reproductive options available to the individual/couples, such as:

- Discriminatory pairing (selective choice of partners)
- Not having children
- Changing partners (recessive disorders)
- Selective abortion through prenatal diagnosis
- Artificial insemination (unrelated/unaffected donor)
- Ovum transfer (GIFT)
- Pre-implantation genetic diagnosis
- Adoption.

The discussion of prenatal diagnosis must not only include methods but efforts should be made to expose the client to the possible risks associated with each method:

- Infection
- Fetal loss (miscarriage)
- Fetal abnormalities
- Psychological trauma.

The genetic counsellor must have a good understanding of other counselling and support services in the community that could be of benefit to their clients/families.

Specific and sensitive

Using exploratory communication skills of para-phrasing and summarizing, the genetic coun-sellor learns what the client 'thinks' and 'feels' about what is being said and responds to these appropriately. Discussion of the genetics should be specific to the particular diagnosis at hand. In most situations, clients do not come into a genetic counselling situation as tabulae rasae. Quite often they have gathered information from friends, relatives and from the internet only to compare these with the information the counsellor would provide. There is always the danger of dragging the counsellor into uncharted areas that may not be relevant to the condition at hand. However, an experienced counsellor would ensure that clients' questions are correctly answered. Sen-sitivity to cultural implications from the par-ticular client's perspective must be evident from the counselling process, as previously discussed. A report of the Royal College of Physicians [27] strongly recommends that an approach to genetic counselling should be developed for the minority ethnic population in the UK. In fact the report went a step further to recom-mend that 'British Pakistanis and Bangladeshis should be counselled by a female, ideally a Muslim in the appropriate language and at home if necessary'.

Ethical considerations for genetic counselling

The principles of medical ethics suggest that the role of the genetic counsellor is to provide clear, accurate and comprehensive information to clients in recog-nition of the following ethical concepts.

Respect for the autonomy of the individual client/couple

The client should be seen as an individual and, according to Brookins [cited in 28], the focus of culturally sensitive nursing care should be on the

individual in the context of his or her culture, and this focus should be on the strengths they bring into the situation. The same should be said for the culturally sensitive counselling service rec-ommended for haemoglobinopathy. The ultimate decision on whether to take the risk of having an affected child with a haemoglobin disorder must rest with the individual/couple.

Confidentiality

Every health-care professional has a code of conduct that demands confidentiality of infor-mation about clients under their care. This is also essential in genetic counselling, as very per-sonal and sensitive information, feelings and views will be shared during the interaction. This applies to storage and sharing of details between carers.

Right to full and comprehensive information

The client has a right to receive accurate, clear and comprehensive information relevant to their partic-ular diagnosis.

Veracity – right to the truth

Avoid false reassurance or falsifying information to appease the client. Doing so negates the principle of beneficence and the moral duty of care by the practitioner.

Informed consent

The issue of informed consent in genetic coun-selling relates to the quality of information given to the client that will enable them to decide on a choice of action that they are ready to live with. How explicit this consent should be has remained controversial in the field of haemo-globinopathy [2, 24]. However, as most qualified nurses, doctors, midwives and health visitors are accountable for their interventions, and in line with the concept of clinical governance, it is be-coming increasingly necessary that informed con-sent for genetic screening and counselling should be made more explicit and not accepted as a fait accompli.

Special challenges of genetic counselling

Many authors have commented on the problems that can be encountered in genetic counselling [10, 11]. Some real-life problems encountered during genetic counselling for haemoglobinopathies will be included in this discussion.

Inaccurate/inappropriate diagnosis

It is advisable to rearrange the session. Obtain a fresh sample and repeat the test.

Communication barriers

This may be due to differences in literacy/ educational status, language/accent and cultural communication evident in non-verbal communication cues. As English is the usual mode of communication in UK, good listening skills are necessary to decipher the intended meaning of things said or not voiced!

Questionable paternity

This is the most challenging of the problems encountered during genetic counselling. It should be dealt with sensitively and humanely. It may be necessary to repeat the test and do more expensive genetic analysis of the family. A private session with the mother may be interestingly revealing! As there is still a lot to be fully understood in terms of genesis, introduction of the probability of a new mutation may be reassuring to all concerned. The ultimate desire of the genetic counsellor is to keep the family unit together to enhance their coping abilities.

Use of interpreters and advocates

It can be problematic to use interpreters to explain genetic information to clients, as verification of information relayed may not always be possible. The knowledge base of some inter-preters on genetics of thalassaemia can sometimes pose a challenge to the genetic counsellor. Regular update sessions should therefore be planned and implemented for health advocates and interpreters. Use of translated leaflets may sometimes help, provided that clients can actually read them!

Time constraints

Adequate time should be set aside for genetic counselling. Harper [10] suggests 1 hour as the usual time it takes to obtain full pedigree details and discuss genetic risks. No counselling session should be rushed or dragged beyond the time needed. Beware of information overload and if necessary arrange a follow-up session to meet the client's needs.

Dealing with bereavement

Although I have experienced personal loss through SCD, prior to that, very little prepared me for the demand made on me by my clients following termination of affected pregnancy or loss of a young one from SCD or thalassaemia. Genetic counsellors in the field of haemoglobinopathy must begin to address clients' need for support following death or termination of an affected pregnancy. Having established a relationship with the family antenatally or over the years, it is not surprising that the counsellor becomes the 'helper' that the family relies upon as they try to deal with a combination of grief and guilt. Referral to a more specialist bereavement counselling is seldom required, as the client group in these conditions has very good community support network at times of crisis. It may help if the counsellor has an understanding of the rudiments of bereavement counselling.

Counselling the parents of a newborn with haemoglobinopathy

Every pregnant woman anticipates the birth of a healthy and perfect baby; however, this is not always the case. The birth of an affected child evokes a lot of emotions that should be recognized and dealt with if the coping strategies of the family are to

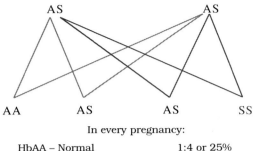

In every pregnancy:

HbAA – Normal   1:4 or 25%

HbAS – Sickle cell trait   1:2 or 50%

HbSS – Sickle cell anaemia   1:4 or 25%

Fig. 24.2 Inheritance of sickle cell.

be enhanced. The feelings include shock, confusion, anxiety, anger, fear and guilt, as evident in the literature [1, 29, 30]. Early diagnosis is a key factor in survival for haemoglobinopathies. Research has shown that thalassaemics die before the age of 2 years without treatment, while up to 30% of deaths in SCD occur before diagnosis [31]. The advent of neonatal screening for haemoglobinopathies has greatly reduced the mortality rates, as this provides an opportunity for early enrolment into a comprehensive disease management programme and commencement of penicillin prophylaxis. Children's illness has a tendency to alter the family dynamics of parent–child relationship, hence a family approach is best adopted from the onset [32]. There is sufficient evidence in the literature to suggest that families require a collection of social, behavioural and psychological support to cope with and adjust to the child's chronic disease [28, 30, 32]. Counselling should therefore be aimed at enhancing long-term adjustment to the disease.

The first contact with a family with an affected newborn is crucial to facilitating their involvement in the comprehensive disease management programme and establishing a therapeutic relationship with the counsellor. In view of the diverse emotions raised by the diagnosis, the counsellor must adopt a sensitive and supportive approach, showing empathic understanding while adopting a non-judgemental stance during this first contact. Opportunity should be given for parents to verbalize their feelings and these should then be explored with them. Counselling at this point must acknowledge these

feelings and reassure parents that those feelings are perfectly normal and natural and that they are similar to feelings expressed by parents facing other types of inherited disorders. Counselling the parents of a newborn must include discussion on the genetic implications of the condition, offering a simple but clear description of the inheritance pattern. If the parents were counselled during the antenatal period, it does no harm to revisit the issue (Fig. 24.2).

Parental education

The focus for parental education must be to teach parents to avoid, anticipate and recognize haemoglobinopathy-related problems in the child. It is important to discuss the family's experience with the disease or trait to establish a baseline. All teaching must be geared to the client's level of understanding. Encourage bonding from a very early stage between the newborn and every member of the family. Parental education includes giving them basic information on the signs and symptoms of the condition; stressing the importance of healthcare maintenance such as immunization, diet, hygiene and compliance with prescribed penicillin prophylaxis. The education should also include basic instruction on how to use the thermometer, as well as teaching parents how to palpate the spleen. Parents should be encouraged to avoid overprotection of the affected child from a very early stage but to treat the child as normal, while recognizing that the child may have special needs for warmth, extra fluid and vigilance for medical emergencies, and regular medical surveillance and follow-up in the hospital. This will ensure normal functioning of the family.

Literature should be provided for the family to keep and refer to as and when required. Simple and concise handbooks are available as backup for counselling [33–35]. All parents of affected newborns should be made aware of the resources available to them in the community, such as the local sickle cell and thalassaemia centre and social services. Encourage active participation in social activities involving the local support groups, parent-user associations and voluntary agencies, such as sickle cell and thalassaemia societies. The family should be introduced to other affected families. This reduces the feeling of isolation experienced by families with newly diagnosed individuals.

Social support is an important factor in facilitating compliance and improving health behaviour. Counselling for parents of the newborn should be an ongoing process involving several sessions. Subsequent visits must begin to address issues affecting other members of the family to enable them cope with the demands and challenges of the condition of the affected child. The counsellor must ensure her availability by making herself accessible to clients/families. The involvement of a psychotherapist or child psychologist provides a useful service for the family, addressing the many psychological challenges faced by some families that the haemoglobinopathy counsellor is professionally ill-equipped to meet. Muncey and Parker [36] stress that attention should be given to the physiological and psychological needs of patients and families with chronic diseases to enable them to live a full and happy life within the constraints of their condition. Nash [32] acknowledges the importance of early emotional, social and cognitive support for families with SCD; it minimizes the burden of the disease.

Counselling support for the young adult with haemoglobinopathy

Adolescence is a turbulent period in the life of an individual. The turbulence increases with a chronic genetic condition like the haemoglobinopathies. Adolescence is also a time of exquisite body image sensitivity, peer group recognition, acceptance, autonomy and comparison [28]. It is usually a time when the child is becoming self-aware and the sudden realization of the nature and implications of having sickle cell or thalassaemia can be rather daunting and overwhelming. For some young adolescents, having grown up with SCD/thalassaemia could have made them more resilient and emotionally mature than their peers. As the young adult with thalassaemia or SCD suddenly confronts the realization of having to face a life-threatening condition on a regular basis, they are also expected

to begin taking on some responsibilities for their own disease management.

Developmental issues in adolescents with haemoglobinopathy

Independence
Dependence is increased as the young adolescent experiences physical vulnerability due to the crippling pain of the condition and past parental over-protection.

Peer group
Acceptance and recognition by peer group becomes a challenge as the young child battles with frequent hospitalization and delayed puberty, which makes them feel different from their peer group due to altered body image. The feelings of isolation, loneliness, rejection and non-verbalization for fear of being rejected are all evident in the maladjusted adolescent [32].

Self-concept
Delayed puberty and leg ulcers may cause problems of altered body image resulting in low self-esteem as social relationships become problematic. The stigma attached to SCD further complicates the picture. The unpredictable onset of sickle cell crisis causes loss of control over personal life, resulting in helplessness and hopelessness. The feelings often expressed by young adults with haemoglobinopathy include:
• Anxiety and frustration
• Anger and resentment
• Blame for parents
• Fear of death/pre-occupation with death
• Unfulfilment, apathy and resignation; this leads to non-compliance with disease management.

It was in recognition of these manifestations that the WHO Working Party on Psychosocial Problems [23] recommended that psychosocial support must be an integral part of the total management of patients with haemoglobin disorders. Studies have shown that young people who have supportive families do better psychologically than those with minimal support [31, 32]. Counselling for the adolescent with haemoglobinopathies should aim to optimize integration of patients into society, enhance disease management and maintain a state of wellness. Counselling should enable the client to develop and adopt coping strategies that will lead to the resolution of feelings often expressed. Counselling intervention should therefore be supportive, educative and sensitive to the needs of this age group. The haemoglobinopathy counsellor should provide opportunities for young adults with haemoglobinopathies to express their feelings by facilitating communication, and providing a safe space for verbalization. Cognitive support from the counsellor helps the patient to understand their condition, and enhance compliance with therapeutic regimes. The client is encouraged to take responsibility for their condition by arranging their own hospital appointment, collecting prescribed medicines, and avoiding the factors that precipitate sickle cell crises.

Social support should include emotional support through reflective listening, exploration of personal circumstances like finances, employment, education and living arrangements. The young adult should be encouraged to participate in user groups where they can meet other affected people who are doing well educationally and career-wise, in spite of the haemoglobinopathy. Liaison with other professionals to find reinforcement and stimulants for the maladjusted adolescent, and referral to specialist services like career advice, a psychologist, psychotherapist or specialist social worker may be beneficial. Visits by the counsellor to clients during hospitalization can be therapeutic for the client. Wherever possible, the family should be involved in the continued support for young adults with haemoglobinopathy. Parents and families play a major role in the adjustment process of children and adolescents. Informational support is provided by ensuring that the client receives materials that they can refer to. This helps to reinforce any instructions given by the doctors. A health record checklist or diary could be provided. Patient education should be given to enable the client to understand the nature, inheritance, manifestations and management of his condition. Empowerment is achieved as competence in self-care activities is fostered.

Haemoglobinopathy counselling and clinical governance

Documentation/record keeping

A counselling checklist will provide an efficient method of counselling documentation.

Existence of standards for practice

Counselling protocols and manual will serve as a framework for counselling activity. This ensures uniformity and a high quality counselling service.

Information leaflets and posters

These are supportive adjuncts to the counselling process for clients to refer to when the counselling process is concluded. Translated versions in relevant languages will enhance the quality of services provided.

Audit tools

Audit tools include user questionnaires after counselling interactions (satisfaction surveys) exploring the clients' experience of the counselling interaction. Also, monitoring access to counselling service through effective record keeping, record of uptake of prenatal diagnosis, number of affected newborns and number of terminations of affected pregnancies.

Self-evaluation questionnaire for counsellors

This is to assess the quality of services being provided and to ensure continued improvement of services.

Staff update

Provision of haemoglobinopathy educational sessions for acute and community staff as part of their continued professional update will greatly improve care provision. This can take the form of study days, conferences or ward/unit teaching sessions.

Multidisciplinary team approach

The nature of the haemoglobinopathies demands that a multidisciplinary team approach is best adopted for the management of these conditions. Members should therefore aim to work collaboratively in recognition of the significant contribution each member makes to the disease management. Regular team meetings involving users enhance the quality of service.

Conclusion

Organization and implementation of community-based counselling services for haemoglobinopathy are essential if the objective of reaching the affected community and ethnic groups is to be achieved. As the problems under discussion may be complex and emotionally laden for the client, the counsellor must possess the necessary skills and expertise to enable and empower the client to develop their own coping strategies for the condition and the many challenges they face. Counsellors need courage, self-awareness and confidence to be effective. To make a commitment to assist another person carries with it many responsibilities and uncertainties. The health-care practitioner who seriously intends to become an effective counsellor must be willing to accept these responsibilities and uncertainties and have a readiness to function as a real person rather than as a performer acting within safely prescribed limits. Counselling in haemoglobinopathies demands sound knowledge of the conditions, genuineness, empathy and honesty, as well as understanding and appreciation of the many cultural differences of the client population. In summary, counselling enables individuals/people:

1 To make informed decisions.
2 To come to terms with their or their family's disorder.

Furthermore, counselling demands:

1 Sensitivity empathy, honesty.
2 Commitment and time.
3 Understanding and appreciation of cultural differences.

Dedication

This chapter is dedicated to my son Kachy who succumbed to sickle cell anaemia at the tender age of five and half years; and my haemoglobinopathy clients and families whose resilience and courage inspired my writing of this chapter.

References

1. Department of Health. *Report of a Working Party of the Standing Medical Advisory Committee on Sickle Cell, Thalassaemia and other Haemoglobinopathies*. London: HMSO, 1993.
2. Anionwu EA, Atkin K. *The Politics of Sickle Cell and Thalassaemia*. Buckingham: Open University Press, 2001.
3. Hurd J, Rowland N. *Counselling in General Practice. A Guide for Counsellors*. Oxford: BAC, 1987.
4. British Association of Counselling. *Code for Ethics and Practice for Counselling*. Rugby: BAC, 1992.
5. Anionwu EN, Patel N, Kamji G *et al.* Counselling for prenatal diagnosis of sickle cell disease and thalassaemia. *J Med Genetics* 1988; **25**: 769–72.
6. Grace NE, Zola IK. Multiculturalism, chronic illness and disability. *Pediatrics* 1993; **91**: 1048–35.
7. Kleinman A; cited in Lubkin IM. *Chronic Illness Impact and Interventions*, 3rd edn. London: Jones & Bartlett, 1995.
8. Richards MPM. The new genetics: some issues for social scientists. *Sociol Health Illness* 1993; **15**: 567–86.
9. Konotey-Ahulu F. *The Sickle Cell Disease Patient*. London: Macmillan Press, 1991.
10. Harper P. *Practical Genetic Counselling*, 5th edn. Oxford: Butterworth Heinemann, 1998.
11. Modell B, Modell M. *Towards a Healthy Baby: Congenital Disorder and the New Genetics in Primary Health Care*. Oxford: Oxford University Press, 1992.
12. Kenworthy N, Snowley G, Gilling C. *Common Foundation Studies in Nursing*, 3rd edn. Edinburgh: Churchill Livingstone, 2001.
13. Macleod-Clarke J, Hooper L, Jesson A. Progression to counselling. *Nurs Times* 1991; **87**: 41–3.
14. Watson O. *Proxemic Behaviour: A Cross-Cultural Study*. The Hague, Netherlands: Monitor, 1980.
15. Murray R, Huelskoetter M. *Psychiatric/Mental Health Nursing*. CA: Appleton & Large, 1991.
16. Witcher S, Fisler J. Multidimensional reactions to therapeutic touch in a hospital setting. *J Personal Social Psychol* 1979; **37**: 87–96.

17. Heron J. *Helping the Client: A Creative Practical Guide*. London: Sage, 2001.
18. May R. *The Art of Counselling – A True Classic in the Literature of the Helping Professions*. London: Souvenir Press, 1992.
19. Byrne C, Sebastian L. The defining characteristics of support. *J Psychol Nurs* 1994; **32**: 33–8.
20. Corey G. *Theory & Practice of Counselling & Psychotherapy*. Pacific Grove, CA: Brooks Cole, 1986.
21. Miller JF. *Coping with Chronic Illness: Overcoming Powerlessness*. Philadephia: FA Davis, 1992.
22. Murray R. *Unsolved Mysteries in Genetic Counselling*. New York: Academic Press, 1975.
23. World Health Organization. *The Psychosocial Aspects of Patients and their Families with Beta Thalassaemia Major and Sickle Cell Disease*. A Report from the WHO sponsored working group – Regional Office for Maternal and Child Health, 1991.
24. Procter AM. The ethics of genetic testing of families. *Curr Paediatr* 2002; **12**: 453–7.
25. Rogers C. *On Becoming a Person*, 4th edn. London: Constable, 1974.
26. Wonke B, Modell B. Impact on future of screening for haemoglobin disorders. *Curr Paediatr* 1998; **8**: 55–61.
27. Royal College of Physicians Report. *Prenatal and Genetic Screening: Community and Service Implications*. London: RCP, 1989.
28. Lubkin IM. *Chronic Illness Impact and Interventions*, 3rd edn. London: Jones & Bartlett, 1995.
29. Black J, Laws S. *Living with Sickle Cell Disease: An inquiry into the Need for Health and Social Service Provision for Sickle Cell Sufferers in Newham*. London: Sickle Cell Society, 1986.
30. Whitten C, Fischoff J. Psychosocial effects of sickle cell disease. *Arch Intern Med* 1974; **133**: 681–9.
31. Midence K, Elander J. *The Psychosocial Aspects of Sickle Cell Disease*. Oxford: Medical Radcliffe Press, 1994
32. Nash K B. *Psychosocial Aspects of Sickle Cell Disease: Past, Present and Future Directions of Research*. New York: Haworth Press, 1994.
33. Oni L, Dick M, Smalling B, Walters J. *Care & Management of Your Child with Sickle Cell Disease – A Parent's Guide*. London: Brent Sickle Cell & Thalassaemia Centre, 1997.
34. Vullo R, Modell B. *What is Thalassaemia? – A Guide to Help Thalassaemics & their Parents to Understand Thalassaemia*. London: UK Thalassaemia Society, 1997.
35. Anionwu E, Jibril H. *Sickle Cell Disease: A Guide for Families*. London: Collins International Textbooks, 1986.
36. Muncey T, Parker A. *Chronic Disease Management: A Practical Guide*. Basingstoke: Palgrave, 2000.

Further reading

Bor R, Miller R, Latz M, Slat H. *Counselling in Health Care Settings*. London: Cassell, 1998.
Burnard P. *Counselling Skills for Health Professionals*. Cheltenham: Stanley Thornes, 1999.
Culley S. *Integrative Counselling Skills in Action*. London: Sage, 1991
Chauhan G, Long A. Communication is the essence of nursing care 1: breaking bad news. *Br J Nurs* 2000; **9**: 979–84.
D'Ardenne P, Mahtani A. *Transcultural Counselling in Action*. London: Sage, 1999.
Egan G. *The Skilled Helper: A Systematic Approach to Effective Helping*. Pacific Grove, CA: Brooks/Cole, 1990.
McLeod J. *An Introduction to Counselling*. Buckingham: Open University Press, 1998.
Nelson-Jones R. *Human Relationship Skills*. London: Cassell, 1990.
Wright B. *Caring in Crisis: A Handbook of Intervention Skills for Nurses*. Edinburgh: Churchill-Livingstone, 1993.

Chapter 25

Sickle cell disorders and thalassaemia: the challenge for health professionals and resources available

Elizabeth N Anionwu

Sickle cell disease (SCD) and thalassaemia constitute some of the commonest inherited disorders that affect mankind. There is increasing appreciation of the challenges that haemoglobinopathies present to health-care professionals across the world. In Britain, for example, the significance of SCD and thalassaemia for the National Health Service (NHS) has begun to be recognized with the inclusion in the NHS Plan [1] of a linked antenatal and neonatal screening programme by 2004 (see http://www-phm.umds.ac.uk/haemscreening/). While this is a heartening development there is also an urgent need to address the care of affected individuals, as health professionals have consistently identified a variety of challenges in the delivery of both screening and management of sickle cell and thalassaemia disorders [2]. It has been estimated that there may be over 12 000 patients with SCD [3] and the UK thalassaemia register has details of approximately 800 affected individuals [4]. In respect to the number of affected births per year, in 2002 Gill and Klynman [5] identified that there were three babies diagnosed with thalassaemia major and over 150 with SCD in Greater London (the latter figure excludes areas that had no statistics). The authors note that this is in contrast to the previous national estimates of a total of 175 births for both thalassaemia major and SCD [6, 7].

Rather than an in-depth analysis of the challenges faced by health professionals (for such a review see Anionwu and Atkin [2]) this chapter aims to provide practical ideas of some of the resources that are available to support them. It will draw upon the examples of dilemmas identified for the author by a range of practitioners (Tables 25.1–25.4) attending the annual haemoglobinopathy course that was held at St Thomas' Hospital in London. While it is recognized that those attending specialist courses cannot be expected to be a representative sample of health professionals, the participants have always been drawn from a wide range of disciplines. These have included nurses, doctors, midwives, medical laboratory scientific officers, social workers and psychologists in different specialties such as accident and emergency, haemoglobinopathy counselling, paediatrics, haematology and primary health care.

The participants were put into multidisciplinary groups and each person was asked to identify a key challenge that they had encountered in the delivery of services to those affected by sickle cell and/or thalassaemia disorders (see Tables 25.1–25.4). Every group then selected one topic from the list that had been generated in order to discuss it in more detail and share ideas of how they would try to resolve the problem. A very lively general feedback session then enabled a wider dissemination of the varied difficulties encountered within each group, the type of solutions proposed and the obstacles that still remain. Particular emphasis was given to how a multidisciplinary and interdisciplinary approach [8, 9], undertaken in collaboration with affected individuals and user groups, can assist practitioners in developing creative solutions to both reduce tensions and improve the quality of health care. As with previous courses, many participants were unaware of readily accessible resources, including guidelines, published papers, useful networks and informative websites. Examples of these will be described so as to provide practitioners with support to meet the different challenges they encounter in respect to SCD and thalassaemia. Prominence will be afforded to online resources and UK professional networks.

Types of challenges

The responses were varied but it was possible to group them into four themes, many of which had been cited by previous course participants. While they cannot cover every type of challenge, the examples nevertheless provide useful insights into issues that generate unease among health professionals. They also mirror many of the concerns that have previously been identified in the literature, at conferences and by user groups [2]. The four themes are:

1 Awareness, attitudes and behaviour of health professionals and patients
2 Specific diagnostic and management issues
3 Screening and genetic counselling
4 Socio-political issues in providing an equitable service.

Discussion

In examining the challenges that are set out in Tables 25.1–25.4 it is of interest to note that, as with previous courses, more were cited for SCD than for thalassaemia. Indeed, course participants in the year 2000 were of the opinion that there was a need for 'a better deal for clients with SCD'. This is not to undermine the concerns that health professionals experience in providing screening and care services for thalassaemia [10–12] and pertinent resources are included further on. Many of the specific issues identified in Tables 25.1–25.4 – such as low levels of awareness and interest, difficulties concerning venous access and blood transfusions and the challenges encountered in screening and genetic counselling – relate to both SCD and thalassaemia. Nevertheless, there are various reasons why professionals might identify a greater number of dilemmas related to SCD in comparison with thalassaemia. Practitioners have a higher probability of encountering individuals with SCD as, having

noted earlier, there are considerably more patients in the UK with this condition than with thalassaemia major or intermedia. In addition, complications of SCD affect many more parts of the body, are usually very acute in onset, variable, unpredictable and some can be unexpectedly life-threatening.

The disorder is often seen in young black individuals and tensions exist in many urban areas, some emanating from the impact of racism on issues such as educational attainment, health and employment prospects [13]. Practitioners should therefore not be surprised if conflicts flare up from time to time within the health-care setting. Shapiro and Ballas [14] from the USA commented in a paper on the painful sickle cell crisis that 'in the English-speaking countries, the majority of people affected are of African descent, whereas the majority of health care professionals are not. Additionally, socio-economic and cultural disparities often exist. Cross-racial and cross-cultural communications have been historically fraught with difficulties. The tensions that permeate our society inevitably affect the very human transactions surrounding the care of patients with pain'.

A UK study on the experiences of hospital care and treatment for SCD pain [15] identified a range of behaviours in patients who experienced frequent admissions. These included an attempt to develop long-term relationships with their carers, becoming either passive or aggressive in their interactions with health professionals or they may regularly attend different hospitals. Health professionals have continually articulated that there is need for greater knowledge, more positive attitude and increased resources for the care of those affected by SCD and thalassaemia.

Resources available

Before focusing on the specific themes, it is apparent from the examples contained in Tables 25.1–25.4 that health professionals would benefit from joining a network of those involved in similar activities; for example, the UK Forum on Haemoglobin Disorders (http://www.haemoglobin.org.uk). This network was established in 1995 and comprises a multidisciplinary group of those involved in various aspects of sickle and thalassaemia services. Members include haemoglobinopathy counsellors, haematologists, paediatricians, nurses, midwives, medical laboratory scientific staff, obstetricians, representatives from the voluntary sector, public health doctors, psychologists, sociologists, social workers and molecular geneticists.

The aims of the forum include promoting optimal and equitable services for haemoglobin disorders and facilitating collaborative research, developing a network of interdisciplinary contacts and acting as an advisory group to relevant agencies. They hold two meetings a year, one of which is in a venue outside London. The topics covered are informed by the wishes of members and provide an opportunity for continuing updates and specialist professional development. The meetings are usually attended by up to 200 people and it is clear that they provide a very useful and supportive network for any health professional involved with sickle cell and thalassaemia services. Another group is the Sickle and Thalassaemia Association of Counsellors (STAC) established in 1986. While the majority of members are specialist nurses employed and working within the NHS-funded centres, others include social workers, lecturers and community project workers. Their website (www.stacuk.org) includes the contact details of sickle cell and thalassaemia counsellors and clinical nurse specialists in the UK, and specialist educational courses. A future and much needed resource will be the 4 Training Centres for Sickle Cell and Thalassaemia Counsellors that have been commissioned by the NHS Sickle and Thalassaemia Screening Programme. Their remit will be to develop modular-based multidisciplinary training programmes for health professionals in England (http://www-phm.umds.ac.uk/haemscreening/).

The four themes

Information about SCD and thalassaemia
(Table 25.1)

There has been a welcome increase in the amount of electronic information that health professionals can utilize to improve their understanding about SCD and thalassaemia. The strength of these

Table 25.1 Awareness, attitudes and behaviour of health professionals and patients

Health-care professionals

'Working with health-care professionals who do not have knowledge/interest in caring for clients with sickle cell disorders' (Specialist nurse, haemoglobinopathies).

'Lack of interest of other clinicians due to sickle patients being seen as trouble makers or awkward people' (Doctor).

'Sickle patients seen as junkies and trouble makers' (Doctor).

'Biggest challenge for me – understanding complexity of disease. For my team – managing diversity in patient needs' (Doctor).

'Learning and understanding the disease, learning management of the disease and the impact on patients' lives' (Doctor).

'Understanding the pathology, management and long-term complications of the disease and dealing with social impact on the patient' (Doctor).

'Lack of understanding of the disease' (Nurse, Accident and Emergency Unit).

'Promoting awareness of client concerns in haematology wards' (Sickle Cell and Thalassaemia Nurse).

Patients and families

'Antisocial behaviours/attitudes by some patients and the disproportionate effect on health-care providers and provision' (Nurse).

tools is that they have been produced locally and internationally by both specialist voluntary and professional organizations, and most are constantly updated. The Sickle Cell Society (www.sicklecellsociety.org) and the UK Thalassaemia Society (www.ukts.org) are both UK-based support organizations and their websites are a useful first port of call for affected individuals and their families, professionals and the general public. They each contain information on the respective disorders, some of which is specifically aimed at health professionals. Topics covered include the inheritance pattern, symptoms and complications, diagnosis, management, psychosocial aspects, personal experiences, research, suggestions for further reading and links to other relevant sites.

Internationally, the Georgia Comprehensive Sickle Cell Information Centre (www.scinfo.org) is an online resource from the USA, the mission of which is to 'provide sickle cell patient and professional education, news, research updates and world wide sickle cell resources'. There is an excellent section on problem-oriented clinical guidelines and topics include pregnancy, priapism and chest syndrome. In addition there is an archive, personal accounts, PowerPoint® presentations, online books and resources as well as streaming videos on a huge number of topics. It has weekly sickle news updates and also facilitates links to a considerable range of relevant websites. It is also possible to obtain a free monthly email update that provides details of recent sickle cell news by contacting aplatt@emory.edu. There is also the site of the Sickle Cell Disease Association of America, Inc. (www.sicklecelldisease.org), which incorporates a section on research updates as well as webcasts that enable the viewer to see and hear conference presentations on SCD by eminent international speakers. There are also sites that contain information about SCD in languages other than English. As an example, the following sites may be useful for those UK practitioners trying to obtain information in French for families who have originated from countries such as the Democratic Republic of Congo (formerly Zaire). These include the African Francophone network for SCD (http://www.drepanet.org) and the site of the Sickle Cell Centre in Guadeloupe in the French West Indies (http://www.pixeldress.com/drepano/). In respect to thalassaemia, a vast array of information about the condition can be downloaded from the site of the Cyprus-based Thalassaemia International Federation (TIF) (http://www.thalassaemia.org.cy/) and the US Cooley's Anemia Foundation (http://www.cooleysanemia.org/).

Specific diagnostic and management issues
(Table 25.2)

In addition to the above, the following are examples of sites that offer more specific information for those involved in health-care services for SCD and thalassaemia. Identification of various haemoglobin variants [16] is a crucial component of sickle cell and thalassaemia services and particular challenges have been identified by some course participants. Useful online resources include the British Committee for Standards in Haematology (1998) guidelines on laboratory diagnosis of haemoglobinopathies [17], which can be downloaded via www.bcshguidelines.com/pdf/bjh809.pdf, as well as

Table 25.2 Specific diagnostic and management issues

Diagnostic issues

'Finding very rare mutations of haemoglobins and the need for better molecular methods of detection becoming easily available' (Biomedical scientist).

'Differentiation of sickle beta thalassaemia and HbSS' (Biomedical scientist).

Pain control

'Recurrent admission to hospital with pain crisis. Pain and opiate dependence' (Doctor).

'Pain control crisis is the biggest challenge' (Doctor)

'Pain control, doctor versus patient's ideas' (Doctor)

Blood transfusions

'We had a 7-year-old boy, known SCD who had a stroke. We could not start the exchange blood transfusion as the father was abroad and the mother would not consent until he returned' (Haematologist).

'Poor venous access' (Doctor).

'Persuading a 30-year-old male with SCD to embark on exchange transfusion programme following a CVA' (Doctor).

'Family refusing blood transfusion for a child of 8 months with beta thalassaemia major' (Haematologist).

Hydroxyurea

Crises in sickle patient and decision re hydroxyurea therapy in days when there are fears of its "possible" carcinogenetic effect' (Doctor).

'Managing a patient on hydroxyurea' (Doctor).

'Use of hydroxyurea in young children with SCD – ethics of the treatment in infants' (Paediatric haematologist).

Pregnancy

'Management of pregnancy' (Doctor) .

Death of patients

'How to tell a patient that another one has died of SCD' (Doctor).

'Dealing with the loss of a friend's 24-year-old son with the disease' (Nurse).

the Globin Gene Server http://globin.cse.psu.edu/, which contains a database of human haemoglobin variants. The British Committee for Standards in Haematology guidelines on the management of the acute painful crisis in SCD [18] is available online: www.bcshguidelines.com/pdf/SICKLE.V4_0802.pdf.

In the USA, a useful site for SCD is the Medlineplus for sickle cell anaemia, which includes information about latest research findings and clinical trials including those related to hydroxyurea in children and adults (www.nlm.nih.gov/medlineplus/sicklecellanemia.html). Resources relating to sociological perspectives on SCD and thalassaemia are accessible via the Centre for Research into Primary Care at the University of Leeds (http://www.leeds.ac.uk/crpc/). The centre provides details of relevant publications and ongoing research. The website of the TASC Unit for the Social Study of Thalassaemia and Sickle Cell at de Montfort University in Leicester (http://tascunit.com/) includes details of courses, research and publications relevant to sociological and social studies of the conditions. The Brent Sickle and Thalassaemia Centre has a dedicated Psychology website (www.sickle-psychology.com/) that provides information on a self-help approach to cognitive behavioural therapy for managing SCD. The Cochrane Library is an electronic publication designed to supply high quality evidence to inform people providing and receiving care, and those responsible for research, teaching, funding and administration at all levels and is freely available to NHS staff, patients and the public in England through the National electronic Library for Health (NeLH) at www.nelh.nhs.uk/cochrane.asp. Reviews on various aspects of management of sickle cell and thalassaemia can be accessed via the Topics button and then clicking on the group entitled Cystic Fibrosis and Genetic Disorders. Examples include neonatal screening for SCD, pneumococcal vaccines for SCD, psychological therapies for thalassaemia and SCD and pain, hydroxyurea and blood transfusions.

The dilemmas associated with treatment regimens such as regular blood transfusions are clearly articulated in Table 25.2. While the reasons for refusal will be varied and each case will be unique, practitioners can best serve the needs of the patient and family by incorporating a multidisciplinary approach and identifying the possible relevance of religious, cultural and health beliefs together with a possible needle phobia.

Young people still die of complications associated with SCD and thalassaemia and concerns related to the impact of death and dying on patients, carers, families and health professionals are illus-

trated in Table 25.2. The author has developed an online information resource aimed at supporting student nurses and midwives to become more competent and confident in addressing these and other issues within a multi-ethnic health-care setting. Entitled Multi-Ethnic Learning and Teaching In NursinG (MELTING), it includes a case scenario featuring a young man with SCD and can be accessed via www.maryseacole.com/maryseacole/melting.

Screening and genetic counselling (Table 25.3)

As noted previously, the NHS Plan [1] incorporated a commitment to creating a nationally linked antenatal and neonatal screening programme for SCD and thalassaemia by 2004. This has resulted in the establishment of the NHS Sickle and Thalassaemia Screening Programme, and their website http://www-phm.umds.ac.uk/haemscreening/ provides a vital resource for health professionals. The publication section includes reports of the outcome of various national and international workshops as well as commissioned projects. One useful example of the latter is the report on the Care Pathways for Antenatal and Neonatal Haemoglobinopathy Screening in London by Gill and Klynman [5], as it includes both a detailed review of the issues as well as the findings of the survey. The site contains helpful links relating to antenatal and child health screening and policy.

Health professionals may find it difficult to obtain funding for information and handouts to support them and their clients in the provision of genetic counselling for the haemoglobinopathies. Such materials need to take into account the huge array of possible combinations, such as the couple cited in Table 25.3 where one is a carrier for

Table 25.3 Screening and genetic counselling

'The main challenge is counselling sickle cell patients, especially pregnant ladies who are approaching childbirth' (Doctor).
'Counselling in pregnancy, e.g. a young couple where one is a carrier for HbE and the other is a carrier for beta thalassaemia trait' (Doctor).
'The need to improve sickle and thalassaemia screening'. (Doctor).

Hb E and the other is a carrier for beta thalassaemia trait. An ideal online resource, that is also available on a CD format, is Accessible Publishing of Genetic Information (ApoGI). Located at www.chime.ucl.ac.uk/APoGI/, APoGI supplies data on nearly all the haemoglobin disorders. It provides information and handouts that professionals can print out and give to individuals or couples found to have sickle, thalassaemia or other haemoglobin variant carrier states or disorders.

Information about the provision of genetic services in the UK can be accessed via the British Society for Human Genetics (http://www.bshg.org.uk/) and details of genetic counselling courses are contained in the site of the Association of Genetic Nurses and Counsellors (http://www.agnc.co.uk/). The NHS National Screening Committee (www.nsc.nhs.uk) determines policy on screening and their site includes information sheets on many conditions plus details about the activities of the Antenatal and Child Health Screening subgroups. Policy positions on screening for various conditions can be found on www.nelh.nhs.uk/screening/. The NHS National Co-ordinating Centre for Health Technology Assessment provides access to executive summaries of their reports by downloading them from their website www.hta.nhsweb.nhs.uk/. These include the two undertaken on screening for SCD and thalassaemia [7, 19], as well as reviews concerning informed decision making and screening for other conditions such as cystic fibrosis and Fragile-X.

Finally, on the wider ethical issues the Human Genetics Commission (www.hcg.gov.uk) is the UK advisory body on how new developments in genetics might impact on people and health care. Their site includes opportunities to become involved in their consultation exercises on ethical issues (examples include Genetics and Reproduction) and access to publications on completed ones. Two examples of the latter are the uses of genetic information and supplying genetic tests directly to the public. It also provides details about the venue of forthcoming quarterly public plenary sessions, and health professionals involved with sickle cell and thalassaemia might find attending such sessions very informative.

Socio-political issues in providing an equitable service (Table 25.4)

The final theme draws together instances of the challenges that relate to constraints identified in the provision of health-care services for conditions primarily impacting upon black and minority ethnic communities. At an institutional level, course participants often expressed frustrations about perceived lack of power to influence their local NHS Trusts to position SCD and thalassaemia services higher on their agendas and thereby increase resources and improve equity of access. NHS Trusts are public bodies that are legally bound by the Race Relations (Amendment) Act 2000, which includes a statutory general duty to promote race equality and that they have 'a due regard to the need to eliminate unlawful racial discrimination, promote equality of opportunity and promote good relations between people of different racial groups'. To assist in delivering the general duty, specific duties have been imposed on public bodies such as NHS Trusts. One that is relevant to the provision of sickle cell and thalassaemia services relates to the policy/service delivery side. Here there is a requirement to set out, in a Race Equality Scheme, information on a number of actions that will help deliver non-discriminatory services to local people. NHS organizations were required to publish a 'race equality scheme' by May 2002 that sets out their arrangements for meeting the duties and this has to be reviewed every 3 years. The Commission for Racial Equality has enforcement powers where public bodies are failing in these duties.

Health professionals in the UK may find out about the Race Equality Scheme in their own NHS

Table 25.4 Socio-political issues in providing an equitable service

'Cultural differences and effects on accessing health care. Refugees' (Nurse).
'Facilities are not available or difficult to access' (Doctor).
'Tackle poverty. Educate. Improve specialist care for sickle/thal – by providing more doctors and nurses specializing in care of HB disorders' (Doctor).
'Providing equitable care for SCD and thalassaemia clients' (Sickle Cell and Thalassaemia Nurse).

Trust, and how it affects services for SCD and thalassaemia. Details about the implications of this legislation can be found on the websites of the Commission for Racial Equality (www.cre.gov.uk), the Department of Health (www.doh.gov.uk/raceequalityresource/index.htm), and the Home Office: www.hmso.gov.uk/acts/acts2000/20000034.htm. There may be issues with providing health services for refugees and asylum-seekers. A helpful resource in the UK [20] can be down-loaded via: www.london.nhs.uk/newsmedia/publications/Asylum_Refugee.pdf. The impact of cultural differences and effects on accessing health care in general may present a challenge to health professionals. An online educational resource mentioned earlier is Multi-Ethnic Learning and Teaching In NursinG (MELTING) at: www.maryseacole.com/maryseacole/melting. It explores the concepts of cultural diversity, transcultural nursing and cultural assessment models and essential aspects of care such as communication and spiritual needs. Extensive references and links to a range of relevant sites are also included.

Those with a general interest in being kept up-to-date and discussing issues related to the health of minority ethnic communities within the UK may wish to join an emailing list for like-minded NHS staff and academics. To find out about joining visit: www.jiscmail.ac.uk/lists/MINORITY-ETHNIC-HEALTH.html.

Conclusion

Health professionals involved in the delivery of sickle and thalassaemia services are situated in every part of the UK, in high-, mid- and low-prevalence areas. Some may have a great deal of experience because they are working in a specialist unit in a metropolitan area, whereas others may be based in rural areas and only see a few cases a year. Practitioners from all these locations face similar challenges. They include being knowledgeable, empathetic and having adequate resources to provide a quality health service that is culturally and linguistically appropriate. The resources identified in this chapter to support busy health practitioners cannot possibly be a complete catalogue of what is currently available. Nevertheless it is to be hoped that the examples cited will provide a cheap and accessible foundation for anybody who can log on to a PC, as well as provide opportunities to network and keep up-to-date with similarly interested colleagues.

References

1. Department of Health. *The NHS Plan. A Plan for Investment. A Plan for Reform*. London: The Stationery Office, 2000.
2. Anionwu EN, Atkin K. *The Politics of Sickle Cell and Thalassaemia*. Buckingham: Open University Press, 2001.
3. Streetly A, Maxwell K, Mejia A. *Sickle Cell Disorders in Greater London: A needs assessment of screening and care services, The Fair Shares for London Report*. London: Department of Public Health Medicine, UMDS and St Thomas's Hospital, 1997.
4. Modell B, Khan M, Darlison M. Survival in beta thalassaemia major in the United Kingdom: data from the UK thalassaemia register. *Lancet* 2000; **355**: 2051–2.
5. Gill C, Klynman N. *Care Pathways for Antenatal and Neonatal Haemoglobinopathy Screening in London*. NHS Haemoglobinopathy Screening Implementation Programme working in collaboration with the London Health Observatory, 2003. http://www.phm.umds.ac.uk/haemscreening/publications.htm.
6. Hickman M, Modell B, Greengros P *et al*. Mapping the prevalence of sickle cell and beta thalassaemia in England: estimating and validating ethnic-specific rates. *Br J Haematol* 1999; **104**: 860–7.
7. Davies SC, Cronin E, Gill M *et al*. *Screening for sickle cell disease and thalassaemia: a systematic review with supplementary research*. Health Technology Assessment Report 4 (3) Executive summary, 2000.
8. Vichinsky EP, Johnson RJ, Lubin BH. Multidisciplinary approach to pain management in sickle cell disease. *Am J Pediatr Hematol Oncol* 1982; **4**: 328–33.
9. Okpala I, Thomas V, Westerdale N *et al*. The comprehensive care of sickle cell disease. *Eur J Haematol* 2002; **68**: 157–62.
10. Lakhani N. Thalassaemia among Asians in Britain (letter). *BMJ* 1999; **318**: 873.
11. Modell B, Harris R, Lane B *et al*. Informed choice in genetic screening for thalassaemia during pregnancy: audit from a national confidential inquiry. *BMJ* 2000; **320**: 337–40.
12. Atkin K, Ahmad WIU, Anionwu E. Service support to families caring for a child with a sickle cell disorder or thalassaemia: the experience of health professionals,

service managers and health commissioners *Health* 1998; **2**: 305–27.

13. Parekh B. *The Future of Multi-Ethnic Britain.* London: Profile Books, 2000.

14. Shapiro BS, Ballas KB. The acute painful crisis. In: Embury SH, Hebbel RP, Mohandas N, Steinberg MH, eds. *Sickle Cell Disease: Basic Principles and Clinical Practice.* New York: Raven Press, 1994.

15. Maxwell K, Streetly A, Bevan D. Experiences of hospital care and treatment seeking for pain from sickle cell disease: qualitative study. *BMJ* 1999; **318**: 1585–90.

16. Bain J. *Haemoglobinopathy Diagnosis.* Oxford: Blackwell Science, 2001.

17. British Committee for Standards in Haematology. Guidelines on the laboratory diagnosis of haemoglobinopathies. *Br J Haematol* 1998; **101**: 783–92.

18. Rees D, Olujohungbe AD, Parker NE *et al.* on behalf of the British Committee for Standards in Haematology. Guidelines for the management of the acute painful crisis in sickle cell disease. *Br J Haematol* 2003; **120**: 744–52.

19. Zeuner D, Ades EA, Karnon J *et al. Antenatal and neonatal haemoglobinopathy screening in the UK: review and economic analysis.* Health Technology Assessment Report, 3(11) Executive Summary, 1999.

20. Burnett A, Fassil Y. *Meeting the Health Needs of Refugee and Asylum Seekers in the UK.* Directorate of Health and Social Care, London: Department of Health, 2002.

Networks

UK Forum on Haemoglobin Disorders: www.haemoglobin.org.uk

Sickle and Thalassaemia Association of Counsellors (STAC) www.stacuk.org

Websites

Accessible Publishing of Genetic Information (APoGI): www.chime.ucl.ac.uk/APoGI/

African Francophone network for SCD: http://www.drepanet.org

Association of Genetic Nurses and Counsellors: http://www.agnc.co.uk/

Brent Sickle and Thalassaemia Centre's Psychology website: www.sickle-psychology.com/

British Committee for Standards in Haematology guidelines on the management of the acute painful crisis in SCD: www.bcshguidelines.com/pdf/SICKLE.V4_0802.pdf

British Committee for Standards in Haematology (1998) guidelines on laboratory diagnosis of haemoglobinopathies: www.bcshguidelines.com/pdf/bjh809.pdf

British Society for Human Genetics: http://www.bshg.org.uk/

Centre for Research into Primary Care at the University of Leeds: http://www.leeds.ac.uk/crpc/

Cochrane Library Cystic Fibrosis and Genetic Disorders topics via the National electronic library for health (NeLH): www.nelh.nhs.uk/cochrane.asp

Commission for Racial Equality: www.cre.gov.uk

Cooley's Anemia Foundation, USA: http://www.cooleysanemia.org/

Department of Health race equality issues: www.doh.gov.uk/race_equalityresource/index.htm

Georgia Comprehensive Sickle Cell Information Centre, USA www.scinfo.org plus free monthly email update via aplatt@emory.edu

Globin Gene Server database of human haemoglobin variants: http://globin.cse.psu.edu/

Human Genetics Commission: www.hcg.gov.uk

Medlineplus for sickle cell anaemia: www.nlm.nih.gov/medlineplus/sicklecellanemia.html

Minority ethnic communities and health email group site: www.jiscmail.ac.uk/lists/MINORITY-ETHNIC-HEALTH.html

Multi-Ethnic Learning and Teaching In NursinG (MELTING) resource: www.maryseacole.com/maryseacole/melting

NHS Sickle and Thalassaemia Screening Programme: http://www-phm.umds.ac.uk/haemscreening/

NHS National Co-ordinating Centre for Health Technology Assessment: www.hta.nhsweb.nhs.uk/

NHS National Screening Committee: www.nsc.nhs.uk

NHS screening policies: www.nelh.nhs.uk/screening/

Race Relations (Amendment) Act 2000 Home Office site: www.hmso.gov.uk/acts/acts2000/20000034.htm

Refugee and asylum seekers in the UK and their health needs: www.london.nhs.uk/newsmedia/publications/Asylum_Refugee.pdf

Sickle Cell Centre, Guadeloupe, French West Indies: http://www.pixeldress.com/drepano/

Sickle Cell Disease Association of America, Inc: www.sicklecelldisease.org

Sickle Cell Society: www.sicklecellsociety.org

TASC Unit for the Social Study of Thalassaemia and Sickle Cell: http://tascunit.com/

Thalassaemia International Federation (TIF): http://www.thalassaemia.org.cy/

UK Thalassaemia Society: www.ukts.org

Index